Multidrug-resistant Tuberculosis

Resurgent and Emerging Infectious Diseases

Volume 1

Multidrug-resistant Tuberculosis

Edited by

Ivan Bastian

Mycobacterium Reference Laboratory,
Institute of Medical & Veterinary Science,
Adelaide, Australia

and

Françoise Portaels

Mycobacteriology Unit,
Institute of Tropical Medicine,
Antwerp, Belgium

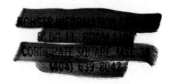

KLUWER ACADEMIC PUBLISHERS
DORDRECHT / BOSTON / LONDON

A C.I.P. Catalogue record for this book is available from the Library of Congress.

ISBN 0-7923-6169-5

Published by Kluwer Academic Publishers,
P.O. Box 17, 3300 AA Dordrecht, The Netherlands.

Sold and distributed in North, Central and South America
by Kluwer Academic Publishers,
101 Philip Drive, Norwell, MA 02061, U.S.A.

In all other countries, sold and distributed
by Kluwer Academic Publishers,
P.O. Box 322, 3300 AH Dordrecht, The Netherlands.

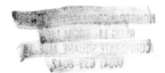

Printed on acid-free paper

Printed in the Netherlands.

This book is dedicated to all those suffering from tuberculosis, who battle with body and spirit against the disease. Among these are the patients, particularly those in penitentiary hospitals in Siberia, who watch helplessly as their illness is rendered more severe, and often fatal, under the weight of multidrug-resistance.

This book also recognises the players in the fight against tuberculosis: the doctors and nurses, health professionals, researchers, and laboratory personnel.

Lastly, IB would like to thank Stephanie, who left home for two years though she didn't know why, and Carmela, who knew why but still came.

During the preparation of this book, Ivan Bastian was supported by a Neil Hamilton Fairley Fellowship (987069) from the National Health and Medical Research Council of Australia.

Many of the contributors to this book participated in a Colloquium entitled "Tuberculosis, the real millennium bug: addressing the threat in developing and industrialised countries", which was held in Antwerp between 14-17 December 1999 through the auspices of the Institute of Tropical Medicine.

The word of a woman seems simple enough
But nothing is ordinary
Upon reflection, we see that it is sacred
It radiates the joy of the world

Most things in life are sacred
Many people kneel before the Gods
I wish for you a simple happiness
And that your dreams come true often

The sun comes and goes
Thank you for your aid
You see, we are given but one life

The entire world is shroud in a thick smoke
It is a bad omen
But we must believe in the forces of good
If we are to protect our house

From so far away
You came to our side
You saved us from death
And we kneel before you
For life is a precious gift from God

Written by a tuberculosis patient in a penitentiary hospital in Siberia

Translated from Russian by A Disu and B Antoine

Table of Contents

Chapter 1

Introduction

Multidrug-resistant tuberculosis: past, present and future

Ivan Bastian and Françoise Portaels
Mycobacteriology Unit, Institute of Tropical Medicine, Antwerp, Belgium

The Lord hath created medicines out of the earth and he that is wise will not abhor them. Ecclesiasticus 38:4, quoted by Selman Waksman when accepting the 1952 Nobel Prize for Medicine that was awarded for the discovery of the first effective antituberculosis drug, streptomycin, which was derived from the soil bacterium, *Streptomyces griseus*.

1. HISTORICAL PERSPECTIVE

This book has been published at the close of the twentieth century when the medical profession and the general community are increasingly concerned about the threat of multidrug-resistant tuberculosis (MDRTB)[1,2]. However, at this epoch, it is enlightening to move back from our immediate concerns about MDRTB 'hot spots' in Asia, South America, and the former Soviet Union [3], and to place our current predicament in an historical context. If the results of the global survey of antituberculosis drug resistance conducted by the World Health Organisation (WHO) and the International Union against Tuberculosis and Lung Disease (IUATLD) can be extrapolated, only 2.2% of TB cases worldwide are due to multidrug-resistant strains [3]. At the beginning of the 20th century, all TB cases were refractory to all available therapies.

Great advances had been made during the 19th century in the understanding of the epidemiology and pathogenesis of TB, and in the diagnosis of the disease (reviewed in references 4-7). Laënnec and the other unitarians, who believed that the numerous clinical manifestations of TB represented a single disease entity, had prevailed over those who considered scrofula, tubercles, and phthisis as separate diseases. Villemin had

1

I. Bastian and F. Portaels (eds.), Multidrug-Resistant Tuberculosis, 1-15.
© 2000 *Kluwer Academic Publishers. Printed in the Netherlands.*

demonstrated in 1865 that TB was caused by a transmissible agent. Koch's famous studies, which were reported in 1882, had found the agent, *Mycobacterium tuberculosis*, and his 'tuberculin' extract, though a therapeutic failure, proved useful for detecting infected individuals. Ehrlich, Neelsen, Rindfleisch, and Ziehl had improved Koch's original staining method into a practical diagnostic test [8], while Röntgen's discovery of X-rays in 1895 completed our diagnostic armamentarium for TB.

Unfortunately, the 19th century did not see similar advances in TB treatment. Patients in the early 1800s received antiphlogistic and counterirritant therapies such as emetics, cathartics, bleeding, and dietary manipulation. More supportive treatments became fashionable in the 1850s when Brehmer founded the first sanatorium in Göbersdorf, Germany. Similar institutions were established across Europe and in the United States (US) over the following decades. The sanatoria relied on strict regimens of enforced rest, fresh air, and good diet to increase the likelihood of self-healing. Though many in-patients responded to such treatment, the long-term results remained depressing. Over 60% of discharged patients died of TB within six years (ie. 17% of the "cured", 51% of the "arrested", and 72% of the "improved")[5]. The results were improved somewhat in the early 20th century when sanatorium treatment was supplemented by various surgical procedures (eg. pneumothorax, thoracoplasty) that aimed to collapse diseased and/or bleeding lung segments.

The chemotherapeutic breakthrough finally came in the 1940s with the discovery of streptomycin (S) by Waksman and Schatz and the production of para-aminosalicylic acid (PAS) by Lehmann and Rosdahl. However, the problem of acquired drug resistance was recognised even during the early treatment trials with these new drugs [6,9]. Drug-resistant organisms could be detected in 90% of patients after four months of monotherapy, and the 5-year survival after streptomycin monotherapy was no better than that obtained by sanatorium treatment [6]. Combined S-PAS trials were then performed in Britain and the US that proved that multidrug chemotherapy prevented the development of drug resistance and effectively treated TB.

The 1950s and 1960s saw the development of numerous antituberculosis drugs: isoniazid (H), the aminoglycosides, viomycin, capreomycin, pyrazinamide (Z), ethionamide, cycloserine, and ethambutol (E). The last major advance was the discovery of rifampicin (R), which was derived from another soil micro-organism, *Nocardia mediterranea*, and was first used in clinical trials in 1967 [10]. Regimens containing various selections of these antituberculosis drugs were evaluated and optimised in a succession of clinical trials conducted by the British Medical Research Council (BMRC) and others [11,12]. For patients with pulmonary disease caused by fully-susceptible organisms, a combination of H, R, and Z for two months followed by H and R for four months (ie. 2 HRZ/4 HR) proved the shortest, best tolerated, and most effective regimen (producing cure rates >97%)[13,14]. WHO, the American Thoracic Society (ATS), and the Centres for Disease Control (CDC) all recommend this short-course chemotherapy (SCC) but with the addition of E or S in the initial phase pending the results of susceptibility tests [15-17]. Finally, operational studies performed by Karel Styblo and the IUATLD demonstrated that SCC given under direct observation could succeed 'in the field'.

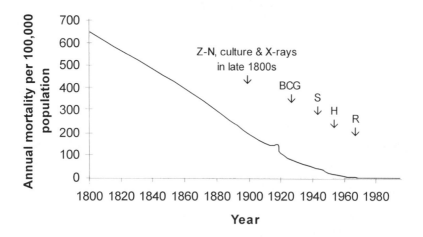

Figure 1. Mortality from tuberculosis (TB) in the United States, 1800-1995. Data were derived from the World Health Statistics Annual and from [18]. The significant decline in TB mortality prior to the introduction of various technologies is shown. Z-N, Ziehl-Neelsen stain; S, streptomycin; H, isoniazid; R, rifampicin.

Hence, in the final decade of the 20th century, WHO was able to recommend a package of diagnostic, therapeutic, and operational interventions, which was 'brand-named' "directly observed treatment, short-course" (DOTS), that could effectively control TB [19,20]. Interestingly, the burden of tuberculosis was declining sharply in industrialised countries well before the advent of these effective regimens and programs (Figure 1). This decrease has been attributed to gradual selection for innate immunity (ie. 'herd resistance') in exposed populations [21], improved nutrition and living conditions, and reduced disease transmission through the segregation of consumptives in infirmaries and sanatoria [22].

This brief historical overview has been given to highlight three points. Firstly, numerous epidemiological factors influence the progress of a TB epidemic. For example, in addition to showing the decline in TB mortality in the US during this century, figure 1 also shows the effect of the crowding and deprivations caused particularly by World War I. The incidence of TB cases is predicted to increase from 7.5 million cases in 1990 to 11.9 million in 2005-an increase of 58% [23,24]. Of this predicted increase in TB incidence, 77% has been attributed to demographic factors (eg. population growth and changing age structures within populations) while epidemiological factors, such as MDRTB, human immunodeficiency virus (HIV) infection, and poverty, will account for only 23%. Hence, while emphasising that drug resistance presents a significant risk to the success of TB control efforts, a book on MDRTB must recognise that drug resistance is only one (minor) factor contributing to the current global TB problem.

The second point to highlight from this historical overview is that numerous disciplines have contributed to TB control (Figure 1). Microbiologists and radiologists had provided accurate means of TB diagnosis by the end of the 19th century; immunologists had provided the (imperfect) vaccine, BCG, by 1928; scientists and clinicians had produced and evaluated various antituberculosis treatments during the 1940s-1980s; and the greatest contribution to TB control may actually have come from the on-going efforts of public health specialists throughout the 19th and 20th centuries. In short, TB control has been a multi-disciplinary undertaking and must continue to be so. This book has therefore gathered contributions from authorities in multiple disciplines (eg. epidemiologists, clinicians, pharmacologists, molecular biologists, and public health specialists) to address all aspects of MDRTB.

Thirdly, this historical overview demonstrates that mankind has had at least two opportunities to effectively control TB but has failed on both occasions. The availability of various chemotherapeutics in the 1940s-1960s suggested that the battle against TB was won [4]. Strains of *M. tuberculosis* resistant to H, S and/or PAS soon appeared representing the failure of our first attempt. The discovery of R, and the success of SCC in treating strains with H and/or S resistance [25], allowed the medical community to continue to ignore the underlying factors that promote drug resistance (eg. limited healthcare funding, ineffective TB control programs, physician mismanagement, and patient non-adherence). The MDRTB of the 1980s-1990s (which now represents *M. tuberculosis* strains resistant to at least H and R) embodies our second failure to address the underlying causes of drug resistance, which also happen to be the problems bedevilling TB control in general.

2.   THE DEFINITION OF MDRTB

The historical overview also shows that MDRTB has meant different things to different people during this century. Until the late 1940s, all TB was equivalent to MDRTB (ie. effectively untreatable). In the 1950s-1970s, MDRTB came to represent *M. tuberculosis* strains resistant to H, S and/or PAS. Then in the 1980s-1990s, after the introduction of R, MDRTB was strictly classified as *M. tuberculosis* strains resistant to at least H and R [26-29].

2.1   Rationale for the current definition of MDRTB

Isoniazid and R are the key drugs in SCC [15-17,28,29]. Isoniazid is potently bactericidal, inexpensive, orally active, and has few adverse reactions [16]. Isoniazid is therefore used for the duration of any treatment regimen unless contraindicated or resistance is documented. Rifampicin is also bactericidal, has excellent sterilising activity, prevents emergence of resistance to other drugs, is rapidly absorbed from the gastrointestinal tract, and is relatively non-toxic [16,30].

Drug-susceptible pulmonary TB can be effectively treated with just H and R for 9 months (ie. 9 HR) [16,31]. The addition of Z during the first two months shortens the duration of treatment to six months [32-34]. Short-course regimens containing four or five drugs (eg. 2 HRZE/ 4 HR) are still effective in the presence of H (and/or S) resistance [16,25,35]. For example, a review of 12 BMRC trials found only four (2.6%) failures among 154 patients infected with strains resistant to H and/or S who were treated with regimens containing four or five drugs [25]. However, to avoid the few failures and relapses who may acquire additional R resistance, Z should be continued for the entire six months of a four-drug short-course regimen in patients who have confirmed H-resistance [16]. Alternatively, R and E can be given for 12 months [16]. In patients with R mono-resistant TB, nine months treatment with H, S, and Z will achieve sputum conversion in 95%-100% of patients and only 5%-6% will relapse after 30 months [36].

In sharp contrast to H- or R- mono-resistance that can be treated easily and effectively with first-line drugs, combined H and R resistance (ie. MDRTB) requires treatment with at least four agents, including a quinolone and an injectable agent (ie. an aminoglycoside or capreomycin)[27,37,38]. These regimens must last for 18-24 months, have multiple adverse effects, cost US$1,850-US$9,190 [39], and are less effective. For example, Goble et al reported that, despite prolonged intensive and optimal treatment, only 56% of 171 HIV-negative MDRTB patients were cured. These patients had chronic disease and were resistant to a median of six drugs [40]. Fortunately, later series of patients with less severe disease (eg. primary MDRTB, or acquired MDRTB with previous exposure to fewer antituberculosis drugs) have produced better results (eg. cure rates of 82.5%-96%)[41,42]. Nonetheless, combined resistance to H and R still has an enormous impact on the duration, ease and cost of antituberculosis chemotherapy, thereby justifying the definition of MDRTB as resistance to at least these two drugs [26-29]. This strict definition will be used throughout this book.

2.2   Importance of a strict definition for MDRTB

A recent debate demonstrates the importance of accurately sub-classifying "drug-resistant" TB into MDRTB and other-drug-resistant tuberculosis (ODRTB, being mono- or poly-resistance not including both H and R) when reviewing treatment outcomes and programmatic interventions. Rifampicin-containing SCC regimens employed within effective DOTS programs have been shown to reduce the prevalence of "drug resistance" in several different countries [43-45]. However, Farmer and Kim have recently asserted that SCC/DOTS has reduced the prevalence of ODRTB but not MDRTB, and has done so only in settings without pre-existing high levels of MDRTB [46].

One example used in this debate is the Beijing Tuberculosis Programme, which introduced fully supervised chemotherapy in 1978 and which has used R extensively since 1988 [43]. Random surveys were conducted biannually between 1978-79 and 1991-92. During this time period, the number (and rate) of cases with initial resistance to H, S, and PAS declined, but R resistance had become established at a rate of 1.7%. Similar experience has been reported from Korea and Algeria [44,45]. Hence, in settings where MDRTB is not established, SCC/DOTS appears to lower the prevalence of "drug resistance" by reducing the absolute number and prevalence of patients with ODRTB but may leave a small (perhaps increasing) 'residue' of MDRTB cases.

There is little experience with using SCC/DOTS in areas with established high levels of MDRTB, when MDRTB is strictly defined as resistance to at least H and R. Establishment of a DOTS program in New York City was associated with a reduction in MDRTB levels [47,48]. However, numerous other interventions were also instituted: expedited laboratory diagnoses, individualised treatment of prevalent MDRTB cases, extensive use of chemoprophylaxis, and optimised infection control procedures [47]. Hence, the individual contribution of the DOTS program to the reduction of MDRTB levels cannot be determined.

DOTS programs have also been trialed in two MDRTB-endemic prison populations in the former Soviet Union and have produced dismal results [49-51]. The rates of MDRTB among prisoners commencing treatment in Baku, Azerbaijan, and Mariinsk, Siberia, were 23% and 22.6%, respectively. After fully-supervised treatment with WHO-recommended regimens, the respective cure rates were only 54% and 46%; the mortality rates were 11%

and 4%, but the default rates were also high (ie. 13% and 6%, respectively), mainly due to inter-prison transfers, release or re-trial. Nonetheless, the cure rate of Category I (ie. 2 HRZE/ 4 HR) and II (2 HRZES/1 HRZE/5 HRE) regimens in these MDRTB-endemic populations was well short of the 85% target set for TB control programs [17]. Treatment regimens may therefore need to be adjusted in populations where a significant proportion of the "drug-resistant" TB is MDRTB.

3.   VIRULENCE AND OTHER QUESTIONS ABOUT MDRTB

The above section not only highlights the importance of accurately defining "drug-resistant" TB but also shows how little is known about MDRTB. There are many unanswered questions. What is the natural history of MDRTB? What is the true global extent of the MDRTB problem? Do TB control programs need to adjust their strategies and treatment regimens to address MDRTB? At what prevalence of MDRTB are these adjustments warranted? Can TB control programs in low- and middle-income countries treat MDRTB patients? If so, should these patients receive a standardised MDRTB treatment regimen or should their therapy be individually tailored? What laboratory facilities do MDRTB treatment programs require? What chemoprophylaxis should contacts of MDRTB patients receive? What is the place of BCG? What practical cost-effective measures can hospitals, laboratories and other institutions adopt to limit the transmission of MDRTB?

One other basic question about "drug-resistant" *M. tuberculosis* remains unresolved and the answer has implications for our response to MDRTB — are "drug-resistant" strains as virulent as drug-susceptible strains? This issue arose in the 1950s and 1960s when strains of *M. tuberculosis* resistant to H and/or S were reported to grow poorly *in vitro*, and to have attenuated infectivity and pathogenicity in animal models [52-54]. The subsequent evidence has been contradictory. Some recent cellular and molecular studies support the assertion that H-resistant strains are less virulent while others do not. KatG, the mycobacterial catalase-peroxidase protein that protects *M. tuberculosis* from intracellular killing by hydrogen peroxide (H_2O_2) and other reactive oxygen intermediates, also activates H [55,56]. The majority of H-resistant strains have point mutations in the gene encoding KatG and some of these mutants entirely lose KatG expression and catalase activity. Isoniazid-resistant strains with reduced/absent catalase and peroxidase activity have shown reduced *in vitro* resistance to H_2O_2 in liquid medium and human monocyte cultures [56]. Similarly, an H-resistant strain of *M.*

bovis lacking catalase activity was shown to be significantly less virulent in guinea pigs than the parent H-sensitive strain [57]. Introduction of a functional *katG* into the resistant avirulent strain restored virulence and H-susceptibility. Van Soolingen et al have also argued that H-resistant strains are less transmissible or virulent based on molecular epidemiological evidence. They have studied the 'molecular fingerprints' of 4,266 TB cases in the Netherlands between 1993-1997 (ie. 78% of culture-positive cases caused by *M. tuberculosis* in the study period)[58]. Isoniazid-resistant strains were less likely to be in a cluster than H-sensitive strains (OR, 0.7; 95% CI, 0.5-0.9), suggesting that some H-resistant strains are less likely to produce secondary cases.

Unpublished experience from our own laboratory has shown that some MDRTB strains are extremely difficult to cultivate *in vitro* (eg. 10^6 bacilli from fresh sub-cultures are required to obtain one colony forming unit on Löwenstein-Jensen media). Similarly, detection of R-resistant *M. tuberculosis* in 139 sputa from Bangladesh using a molecular method [59] has demonstrated that sputa containing R-resistant strains were less-frequently positive in primary cultures than sputa containing R-susceptible strains (χ^2=5.89; p=0.015).

Nonetheless, ample evidence has accumulated over the last 10-15 years that MDRTB is transmitted and is pathogenic in immunocompetent, as well as immunocompromised, populations [49,50,60-63]. Epidemiological studies and animal models have found that drug-sensitive and drug-resistant strains of *M. tuberculosis* demonstrate a range of infectivity and pathogenicity [60,64]. In fact, the original studies of H-resistant strains in the 1950s reported the same findings. While Wolinsky et al found that H resistance correlated with loss of catalase activity and avirulence, they also found that four of 20 H-resistant strains were fully virulent or only "slightly attenuated" [52]. Furthermore, the molecular epidemiological studies of van Soolingen et al suggest that particular genotypes of H-resistant *M. tuberculosis* are transmissible and virulent. Finally, Billington et al have recently found that some mutations in the *rpoB* gene that confer R resistance in *M. tuberculosis* occur at little physiological cost to the mycobacterium [65].

Much further work is required to clarify the inter-relationship of drug resistance, virulence, and the host immune response. In the meantime, while the evidence regarding the virulence of drug-resistant *M. tuberculosis* remains conflicting, there is no doubt that some MDR strains are definitely transmissible and fully virulent. Hence, until further data are available, our approach to the current MDRTB problem must assume the 'worst-case scenario' that MDRTB is as virulent as drug-susceptible *M. tuberculosis*.

4. MDRTB IN THE PRESENT AND FUTURE

The chapters in this book address many of the questions currently surrounding MDRTB. Chapters 2 and 3 describe the epidemiology of MDRTB in industrialised countries and in low- and middle-income countries. The true extent of MDRTB is better described now than even a few years ago [66], largely due to the WHO/IUATLD Global Project on Anti-Tuberculosis Drug Resistance Surveillance [3]. However, Espinal highlights in chapter 3 that the prevalence of MDRTB remains undefined in much of Asia and many parts of Eastern Europe.

MDRTB has been linked with HIV infection in some outbreaks in high-income countries. The interaction of HIV and MDRTB is discussed by McCray and Onorato in chapter 4 and they conclude that nosocomial outbreaks largely account for the apparent association. However, they note the unusual incidence of rifampicin mono-resistance among HIV-positive patients and suggest that further research is required into the propensity of HIV/AIDS patients to develop drug-resistance. The practical factors contributing to the development of MDRTB are reviewed by Pablos-Méndez and Lessnau in chapter 5. These causes can be classified under two headings: clinical mismanagement (eg. delayed diagnosis, inadequate initial treatment, failure to recognise pre-existing drug resistance, addition of a single drug to a failing regimen, failure to promote adherence) and programmatic factors (eg. weak political commitment, irregular drug supplies).

Controversy has surrounded the appropriateness and effectiveness of the DOTS strategy in MDRTB-endemic areas [46,49,50]. In chapter 7, Raviglione presents evidence that DOTS prevents the emergence of drug resistance but concludes that standard SCC within a routine DOTS program may not adequately address high pre-existing levels of MDRTB. A later chapter by Dye and Williams on the mathematical modelling of MDRTB comes to a similar conclusion. Both chapters suggest that operational studies must determine the appropriate mix of additional interventions (eg. earlier detection of drug resistance, judicious use of second-line drugs) required in these MDRTB-endemic areas.

MDRTB can be effectively controlled in high-income countries, as shown by the experience in New York City [47,48]. The current methods for detecting and treating MDRTB are reviewed in chapters 8, 10, and 11, by experts from the National Jewish Medical and Research Centre in Denver, who have extensive experience in managing MDRTB patients. In a subsequent chapter, Telzak shows that with prompt institution of this specialised care, which is currently only possible in industrialised countries, the outcome of MDRTB patients can be greatly improved and their mortality significantly reduced, even if they are HIV-positive. The many difficulties (and possibilities) of adapting such treatment programs for use in developing countries are discussed in chapter 12. However, there is also some cause for optimism because Crofton and Van Deun do present some encouraging results from an MDRTB treatment program in Bangladesh that used a standardised treatment regimen and achieved culture conversion rates of 96.1% after 3 months.

Chapters 14 and 15 discuss the appropriate management of health care workers and other individuals exposed to MDRTB patients. Both chapters weigh the advantages and disadvantages of BCG in these circumstances. They also highlight the difficulties of using an unproven prophylactic regimen (eg. Z and ofloxacin) that has appreciable adverse effects. In chapter 18, Richards and Jarvis present recommendations on the administrative measures, engineering controls, and personal respiratory protective devices required to control the spread of *M. tuberculosis*, including MDRTB. The authors also consider the costs of these measures and their applicability and adaptation for low-resource countries.

All of the above chapters show that the diagnostics and therapeutics for managing MDRTB are currently available in high-income countries (but not elsewhere). Three other chapters by Takiff, Palomino, and Barry demonstrate that the research technology also exists to develop cheap rapid simple diagnostics and new effective chemotherapeutics that may be used in low- and middle-income countries.

The final chapter by Farmer and other proponents of "DOTS-Plus for MDRTB" provides a framework for delivering these resources and expertise to MDRTB-endemic populations in low- and middle-income countries. However, their chapter epitomises the current predicament of all MDRTB intervention programs. There is a lack of data on several aspects of MDRTB epidemiology and treatment. For example, Farmer et al discuss the risk of producing resistance to additional drugs if patients with ODRTB or MDRTB receive standard SCC (ie. the 'amplifier effect'). They present evidence that confirms the existence of the 'amplifier effect' but the frequency of this phenomenon remains largely undefined. Extensive studies are in progress comparing pre- and post-treatment isolates from patients with initial drug resistance who fail standard SCC. These studies are employing DNA 'finger-print' analyses to differentiate the 'amplifier effect' from other explanations for finding post-treatment isolates with resistance to additional agents (ie. super-infection, mixed infection, and mis-labelling of specimens).

There are also other unanswered questions about MDRTB. What prevalence of MDRTB justifies institution of a "DOTS-Plus" program? What format should "DOTS-Plus" programs take? Nonetheless, MDRTB cannot be ignored in the 'hot spots' until we know all of the answers. Farmer et al correctly emphasise that on-going operational studies are required to answer these questions. In fact, WHO has established a Working Group to co-ordinate pilot "DOTS-Plus" projects that will answer some of the above questions while assessing the feasibility of MDRTB management within TB control programs [67].

5. "THE PERFECT EXPRESSION OF OUR IMPERFECT CIVILIZATION"

In conclusion, this book affirms that the tools for controlling TB (and MDRTB) are available in industrialised countries but health care professionals, national governments, and international organisations lack the will to make these facilities available in low- and middle-income countries. The current situation regarding TB and MDRTB is encapsulated in a quotation from a book on the history of TB, "Tuberculosis has been called the perfect expression of our imperfect civilization" [68].

The excessive disease burden affecting the world's poor is now worrying economists as well as health professionals [69,70]. Only 18% of the world's population live in high-income countries but they consume >60% of the global non-renewable resources (eg. oil)[69]. WHO estimates that US$56 billion is spent annually on health research but less than 10% of that sum is used to study diseases that afflict 90% of the world's population [71]. The industrialised countries must address this disparity for several reasons [69]:

1. international travel, trade and migration can easily spread emerging and re-emerging infectious diseases (including TB and MDRTB) to industrialised countries;
2. continued neglect of the health needs of the world's poor will result in social dislocation and unrest; and, most importantly,
3. there is a moral imperative to do so.

Novel approaches are urgently required to finance health programs in developing countries, to fund drug and vaccine development, and to recognise intellectual property rights while still providing the new drugs and vaccines where they are needed [70].

TB and MDRTB exemplify the disparity between rich and poor. TB was the seventh leading cause of death in 1990 [72]. This ranking will be unchanged in 2020. Eighty percent of all incident TB cases in 1997 occurred in just 22 low- and middle-income countries, with more than 50% occurring in 5 SE Asian countries [73]. As chapters 2 and 3 in this book show, the MDRTB 'hot spots' also cluster in low- and middle-income countries.

This publication is therefore presented not only as a textbook for health professionals and scientists interested in MDRTB, but also as a prod to governments and international organisations to support and fund an effective response to the problem of drug-sensitive as well as "drug-resistant" TB. We have the technology. Let's 'just do it'!

REFERENCES

1. Heymann SJ, Brewer TF, Wilson ME, Fineberg HV. The need for global action against multidrug-resistant tuberculosis. JAMA 1999; 281: 2138-40.
2. Garrett L. TB surge in former East Bloc. Newsday, March 25, 1998, pA 21.
3. Pablos-Méndez A, Raviglione MC, Laszlo A, et al. Global surveillance for antituberculosis drug resistance, 1994-1997. N Engl J Med 1998; 338: 1641-9.
4. Ryan F. The forgotten plague: how the battle against tuberculosis was won – and lost. Little, Brown & Co., Boston 1992.
5. Ayvazian LF. History of tuberculosis, Chapter 1, 1-20. In: Reichman LB, Hershfield ES (eds.), Tuberculosis: a comprehensive international approach. Marcel Dekker Inc., New York 1993.
6. Rossman MD, MacGregor RR. Introduction and brief history, xvii-xxiii. In: Rossman MD, MacGregor RR (eds.), Tuberculosis: clinical management and new challenges. McGraw Hill Inc., New York 1995.
7. Herzog H. History of tuberculosis. Respiration 1999; 65: 5-15.
8. Bishop PJ, Neumann G. The history of the Ziehl-Neelsen stain. Tubercle 1970; 51: 196-206.
9. McDermott W, Muschenheim C, Hadley SJ, et al. Streptomycin in the treatment of tuberculosis in humans. Ann Intern Med 1947; 27: 769-822.
10. Sensi P. History of development of rifampin. Rev Infect Dis 1983; 5(suppl 3): S402-6.
11. Schluger NW, Harkin TJ, Rom WN. Principles of therapy of tuberculosis in the modern era, Chapter 60. In: Rom WN, Garay SM (eds.), Tuberculosis. Little Brown & Company, Boston, 1996.
12. Iseman M, Sbarbaro JA. Short-course chemotherapy of tuberculosis. Hail Britannia (and friends). Am J Respir Dis 1991; 143: 697-698.
13. Hong Kong Chest Service/British Medical Research Council. Controlled trials of 2, 4, and 6 months of pyrazinamide in 6-month, three-times-weekly regimens for smear-positive pulmonary tuberculosis, including an assessment of a combined preparation of isoniazid, rifampicin, and pyrazinamide, results at 30 months. Am Rev Respir Dis 1991; 143: 700-706.
14. Combs DL, O'Brien PJ, Geiter LJ. USPHS tuberculosis short-course chemotherapy trial 21: effectiveness, toxicity, and acceptability. The report of final results. Ann Intern Med 1990; 112: 397-406.
15. Centers for Disease Control. Initial therapy for tuberculosis in the era of multidrug resistance: recommendations of the Advisory Council for the Elimination of Tuberculosis. MMWR Morb Mortal Wkly Rep 1993 (RR-7): 1-8.
16. American Thoracic Society/Centers for Disease Control. Treatment of tuberculosis and tuberculosis infection in adults and children. Am J Respir Crit Care Med 1994; 149: 1359-1374.
17. Global Tuberculosis Programme. Treatment of tuberculosis: guidelines for national programmes. 2nd ed (WHO/TB/97.220). World Heath Organization, Geneva, 1997.
18. Grigg ERN. The arcana of tuberculosis: with a brief epidemiologic history of the disease in the U.S.A. Am Rev Tuberc Pulm Dis 1958; 78: 151-172.

19. WHO Tuberculosis Programme: framework for effective tuberculosis control (WHO/TB/94.179). World Health Organization, Geneva, 1994.
20. Kochi A. Tuberculosis control - is DOTS the health breakthrough of the 1990s? World Health Forum 1997; 18: 225-247.
21. Stead WW. The origin and erratic global spread of tuberculosis: how the past explains the present and is the key to the future. Clin Chest Med 1997; 18: 65-77.
22. Wilson LG. The historical decline of tuberculosis in Europe and America: its causes and significance. J Hist Med Allied Sci 1990; 45: 366-396.
23. Centers for Disease Control. Estimates of future global tuberculosis morbidity and mortality. MMWR Morb Mortal Wkly Rep 1993; 42: 961-964.
24. Dolin PJ, Raviglione MC, Kochi A. Global tuberculosis incidence and mortality during 1990-2000. Bull World Health Org 1994; 72: 213-220.
25. Mitchison DA, Nunn AJ. Influence of initial drug resistance on the response to short-course chemotherapy of pulmonary tuberculosis. Am Rev Respir Dis 1986; 133: 423-430.
26. Kochi A, Vareldzis B, Styblo K. Multidrug-resistant tuberculosis and its control. Res Microbiol 1994; 144: 104-110.
27. Iseman MD. Treatment of multidrug-resistant tuberculosis. N Engl J Med 1993; 329: 784-791.
28. Pablos-Méndez A, Raviglione MC, Laszlo A, et al. Global surveillance for antituberculosis drug resistance, 1994-1997. N Engl J Med 1998; 338:1641-1649.
29. Antituberculosis Drug Resistance in the World: The WHO/IUATLD Global Project on Anti-Tuberculosis Drug Resistance Surveillance 1994-1997 (WHO/TB/97.229). World Health Organization, Geneva, 1997.
30. Mitchison DA. The action of antituberculosis drugs in short-course chemotherapy. Tubercle 1985; 66: 219-225.
31. Dutt AK, Moers D, Stead WW. Short-course chemotherapy for tuberculosis with mainly twice-weekly isoniazid and rifampin. Am J Med 1984; 77: 233-242.
32. Hong Kong Chest Service/British Medical Research Council. Five-year follow-up of a controlled trial of five 6-month regimens of chemotherapy for pulmonary tuberculosis. Am Rev Respir Dis 1987; 136: 1339-1342.
33. Hong Kong Chest Service/British Medical Research Council. Controlled trial of 2, 4, and 6 months of pyrazinamide in 6-month, three-times-weekly regimens for smear-positive tuberculosis, including an assessment of a combination preparation of isoniazid.rifampin, and pyrazinamide: results at 30 months. Am Rev Respir Dis 1991; 143: 700-706.
34. Combs DL, O'Brien RJ, Geiter LJ. USPHS tuberculosis short-course chemotherapy trial 21: effectiveness, toxicity, and acceptability. The report of final results. Ann Intern Med 1990; 112: 397-406.
35. Singapore Tuberculosis Service/British Medical Research Council. Clinical trial of six-month and four-month regimens of chemotherapy in the treatment of pulmonary tuberculosis. Am Rev Respir Dis 1979; 119: 579-585.
36. Hong Kong Chest Service/British Medical Research Council. Controlled trial of 6-month and 9-month regimens of daily and intermittent streptomycin plus isoniazid plus pyrazinamide for pulmonary tuberculosis in Hong Kong. The results up to 30 months. Am Rev Respir Dis 1977; 115: 727-735.
37. Crofton J, Chaulet P, Maher D, et al. Guidelines for the management of drug resistant tuberculosis (WHO/TB/96.210). World Health Organization, Geneva, 1997.
38. Bastian I, Colebunders R. Treatment and prevention of multidrug-resistant tuberculosis. Drugs 1999; 58: 633-661.

39. Bastian I, Rigouts L, Van Deun A, Portaels F. Directly observed treatment, short-course strategy and multidrug-resistant tuberculosis: are any modifications required? Bull World Health Org (in press).

40. Goble M, Iseman MD, Madsen LA, et al. Treatment of 171 patients with pulmonary tuberculosis resistant to isoniazid and rifampin. N Engl J Med 1993; 328: 527-532.

41. Telzak EE, Sepkowitz K, Alpert P, et al. Multidrug-resistant tuberculosis in patients without HIV infection. N Engl J Med 1995; 333: 907-911.

42. Park SK, Kim CT, Song SD. Outcome of chemotherapy in 107 patients with pulmonary tuberculosis resistant to isoniazid and rifampin. Int J Tuberc Lung Dis 1998; 2: 877-884.

43. Zhang LX, Kan GQ, Tu DH, et al. Trend of initial drug resistance of tubercle bacilli isolated from new patients with pulmonary tuberculosis and its correlation with the tuberculosis programme in Beijing. Tuberc Lung Dis 1995; 76: 100-103.

44. Kim SJ, Bai GH, Hong YP. Drug-resistant tuberculosis in Korea, 1994. Int J Tuberc Lung Dis 1997; 1: 302-308.

45. Boulahbal F, Khaled S, Tazir M. The interest of follow-up of resistance of the tubercle bacillus in the evaluation of a programme. Bull Int Union Tuberc Lung Dis 1989; 64: 23-25.

46. Farmer P, Kim JY. Community based approaches to the control of multidrug resistant tuberculosis: introducing "DOTS-plus". BMJ 1998; 317: 671-674.

47. Frieden TR, Fujiwara PI, Washko RM, Hamburg MA. Tuberculosis in New York City – turning the tide. N Engl J Med 1995; 333: 229-233.

48. Moore M, Onorato IM, McCray E, Castro KG. Trends in drug-resistant tuberculosis in the United States, 1993-1996. JAMA 1997; 278: 833-837.

49. Coninx R, Mathieu C, Debacker M, et al. First-line tuberculosis therapy and drug-resistant *Mycobacterium tuberculosis* in prisons. Lancet 1999; 353: 969-973.

50. Kimerling ME, Kluge H, Vezhnina N, et al. Inadequacy of the current WHO re-treatment regimen in a central Siberian prison: treatment failure and MDR-TB. Int J Tuberc Lung Dis 1999; 3: 451-453.

51. Portaels F, Rigouts L, Bastian I. Addressing multidrug-resistant tuberculosis in penitentiary hospitals and in the general population of the former Soviet Union. Int J Tuberc Lung Dis 1999; 3: 582-588.

52. Wolinsky E, Smith MM, Steenken W. Isoniazid susceptibility, catalase activity, and guinea pig virulence of recently isolated cultures of tubercle bacilli. Am Rev Tuberc 1956; 73: 768-772.

53. Mitchison DA, Wallace JG, Bhatia AL, et al. A comparison of the virulence in guinea pigs of South India and British tubercle bacilli. Tubercle 1960; 41: 1-22.

54. Cohn ML, Davis CL. Infectivity and pathogenicity of drug-resistant strains of tubercle bacilli studied by aerogenic infection of guinea pigs. Am Rev Respir Dis 1970; 102: 97-100.

55. Zhang Y, Heym B, Allen B, et al. The catalase-peroxidase gene and isoniazid resistance of *Mycobacterium tuberculosis*. Nature 1992; 358: 591-593.

56. Manca C, Paul S, Barry CE III, et al. *Mycobacterium tuberculosis* catalase and peroxidase activities and resistance to oxidative killing in human monocytes in vitro. Infect Immun 1999; 67: 74-79.

57. Wilson TM, de Lisle GW, Collins DM. Effect of inhA and katG on isoniazid resistance and virulence of *Mycobacterium bovis*. Mol Microbiol 1995; 15: 1009-1015.

58. van Soolingen D, Borgdorff MW, de Haas PEW, et al. Molecular epidemiology of tuberculosis in the Netherlands: a nationwide study from 1993-1997. J Infect Dis 1999; 180: 726-736.

59. De Beenhouwer H, Lhiang Z, Jannes G, et al. Rapid detection of rifampicin resistance in sputum and biopsy specimens from tuberculosis patients by PCR and line probe assay. Tuberc Lung Dis 1995; 76: 425-430.
60. Snider DE, Kelly GD, Cauthen GM, et al. Infection and disease among contacts of tuberculosis cases with drug-resistant and drug-susceptible cases. Am Rev Respir Dis 1985; 132: 125-132.
61. Kritski AL, Ozorio Marques MJ, Rabahi MF, et al. Transmission of tuberculosis to close contacts of patients with multidrug-resistant tuberculosis. Am J Respir Crit Care Med 1996; 153: 331-335.
62. Victor TC, Warren R, Beyers N, van Helden PD. Transmission of multidrug-resistant strains of *M. tuberculosis* in a high incidence community. Eur J Clin Microbiol Infect Dis 1997; 16: 548-549.
63. Bifani PJ, Plikaytis BB, Kapur V, et al. Origin and interstate spread of a New York City multidrug-resistant *M. tuberculosis* clone family. JAMA 1996; 275: 452-457.
64. Ordway DJ, Sonnenburg MG, Donahue SA, et al. Drug-resistant strains of *Mycobacterium tuberculosis* exhibit a range of virulence for mice. Infect Immun 1995; 63: 741-743.
65. Billington OJ, McHugh TD, Gillespie SH. Physiological cost of rifampin resistance induced *in vitro* in *Mycobacterium tuberculosis*. Antimicrob Agents Chemother 1999; 43: 1866-1869.
66. Cohn DL, Bustreo F, Raviglione MC. Drug-resistant tuberculosis: review of the worldwide situation and the WHO/IUATLD Global Surveillance Project. Clin Infect Dis 1997; 24(Suppl 1): S121-S130.
67. Espinal MA, Dye C, Raviglione M, Kochi A. Rational 'DOTS Plus' for the control of MDR-TB. Int J Tuberc Lung Dis 1999; 3: 561-563.
68. Dormandy T. The White Death: a history of tuberculosis. Hambledon Press, London, 1998.
69. Guerrant RL, Blackwood BL. Threats to global health and survival: the growing crises of tropical infectious diseases—our "unfinished agenda". Clin Infect Dis 1999; 28: 966-986.
70. Sachs J. Helping the world's poorest. The Economist August 14, 1999: p. 17-20.
71. Balms for the poor. The Economist August 14, 1999: p. 63-65.
72. Murray CJL, Lopez AD. Alternative projections of mortality and disability by cause 1990-2020: Global Burden of Disease Study. Lancet 1997; 349: 1498-1504.
73. Dye C, Scheele S, Dolin P, et al. Global burden of tuberculosis: estimated incidence, prevalence, and mortality by country. JAMA 1999; 282: 677-686.

Chapter 2

The epidemiology of multidrug-resistant tuberculosis in the United States and other established market economies

Marisa Moore, Eugene McCray and Ida M. Onorato
Surveillance and Epidemiology Branch, Division of Tuberculosis Elimination, National Center for HIV, STD, and TB Prevention, Centers for Disease Control and Prevention. Atlanta, GA

1.   INTRODUCTION

Mycobacterium tuberculosis resistant to multiple antituberculosis drugs emerged as a serious threat to tuberculosis (TB) control efforts in the United States (US) in the late 1980s and early 1990s. The strains responsible for the extended and large outbreaks in hospitals and correctional facilities, reported primarily from New York, were resistant to at least isoniazid and rifampicin, and the term multidrug-resistant (or MDR) became used to refer selectively to resistance to at least these two key first-line drugs. The outbreaks primarily involved patients with human immunodeficiency virus (HIV) infection and were characterized by high morbidity and mortality, delayed diagnosis, extended infectious periods and multiple generations of source cases [1-5]. Although drug-resistant TB was not a new phenomenon, MDRTB had rarely been encountered in the US [6]. This chapter describes the emergence of MDRTB in the US, the steps that led to improved surveillance for drug-resistant TB, and key characteristics of MDRTB patients during 1993-1998, based on national surveillance data. In addition, a brief summary of the experience of other established market economies is also provided.

I. Bastian and F. Portaels (eds.), Multidrug-Resistant Tuberculosis, 17-28.
© 2000 *Kluwer Academic Publishers. Printed in the Netherlands.*

2.   EMERGENCE OF MDRTB IN THE UNITED STATES

The outbreaks of MDRTB in the late 1980s and early 1990s were associated with a resurgence of TB disease in the US that dramatically reversed the trend of declining numbers of cases and case rates since standardized reporting began in 1953. Between 1985 and 1992, the number of cases increased 20%, resulting in a peak of 26,673 cases (10.5 cases per 100,000) in 1992. Four major factors contributed to this resurgence: increased immigration from countries with a high prevalence of TB, the HIV/AIDS epidemic, a decline in funding and infrastructure dedicated to TB control, and transmission in congregate settings such as hospitals and correctional facilities. In response to this public health crisis, vigorous efforts to rebuild the public health infrastructure for TB control and strengthen the priority activities of state and local TB programs were initiated with the financial support and collaboration of the federal government.

Beginning in the early 1960s, the Centers for Disease Control and Prevention (CDC) monitored anti-TB drug resistance in the US through periodic surveys [6-10]. The surveys had generally found stable or decreasing rates of resistance, and in the setting of increasing funding constraints, the surveys were discontinued in 1986 [6]. Thus, the emergence of MDRTB was not detected through these surveys, but through reported outbreaks. In response, a federal task force developed a National Action Plan for addressing the urgent public health problem posed by these MDRTB outbreaks [11]. An initial objective of the plan was to determine the magnitude and nature of the problem. To assist, CDC conducted interim surveys in the first quarters of 1991 and 1992 and then added initial drug susceptibility test results to the individual TB case report used for national surveillance beginning in 1993. The 1991 and 1992 surveys included initial isolates from the 50 states and the District of Columbia, and 3.5% were resistant to at least isoniazid and rifampicin [12,13]. The overwhelming majority of MDRTB patients (62% in 1991) were reported from New York City.

The primary causes of drug-resistant TB were well established prior to the MDRTB outbreaks. Spontaneous and random mutations result in a low proportion of bacilli with single drug resistance in unselected populations of *M. tuberculosis* ($1:10^6$ for isoniazid; $1:10^8$ for rifampicin) [14]. Bacilli resistant to two drugs as a result of these mutations are even less likely. For example, mutants resistant to at least isoniazid and rifampicin are expected less than once in an unselected population of 10^{14} bacilli. Thus, even in pulmonary cavities that may contain up to 10^9 bacilli, bacilli resistant to these two drugs simultaneously are not likely to be found [15]. Exposure of unselected populations to anti-TB drugs, however, may result in the development of clinical drug resistance. Non-adherence to therapy and use of inadequate treatment regimens are the two major causes of clinical drug resistance, resulting from exposure of bacilli to a single drug for a prolonged period of time. Review of the previous clinical management of patients referred to a specialist MDRTB treatment center found an average of nearly four management errors per patient [16]. The most common errors included addition of a single drug to a failing regimen, initiation of an inadequate primary regimen, and failure to identify and address non-adherence to the prescribed regimen.

To prevent further development of MDRTB, standards of diagnosis and treatment in the US were expanded to include initial drug regimens of at least four first-line drugs and initial drug susceptibility testing for all patients with culture-positive disease to guide further management [17]. The use of directly observed therapy and other adherence promoting strategies were encouraged for all patients, and accountability for ensuring the completion of treatment was emphasized as a key role for health departments [17,18]. Recommendations to improve the use of rapid laboratory methods for diagnosis were also developed and funding was increased to promote their implementation [19].

3. TRENDS IN TB IN THE UNITED STATES, 1992-1998

Since the peak of the resurgence of TB in the US in 1992, the number of reported TB cases and TB case rate steadily decreased each year (Figure 1). During 1998, a total of 18,361 TB cases (6.8 cases per 100,000 population) were reported to CDC from the 50 states and the District of Columbia, a decrease of 8% from 1997 and 31% from 1992 [20]. This sustained overall decline reflected substantial decreases in the seven states (California, Florida, Georgia, Illinois, New Jersey, New York, and Texas) reporting the highest numbers of cases and accounting for 60% of the total number of US cases in 1998. Overall substantial decreases also occurred in 14 other states during the seven-year period. In the remaining 23 states and the District of Columbia, annual case counts fluctuated (e.g., an increase followed by a decrease) or remained relatively stable during 1992-1998. Most of these states had case rates below the year 2000 interim target goal for elimination of TB in the US of 3.5 per 100,000 (17 states) or reported less than 100 cases (16 states) in 1998.

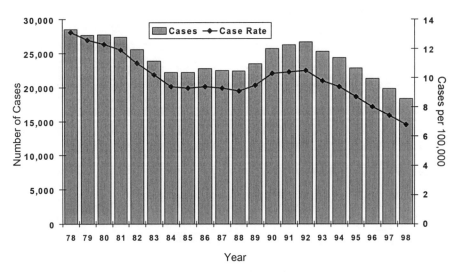

Figure 1. The annual number of reported tuberculosis cases and case rate, United States, 1978-1998.

In 1998, 6% of cases were reported in children under 15 years old, 8% in persons 15-24 years, 35% in persons 25-44 years, 27% in persons 45-64, and 24% in persons 65 years and older. The overall decline in TB cases and case rates during 1992-1998 reflected substantial declines in both the number of cases reported in each of these age groups and the respective TB case rates. The decreases were primarily limited to cases occurring in US-born persons, however. The number of cases among US-born persons decreased 44% during this period, with substantial declines in all age groups. The total number of cases among foreign-born persons increased 4% during this period, reflecting a small increase among adults aged 25-44 years, a larger increase among adults aged ≥45 years, and a substantial decline among children under 15 years old. As a result, the proportion of cases in foreign-born persons increased steadily, from 27% in 1992 to 42% in 1998.

The HIV/AIDS epidemic has had a dramatic impact on the epidemiology of TB, both globally and in the US. More than 30% of excess cases during the TB resurgence in the US were attributed to persons with HIV co-infection [21,22]. Monitoring the impact through the national surveillance system has been limited by incomplete reporting of HIV test results since information about HIV status was added to the TB case report in 1993. Using registry match data to supplement HIV test results submitted on the individual TB case report, minimum estimates of the proportion with HIV co-infection ranged from 15% during 1993-1994 to 10% in 1997 for persons of all ages reported with TB and from 29% to 21%, respectively, for persons aged 25 to 44. Levels of co-infection varied by geographic location, however. For example, in 1997, the proportion in persons aged 25 to 44 ranged from 15% in California to more than 35% in Florida and New York.

4.   MDRTB IN THE UNITED STATES, 1993-1998

A total of 1841 MDRTB cases were reported from the 50 states and the District of Columbia during 1993 through 1998. The number and proportion of reported MDRTB cases decreased each year, from nearly 500 or 3% in 1993 to 150 or 1% in 1998 (Table 1). The decrease in MDRTB was influenced by a substantial decrease in New York City (from 9.1% in 1993 to 2.8% in 1998). As a result, the percentage of MDRTB cases that were reported from New York City dropped from 48% in 1993 to 23% in 1998. During this period, the proportion of MDRTB in areas of the US excluding New York City decreased from 1.7% to 0.9%.

Table 1. Number and percentage of TB patients with MDRTB by year of report and history of prior TB, United States, 1993-1998

Year	No prior TB	Prior TB	Total TB
1993	410 (2.5 %)	76 (7.7%)	487 (2.8%)
1994	352 (2.2%)	75 (7.3%)	431 (2.4%)
1995	251 (1.6%)	70 (7.4%)	325 (1.9%)
1996	206 (1.4%)	42 (4.9%)	249 (1.5%)
1997	158 (1.1%)	39 (5.5%)	199 (1.3%)
1998	125 (1.0%)	24 (3.3%)	150 (1.1%)
All years	1502 (1.7%)	326 (6.2%)	1841 (1.9%)

Chi-square for linear trend by year: p<0.001 for no prior TB, prior TB, and total TB. Chi-square comparison of no prior TB vs. prior TB: p<0.001 for each year and overall.

Previous treatment is an important risk factor for drug-resistant TB. Because treatment history is not collected on the TB case report sent to CDC, prior history of TB is used to estimate primary and acquired anti-TB drug resistance. The proportion of MDRTB in persons who had a known prior TB episode (approximately 5% of all cases), an estimate of acquired resistance, was at least three times that for patients with no prior history of TB, an estimate of primary resistance (Table 1). In multivariate analysis, prior TB and residence in New York City were found to be the strongest predictors of MDRTB [23]. During 1993-1998, the number and proportion of MDRTB cases decreased in patients with and without a prior TB episode.

The distribution of MDRTB cases by age group and birth country, overall and by history of prior TB, is presented in Table 2. Approximately 80% of MDRTB cases were reported in persons 25 through 64 years old. The age groups of persons with TB less than 25 years old and more than 65 years old each accounted for approximately 10% of reported cases. The percentage of persons with MDRTB was lowest in those older than 65 years, and no MDRTB cases were reported in the small number of children less than 15 years old with prior TB (<1%). During 1993-1998, the proportion of MDRTB among persons without a history of prior TB was similar in both US- and foreign-born persons. The proportion of MDRTB among cases in foreign-born persons with prior TB, however, was nearly three times that of US-born persons. Nearly 40% of MDRTB cases in the foreign-born occurred in persons from the three top countries of birth for all foreign-born reported with TB: Mexico, the Philippines, and Vietnam. The number of MDRTB cases in US-born persons decreased more markedly than in foreign-born persons during this period. As a result, the percentage of MDRTB cases that were reported in foreign-born persons increased from 31% in 1993 to 61% in 1998. During 1993-1998, the proportion of foreign-born persons with MDRTB decreased from 3.0% to 1.6%, whereas the proportion for US-born persons decreased from 2.7% to 0.7%.

Table 2. Number and percentage of TB patients with MDRTB by age group and history of prior TB, United States, 1993-1998

Age group (years)	No prior TB	Prior TB	Total TB
0-14	31 (1.8%)	0 (0%)	31 (1.8%)
15-24	123 (1.7%)	24 (13.5%)	148 (2.0%)
25-44	829 (2.3%)	146 (8.8%)	982 (2.6%)
45-64	380 (1.6%)	103 (6.2%)	486 (1.9%)
65 +	139 (0.6%)	53 (3.0%)	194 (0.8%)
Birth Country			
United States	938 (1.6%)	128 (3.8%)	1071 (1.7%)
Foreign	551 (1.7%)	196 (10.6%)	750 (2.2%)

Chi-square for linear trend by age group: p<0.001 for no prior TB, prior TB (excluding age group 0-14), and total TB. Chi-square comparison of U.S.-born vs. foreign-born: p = 0.22 for no prior TB; p<0.001 for prior TB and total TB.

Seven states accounted for approximately 60% of reported TB cases in the US during 1993-1998; however, 56% of MDRTB cases were reported from two states, New York and California. As the proportion of US MDRTB cases reported from New York decreased from 52% in 1993 to 25% in 1998 (primarily reflecting the steady decline in New York City), the proportion of US MDRTB cases reported from California increased from 11% to 24%. The percentage of cases with MDRTB in California decreased from 1.7% in 1993 to 1.3% in 1998, and the percentage did not exceed 2% in the state's two largest cities. The threat of MDRTB, however, existed across the nation. Forty-five states and the District of Columbia reported at least one MDRTB case during 1993-1998. The potential for travel and migration to impact the risk in health jurisdictions nationwide was highlighted by the spread of Strain W, a highly resistant MDR strain responsible for large nosocomial outbreaks in New York in the early 1990s [24]. The overall percentage of MDRTB, however, was 1.0% or less in 24 states (accounting for 7% of the MDRTB cases and 24% of all cases) and less than 2% in 43 states (accounting for 47% of the MDRTB cases and 77% of all cases) during this period.

HIV infection has been identified as a risk factor for MDRTB in some US studies [25-27]. This association appears to have occurred in areas with ongoing transmission of MDRTB and exposure of persons with HIV who are at increased risk for developing TB once infected with *M. tuberculosis*. Based on HIV test results for TB cases submitted to the national surveillance system combined with TB and AIDS registry match data, a minimum of one-third of MDRTB cases reported during 1993-1997 occurred in persons with HIV co-infection. This varied by reporting area, however. For example, the proportion of MDRTB cases occurring in persons with HIV co-infection ranged from 5% in California to more than 50% in New York City. In contrast, the proportion of MDRTB cases occurring in foreign-born persons ranged from 83% in California to 24% in New York City. During this period, a larger decrease in the number and proportion of MDRTB cases occurred in HIV co-infected patients compared with those without co-infection.

During 1993-1998, approximately 90% of MDRTB patients had pulmonary TB (with or without extrapulmonary TB), and 4% were dead at the time of diagnosis. Of those with pulmonary TB, 70% were sputum smear-positive at the time of diagnosis. Based on follow-up data available for 1993-1996 cases, 34% of MDRTB patients died during therapy compared with 11% of non-MDRTB patients. Of those who did not die during therapy, 67% versus 88% completed therapy, respectively. Clinical research studies, designed to specifically describe response to therapy, have reported improved outcomes for both HIV-infected and HIV-negative MDRTB patients compared with the high mortality observed during the initial MDRTB outbreaks at the peak of the TB resurgence in the US [28-31]. For example, in a series of 25 patients without HIV infection, 24 had clinical responses and there were no relapses or treatment failures during a median follow-up of 91 weeks. The remaining patient died prior to receiving appropriate therapy [30]. In a series of 34 MDRTB patients with HIV infection, the overall response rate was 50% [28].

5.   MDRTB IN OTHER ESTABLISHED MARKET ECONOMIES

Other established market economies have reported similar recent experiences with MDRTB, including problems with nosocomial outbreaks, often involving HIV-infected patients [32-35]. The prevalence of MDRTB in such countries appears to have remained relatively low, however. A number of countries participated in the WHO Global Project on Anti-Tuberculosis Drug Resistance Surveillance [36,37]. In this project, countries followed standardized methods to determine population-based prevalence of drug-resistant TB. Participating countries included England and Wales, France, Italy, New Zealand, the Netherlands, Northern Ireland, Portugal, Scotland, and Spain, and reported levels of primary MDRTB were less than 1% in most of these countries. The reported prevalence was consistent with their relatively low rates of TB-notifications. In Italy, a substantially higher estimate was obtained because of a recent extended MDRTB outbreak and the survey focused on an HIV-infected population.

The impact of foreign-born persons from regions with a high prevalence of TB is an increasing concern in a number of these countries [38,39]. Several reports have highlighted the finding that high proportions of MDRTB patients in these countries are also foreign-born. In a ten-year population-based study in Alberta and British Columbia, Canada, a total of 24 (0.7%) MDRTB cases were identified, and 20 occurred in foreign-born patients [40]. All 16 isolates available for DNA fingerprinting had unique fingerprints, suggesting that infection was likely acquired in the birth country and that recent transmission of MDRTB in this Canadian region had not occurred. Two-thirds of the MDRTB was attributed to acquired drug resistance. In population based data from the Netherlands during 1994-1996 and from Denmark during 1993-1995, nearly 90% of MDRTB cases occurred in foreign-born persons [41,42]. During 1992-1994, a survey of laboratories in France detected 146 (0.6%) MDRTB cases, and approximately half occurred in persons born outside Europe [43]. This survey focused on districts that had monitored HIV infection. Among primary MDRTB cases, 11(35%) were in HIV-infected persons, and HIV infection remained associated with MDRTB in a multivariate model.

6.   LESSONS LEARNED

The emergence of MDRTB in the US, associated with an overall resurgence of TB in the mid 1980s and early 1990s, alerted the nation to serious weaknesses in TB control efforts. The effectiveness of the response, however, has been encouraging, and national surveillance data have assisted in evaluating key indicators of improvement. Since the peak of the resurgence in 1992, the annual total numbers of US TB cases and TB case rate have steadily decreased. In addition, during 1993-1998, the number and proportion of MDRTB cases markedly decreased. Ongoing transmission of MDR strains primarily impacted young adults aged 25 to 44, particularly US-born persons and those with HIV co-infection, and the greatest declines in MDRTB occurred in these groups.

The recent experience with MDRTB in the United States was a sobering reminder that extreme vigilance in ensuring that TB patients are treated with appropriate regimens and are fully adherent to these regimens is a first priority of any TB control program. The experience also served to highlight the importance of surveillance for drug-resistant TB as an essential component of TB control. Ideally, local, regional and national systems should provide timely information to enable programs to detect outbreaks; however, the most important role of surveillance for drug-resistant TB is as an evaluation tool. Stable or decreasing primary drug resistance is one measure of successful efforts to reduce ongoing transmission. Increasing drug resistance is a warning signal that ongoing transmission may be occurring. Other explanations include the possibility of imported drug resistance through migration into the region.

MDRTB outbreaks in hospitals and other congregate settings served as another important reminder. Adherence to basic infection control policies and procedures is essential to prevent transmission of *M. tuberculosis* in these settings. Of critical importance are administrative procedures that systematically identify patients with suspected TB, assess their potential infectiousness, and ensure appropriate action (e.g., isolation, prompt treatment) in order to limit exposures of staff and patients [44]. Furthermore, the emergence of MDRTB highlighted that the anti-TB drug armamentarium had not been bolstered by new drugs specifically developed for treating tuberculosis in several decades. Alternative drug regimens designed to treat MDRTB are complex and expensive, require long treatment duration, and are associated with adverse effects.

Valuable lessons from the recent MDRTB experience emphasize that conducting priority TB control activities effectively is critical to sustained success. The potential for the HIV/AIDS epidemic to amplify ongoing transmission of *M. tuberculosis* and the increasing impact of TB in foreign-born populations are also important considerations in directing national public health priorities for countries such as the United States and other established market economies. Finally, as recently suggested by the Advisory Council for the Elimination of Tuberculosis in the United States, support of a research agenda that promotes the development of a new TB vaccine and better diagnostic and treatment methods is essential to contribute to the global battle against tuberculosis and progress toward the ultimate goal of TB elimination [45].

REFERENCES

1.	Edlin BR, Tokars JI, Grieco MH, Crawford JT, Williams J, Sordillo EM, Ong KR, Kilburn JO, Dooley SW, Castro KG, Jarvis WR, Holmberg SD. An outbreak of multidrug-resistant tuberculosis among hospitalized patients with the acquired immunodeficiency syndrome. N Engl J Med 1992; 326: 1514-1521.
2.	Pearson ML, Jereb JA, Frieden TR, Crawford JT, Davis BJ, Dooley SW, Jarvis WR. Nosocomial transmission of multidrug-resistant *Mycobacterium tuberculosis*: a risk to patients and health care workers. Ann Intern Med 1992; 117: 191-196.
3.	Beck-Sague C, Dooley SW, Hutton MD, Otten J, Breeden A, Crawford JT, Pitchenfik AE, Woodley C, Cauthen G, Jarvis WR. Hospital outbreak of multidrug-resistant *Mycobacterium tuberculosis* infections: factors in transmission to staff and HIV-infected patients. JAMA 1992; 268: 1280-1286.
4.	Fischl MA, Uttamchandani RB, Daikos GL, Poblete RB, Moreno JN, Reyes RR, Boota AM, Thompson LM, Cleary TJ, Lai S. An outbreak of tuberculosis caused by multiple-drug resistant tubercle bacilli among patients with HIV infection. Ann Intern Med 1992; 117: 177-183.
5.	Valway SE, Greifinger RB, Papania M, Kilburn JO, Woodley C, DiFerdinando GT, Dooley SW. Multidrug-resistant tuberculosis in the New York State Prison System, 1990-1991. J Infect Dis 1994; 170: 151-156.
6.	Snider DE, Cauthen GM, Farer LS, Kelly GD, Kilburn JO, Good RC, Dooley SW. Drug-resistant tuberculosis. Am Rev Respir Dis 1991; 144: 732.
7.	Doster B, Caras GJ, Snider DE. A continuing survey of primary drug resistance in tuberculosis, 1961 to 1968. Am Rev Respir Dis 1976; 113: 419-425.
8.	Kopanoff DE, Kilburn JO, Glassroth JL, Snider DE, Farer LS, Good RC. A continuing survey of tuberculosis primary drug resistance in the United States: March 1975 to November 1977. Am Rev Respir Dis 1978; 118: 835-842.
9.	Centers for Disease Control. Primary resistance to antituberculosis drugs--United States. MMWR Morb Mortal Wkly Rep 1980; 29: 345-346.
10.	Centers for Disease Control. Primary resistance to antituberculosis drugs-- United States. MMWR Morb Mortal Wkly Rep 1983; 32: 521-523.
11.	Centers for Disease Control. National action plan to combat multidrug-resistant tuberculosis. MMWR Morb Mortal Wkly Rep 1992; 41(No. RR-11): 1-45.
12.	Bloch AB, Cauthen GM, Onorato IM, Dansbury KG, Kelly GD, Driver CR, Snider DE. Nationwide survey of drug-resistant tuberculosis in the United States. JAMA 1994; 271: 665-671.
13.	Bloch AB, Cauthen GM, Onorato IM, Dansbury KG, Kelly GD, Driver CR, Snider DE. Drug resistant tuberculosis (TB) trends in the U.S.: comparison of two nationwide surveys [Abstract]. Presented at the 1994 American Lung Association/American Thoracic Society International Conference; May 21-25, 1994; Boston, Mass.
14.	David HL. Probability distribution of drug-resistant mutants in unselected populations of *Mycobacterium tuberculosis*. Appl Microbiol 1970; 20: 810-814.
15.	Canetti G. The J. Burns Amberson Lecture: Present aspects of bacterial resistance in tuberculosis. Am Rev Respir Dis 1965; 92: 687-703.

16. Mahmoudi A, Iseman MD. Pitfalls in the care of patients with tuberculosis: Common errors and their association with the acquisition of drug resistance. JAMA 1993; 270: 65-68.

17. American Thoracic Society and the Centers for Disease Control and Prevention. Treatment of tuberculosis and tuberculosis infection in adults and children. Am J Respir Crit Care Med 1994; 149: 1359-1374.

18. Centers for Disease Control and Prevention. Essential components of a tuberculosis prevention and control program: recommendations of the Advisory Council for the Elimination of Tuberculosis. MMWR Morb Mortal Wkly Rep 1995; 44(No. RR-11): 1-16.

19. Tenover FC, Crawford JT, Huebner RE, Geiter LJ, Horsburgh CR, Good RC. The resurgence of tuberculosis: Is your laboratory ready? J Clin Microbiol 1993; 31: 767-770.

20. Centers for Disease Control and Prevention. Progress toward the elimination of tuberculosis--United States, 1998. MMWR Morb Mortal Wkly Rep 1999; 48: 732-736.

21. Cantwell MF, Snider DE, Cauthen GM, Onorato IM. Epidemiology of tuberculosis in the United States, 1985 through 1992. JAMA 1994; 272: 535-539.

22. Burwen DR, Bloch AB, Griffin LD, Ciesielski CA, Stern HA, Onorato IM. National trends in the concurrence of tuberculosis and acquired immunodeficiency syndrome. Arch Intern Med 1995; 155: 1281-1286.

23. Moore M, Onorato IM, McCray E, Castro KG. Trends in drug-resistant tuberculosis in the United States, 1993-1996. JAMA 1997; 278: 833-837.

24. Agerton TB, Valway SE, Blinkhorn RJ, Shilkret KL, Reves R, Schluter WW, Gore B, Pozsik CJ, Plikaytis BB, Woodley C, Onorato IM. Spread of Strain W, a highly drug-resistant strain of *Mycobacterium tuberculosis*, across the United States. Clin Infect Dis 1999; 29: 85-92.

25. Frieden TR, Sterling T, Pablos-Mendez A, Kilburn JO, Cauthen GM, Dooley SW. The emergence of drug-resistant tuberculosis in New York City. N Engl J Med 1993; 328: 521-526.

26. Gordin FM, Nelson ET, Matts JP, Cohn DL, Ernst J, Benator D, Besch CL, Crane LR, Sampson JH, Bragg PS, El-Sadr W. The impact of human immunodeficiency virus infection on drug-resistant tuberculosis. Am J Respir Crit Care Med 1996; 154: 1478-1483.

27. Moore M, McCray E, Onorato IM. Cross-matching TB and AIDS registries: TB patients with HIV co-infection, United States, 1993-1994. Public Health Rep 1999; 114: 269-277.

28. Turett GS, Telzak EE, Torian LV, Blum S, Alland D, Weisfuse I, Fazal BA. Improved outcomes for patients with multidrug-resistant tuberculosis. Clin Infect Dis 1995; 21: 1238-1244.

29. Salomon N, Perlman DC, Friedmann P, Buchstein S, Kreiswirth BN, Mildvan D. Predictors and outcome of multidrug-resistant tuberculosis. Clin Infect Dis 1995; 21: 1245-1252.

30. Telzak EE, Sepkowitz K, Alpert P, Mannheimer S, Medard F, El-Sadr W, Blum S, Gagliardi A, Salomon N, Turett G. Multidrug-resistant tuberculosis in patients without HIV infection. N Engl J Med 1995; 333: 907-911.

31. Telzak EE, Chirgwin KD, Nelson ET, Matts JP, Sepkowitz KA, Benson CA, Perlman DC, El-Sadr WM. Predictors for multidrug-resistant tuberculosis among HIV-infected patients and response to specific drug regimens. Int J Tuberc Lung Dis 1999; 3: 337-343.

32. Centers for Disease Control. Multidrug-resistant tuberculosis outbreak on an HIV ward--Madrid, Spain, 1991-1995. MMWR Morb Mortal Wkly Rep 1996; 45: 330-333.

33. Moro ML, Gori A, Errante I, Infuso A, Franzetti F, Sodano L, Iemoli E, the Italian Multidrug-Resistant Tuberculosis Outbreak Study Group. An outbreak of multidrug-resistant tuberculosis involving HIV-infected patients of two hospitals in Milan, Italy. AIDS 1998; 12: 1095-1102.

34. Breathnach AS, de Ruiter A, Holdsworth GMC, Bateman NT, O'Sullivan DGM, Rees PJ, Snashall D, Milburn HJ, Peters BS, Watson J, Drobniewski FA, French GL. An outbreak of multi-drug-resistant tuberculosis in a London teaching hospital. J Hosp Infect 1998; 39: 111-117.

35. Portugal I, Covas MJ, Brum L, Viveiros M, Ferrinho P, Moniz-Pereira J, David H. Outbreak of multiple drug-resistant tuberculosis in Lisbon: detection by restriction fragment length polymorphism analysis. Int J Tuberc Lung Dis 1999; 3: 207-213.

36. Pablos-Méndez A, Raviglione MC, Laszlo A, Binkin N, Rieder HL, Bustreo F, Cohn DL, Lambregts-van Weezenbeek CSB, Kim SJ, Chaulet P, Nunn P. Global surveillance for antituberculosis-drug resistance, 1994-1997. N Engl J Med 1998; 338: 1641-1649.

37. Pablos-Méndez A, Laszlo A, Bustreo F, Binkin N, Cohn DL, Lambregts-van Weezenbeek CSB, Kim SJ, Chaulet P, Nunn P, Raviglione MC. Anti-tuberculosis drug resistance in the world. WHO Global Tuberculosis Programme, Geneva, 1997.

38. Centers for Disease Control. Tuberculosis--Western Europe, 1974-1991. MMWR Morb Mortal Wkly Rep 1993; 42: 628-631.

39. Long R, Njoo H, Hershfield E. Tuberculosis: 3. Epidemiology of the disease in Canada. CMAJ 1999; 160: 1185-1190.

40. Hersi A, Elwood K, Cowie R, Kunimoto D, Long R. Multidrug-resistant tuberculosis in Alberta and British Columbia, 1989 to 1998. Can Respir J 1999; 6: 155-160.

41. Lambregts-van Weezenbeek CSB, Jansen HM, Veen J, Nagelkerke NJD, Sebek MMGG, van Soolingen D. Origin and management of primary and acquired drug-resistant tuberculosis in The Netherlands: the truth behind the rates. Int J Tuberc Lung Dis 1998; 2: 296-302.

42. Viskum K, Kok-Jensen A. Multidrug-resistant tuberculosis in Denmark 1993-1995. Int J Tuberc Lung Dis 1997; 1: 299-301.

43. Schwoebel V, Decludt B, de Benoist A, Haeghebaert S, Torrea G, Vincent V, Grosset J. Multidrug resistant tuberculosis in France 1992-4: two case-control studies. BMJ 1998; 317: 630-631.

44. Centers for Disease Control and Prevention. Guidelines for preventing the transmission of *Mycobacterium tuberculosis* in health-care facilities, 1994. MMWR Morb Mortal Wkly Rep 1994; 43(No. RR-13): 1-132.

45. Centers for Disease Control and Prevention. Tuberculosis elimination revisited: obstacles, opportunities, and a renewed commitment. Advisory Council for the Elimination of Tuberculosis (ACET). MMWR Morb Mortal Wkly Rep 1998; 48(No. RR-9): 1-13.

Chapter 3

Epidemiology of multidrug-resistant tuberculosis in low- and middle-income countries

Marcos A. Espinal
Drug Resistance Surveillance Team, Communicable Diseases Surveillance and Response, World Health Organization, Geneva, Switzerland

1.   INTRODUCTION

Drug-resistant tuberculosis (TB) was reported soon after the introduction of streptomycin [1], although it did not receive major attention until recently [2,3]. It was not considered a major issue in the industrialized world until outbreaks of multidrug-resistant TB (MDRTB), defined as resistance to at least isoniazid and rifampicin, were reported among HIV-infected people [4-7]. There has been an increasing concern on how drug-resistant TB and, more specifically, MDRTB is, or will be, negatively affecting TB control activities [8,9]. Since rifampicin and isoniazid are the most powerful first-line anti-TB drugs, it would be fair to assume that if MDRTB reaches significant levels in a given country, control efforts would fail to achieve their main goal: the decline of TB incidence by reducing *Mycobacterium tuberculosis (M. tuberculosis)* transmission through the cure of TB cases. Administration of standard short-course chemotherapy (SSCC) with first-line drugs (isoniazid, rifampicin, streptomycin, ethambutol, pyrazinamide, and thioacetazone) under directly observed therapy (DOT) is the cornerstone of modern TB control. Unfortunately, data available on the treatment outcome of MDRTB cases under routine programmatic conditions suggest that patients with MDRTB respond poorly to SSCC with first-line drugs [10].

I. Bastian and F. Portaels (eds.), Multidrug-Resistant Tuberculosis, 29-44.

In order to assess the threat that MDRTB poses to the control of TB in low- and middle-income countries, this chapter will provide an overview of the epidemiology of MDRTB in such settings. The transmission dynamics of MDR strains of *M. tuberculosis* in the community, the associated factors, and the latest available data will be reviewed. Countries classified by the World Bank as low- and middle-income according to their gross national product (GNP) per capita will be the subject of this chapter [11].

2.   TRANSMISSION DYNAMICS OF MDRTB

While the transmission dynamics of MDRTB have not yet been fully elucidated, the basic epidemiology of TB has been described and can be used as a starting point. To understand the dynamics of MDRTB, the concepts of 'infection' and 'disease' must be distinguished since each has its own implications for control activities. Recently, there has been increasing concern regarding the number of people infected with MDR strains of *M. tuberculosis*. Because the tuberculin test does not distinguish between resistant and susceptible strains, the number of people infected with MDR strains cannot be measured. Thus, all available estimates are subject to broad scepticism. Yet the importance of these estimates is not how many people are infected, but rather how many of these infected individuals will develop disease.

The epidemiology of TB indicates that only a small proportion of subjects infected with *M. tuberculosis* will develop disease [12]. The lifetime risk of an individual progressing to active TB is estimated to be approximately 10%, if infection has occurred in childhood [13]. The risk is greatest within the first two years of infection; and after about seven years starts to level off, remaining unchanged over the following decade [14-18]. In persons with a long-standing infection without a recognizable predisposing factor (e.g., human immunodeficiency virus infection, diabetes, silicosis), the risk is approximately 1 per 1000 person-years. In the case of infection with MDR or any other drug-resistant strains of *M. tuberculosis*, these risks could be even smaller if such strains are indeed less virulent than drug-susceptible strains, as has been suggested [19,20]. This suggestion is further supported by the molecular basis of multidrug resistance, which is the stepwise acquisition of multiple new mutations [21,22]. The large number of mutations required to produce MDRTB is believed to carry a fitness cost, resulting in less viable and less virulent strains [23,24]. These strains, by definition, have lower capacity to overcome body defences and, therefore, have less capacity to produce disease.

On the other hand, less virulent strains may still cause disease in immunocompromised hosts, such as subjects co-infected with human immunodeficiency virus (HIV) infection. Because of the immunosuppression caused by HIV, subjects co-infected with *M. tuberculosis* are known to be at increased risk of developing active TB by rapid progression to active disease after primary infection and by endogenous reactivation of latent infection [25]. Nosocomial outbreaks of MDRTB associated with HIV infection exemplify the dangerous interaction of these two diseases [26,27], and the importance of nosocomial transmission of MDRTB among HIV-positive patients.

Regardless of how disease in adults is caused by MDR strains (primary infection, re-infection, or reactivation) [28], infectious cases are those who are sputum smear-positive and, therefore, likely to transmit *M. tuberculosis* to others. While transmissibility and infectiousness of MDR strains are still very much a subject of research, transmission certainly still occurs even if subjects with MDRTB are less likely to transmit *M. tuberculosis* than subjects with drug-susceptible TB [29]. As with patients with drug-susceptible TB, a proportion of MDRTB cases may remain alive for some time even without proper treatment and can spread MDR strains in the community before they die or cure spontaneously. Thus, if those who fail to 'sputum convert' are not properly treated, the potential for increased transmission in the community will exist, regardless of the relative level of transmissibility of the infecting agent.

Irrespective of the virulence and transmissibility of MDR strains, MDRTB is associated with poor TB treatment programme conditions and, therefore, with managerial problems [30-32]. Thus, factors related to TB control activities rather than the burden of TB itself are more likely to be explain with the epidemiology of MDRTB. In fact, countries with efficient national TB programmes (NTP) such as Benin and Chile have been able to keep MDRTB at very low levels [33-34]. Furthermore, several countries in Africa are dealing with a high burden of TB (as a result of high levels of HIV) but have very low levels of MDRTB [35,36]. These observations confirm that burden of disease is not the main determinant to the genesis of MDRTB. Rather, lack of DOT and unregulated treatment for TB play a significant role in the emergence and spread of MDRTB, since drug-resistant TB is the consequence of misuse of anti-TB drugs. Chaotic treatment for TB is also directly linked to unregulated availability of drugs on the market [37].

3.   ASSESSMENT OF MDRTB PREVALENCE

While data on the prevalence of *M. tuberculosis* drug resistance have been available for several years, the lack of sound methodological guidelines including proper drug susceptibility testing (DST) made these data inadequate to assess the magnitude of the problem. A ten-year review by the World Health Organization (WHO) concluded that most of the studies conducted in low- and middle-income countries were not representative of the population with TB in these settings [38]. Hence, no clear conclusion could be reached regarding the true scope of the problem. In addition, these studies shared several methodological problems including lack of laboratory quality control, poor or no description at all of the methods of sampling, lack of standardization in the methods of laboratory testing and reporting of results, and no distinction between drug resistance in new (i.e., primary drug resistance) and retreatment (i.e., acquired drug resistance) cases of TB. This last problem is worthy of comment since drug resistance in new and retreatment cases has different meanings and, therefore, should be reported separately.   Resistance found in retreatment cases suggests inadequate treatment in the past, whereas resistance found in new cases indicates the level of transmission that is occurring in the community. However, resistance among retreatment cases could be subject to erroneous interpretation, because it is usually estimated from a small number of cases (unless there is a substantial pool of retreatment/chronic patients). In this regard, countries with efficient NTP could observe an increase in the proportion of drug resistance among retreatment cases as the total number of these cases are reduced over the years due to a rapid reduction of drug-susceptible TB.   As a result of this process, an effective NTP could ultimately have few retreatment cases but all of them might have drug-resistant TB.

The challenge of accurately estimating the level of resistance in new and retreatment cases relies on the ability to prevent misclassification of retreatment cases as new cases. This is a very difficult task, as retreatment cases may deny their previous treatment history because of the misconception that they would not receive treatment otherwise. One option to consider is to report the combined prevalence of drug resistance, which may well reflect the overall number of circulating strains in the community. However, this indicator is also subject to bias because sampling in most surveys is based only upon the pool of new cases. To overcome such a bias, the contribution to the overall level of resistance from retreatment cases should be weighted by the proportion of retreatment cases among all cases registered for treatment in the whole country [39].

Despite the above constraints, efforts should be made to assess and report the level of drug resistance according to the type of patient: new versus retreatment. WHO and the International Union against Tuberculosis and Lung Disease (IUATLD) took this and other issues into account in the global project on anti-TB drug resistance surveillance (DRS) that was launched in 1994. The main goals of this initiative are to collect, in a standardized manner, comparable data on the extent and type of drug resistance at the national level and to monitor trends over time [39,40]. Following standardized methodological guidelines, this project collected data from several low- and middle-income countries and provided an insight into the problem of MDRTB in these settings.

4.   MAGNITUDE OF MDRTB PROBLEM

In the next few pages, data from low- and middle-income countries in Latin America, Africa, Eastern Europe, and Asia will be presented and discussed. High-income countries in any of these geographic areas will not be included, as they are not the purpose of this chapter. Since hospital-based studies would not be suitable to draw conclusions on the magnitude of MDRTB in a given country, due to the inability to generate estimates on representative populations (selection bias), this type of study will not be considered in this chapter.

4.1   Africa

Representative data from Africa have been very limited and few countries have monitored the level of drug-resistant TB over time. One of these countries is Algeria, where drug resistance decreased from 1965 to 1985 after the implementation of sound control measures in 1967. MDRTB among new cases has remained stable at low levels since the introduction of rifampicin in 1969 [41]. Among retreatment cases, however, the proportion of MDRTB increased from 2.7% during 1975-80 to 11% during 1981-85. This result was basically due to a reduction in the total number of retreatment cases from 917 to 145. Representative studies carried out between 1980 and 1994 in Kenya, Western Cape province in South Africa, Karonga District in Malawi, and Tanzania reported very low levels of MDRTB among new cases (Figure 1) [42-45]. Similarly, the WHO/IUATLD global project reported levels of MDRTB among new cases between 0% and 1.9% in Benin, Botswana, Kenya, Lesotho, Swaziland, Sierra Leone, and Zimbabwe [40]. The prevalence of MDRTB among retreatment cases ranged from 0 to 12.8%. Ivory Coast, however, was considered a "hot spot", because of a substantial level of MDRTB (5.3%). Further data collected in nineteen districts of three geographical zones of Uganda have revealed that MDRTB is only 0.7% among new cases and 4.4% among retreatment cases [46]. Likewise, in Mpumalanga Province, South Africa, MDRTB was reported in only 1.5% of the new cases studied [47]. While not representative countrywide, the findings of these latter two studies (which also followed WHO/IUATLD guidelines) suggest that MDRTB is not a problem in these geographical settings.

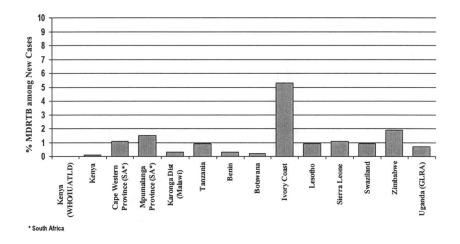

Figure 1. Prevalence of MDRTB among new cases in Africa

The above findings indicate that in Africa, with few exceptions, MDRTB is not a public health problem at present. The low level of MDRTB in Africa has been attributed to the recent introduction of rifampicin into treatment regimens [39]. It appears, however, that lack of MDRTB is more the result of sound control programmes using DOT rather than the time period of rifampicin introduction in these countries. In Benin, for instance, rifampicin was introduced in 1983 and twelve years later there was no MDRTB [33]. This is also the case for Botswana and Kenya. In contrast, Ivory Coast introduced rifampicin in 1985 and MDRTB was found to be a problem in 1995. Importantly, DOT is not widely practiced in Ivory Coast [35] in contrast to Benin, Kenya, and Botswana.

Even if the prevalence of MDRTB in many of these countries is low, its presence should be a wake-up call to continue monitoring its course in addition to promoting the improvement and expansion of control activities. African countries should pursue strategies oriented to preventing MDRTB. This may be achieved not only by adopting DOTS but also by trialing and implementing novel strategies (e.g., active case finding, preventive therapy for TB, enhanced surveillance) to reverse the increasing incidence of HIV-associated TB [25]. Limiting the availability of drugs sold over the counter will also limit the upsurge of MDRTB.

In a region already overburdened by HIV, MDRTB must not become a major public health problem. A substantial level of MDRTB in any one country, as in the case of Ivory Coast, may be all that is needed for it to spread to other countries. Surveillance for drug-resistant TB is currently under way in the Central African Republic, Guinea, Gambia, Morocco, Mozambique, Nigeria, and Uganda (country-wide). The resulting data will contribute to our understanding of the situation of MDRTB in Africa.

4.2   Latin America

In a multi-center study carried out between 1980 and 1990, Laszlo et al. showed that resistance to anti-TB drugs was a cause for concern in ten Latin American countries [48]. Resistance levels of more than 15% to one or more drugs were reported from Bolivia, Colombia, Haiti, Mexico and Peru. The overall level of MDRTB found in this study was 0.5%; however, these data were not representative of the population with TB in these countries. Other studies conducted in Argentina [49] and Chile [34] found levels of MDRTB of less than 0.3% among new cases of TB. The case of Chile is worthy of comment as an impressive example of how the implementation of DOTS for more than 20 years has been able to prevent the upsurge of MDRTB [50]. Chile has experienced a steady decrease in the incidence of TB from 105.6 / 100,000 people in 1971 to 40.7 / 100,000 people in 1994 [51]. MDRTB among new cases between 1981 and 1995 has ranged between 0 and 0.9% in national samples and there is no evidence that this situation will worsen.

In contrast, data released by the WHO/IUATLD global project showed that MDRTB among new cases was a significant problem in Argentina (4.6%), the Dominican Republic (6.6%) and, to lesser extent, in Peru (2.5%) [40] (Figure 2). While the data from Argentina were influenced by nosocomial outbreaks of MDRTB related to HIV (0.8% in HIV-negative subjects compared to 28.3% in HIV-positive subjects) during the time of survey, the high level of MDRTB in the Dominican Republic appeared to be the result of poor programme activities over several years [52]. A recent survey in the Mexican states of Baja California, Oaxaca, and Sinaloa found levels of MDRTB of 2% among new cases [53], which suggests that surveillance efforts need to be expanded to other Mexican states in order to have a clear view of the magnitude of the problem in this country. The situation in other Latin American countries does not appear to be as serious as in the above countries [40,54]. Among retreatment cases, the WHO/IUATLD global project reported levels of MDRTB as low as 4.7% in Bolivia up to 22.2% in Argentina [40].

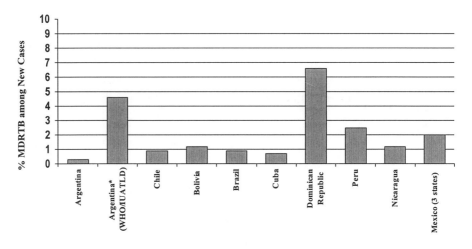

* 0.8% among HIV-negative subjects and 28.3% among HIV-positive subjects

Figure 2. Prevalence of MDRTB among new cases in Latin America

In summary, data from Latin America suggest that in most countries MDRTB among new cases is at very low levels. Trend data will be needed to determine if the increased proportion of MDRTB among retreatment cases is the result of a reduction in the total number of retreatment cases or the result of a true increase in MDRTB cases. The matter should be closely monitored in order to detect changes. Surveillance efforts are currently under way in Venezuela, Uruguay, Colombia, Peru, and Argentina.

4.3   Asia

Urgent DRS data are needed from Asia, as this region is home to 64% of the world's TB cases and contains eleven of the twenty-two countries with the highest burden of TB. Moreover India, China, Indonesia, Bangladesh, and Pakistan are estimated to be five of the six countries with the highest TB incidence in the world [55]. Cohn et al. considered only two of fourteen studies from Asia as representative of the population surveyed [38]. Thus, no conclusion could be drawn regarding the magnitude of drug resistance and MDRTB in this region. Nevertheless, some of the data shed light on this issue. A study in Beijing, China, to assess trends in drug resistance among new cases of TB reported levels of MDRTB between 0.4% in 1981-82 and

0.8% in 1991-92, with a peak of 1.6% in 1987-88 [56] (figure 3). The lack of a significant increasing trend (p = 0.5) was attributed to an increase in the coverage of fully-supervised SSCC among new smear-positive subjects from 62% in 1981 to 98% in 1992. While these numbers suggest low levels of MDRTB, it is also certain that they were not representative of China as a whole. Data collected by the WHO/IUATLD global project on DRS in Henan, the largest province in China, suggest that 16.6% of 916 new cases and 37% of 456 retreatment cases had MDRTB [57]. Misclassification of retreatment cases as new cases and some laboratory limitations were detected in this study. While the investigators implemented measures (e.g., re-interview of patients, record review, re-testing of strains) to correct these deficiencies, a new survey has been recommended in order to confirm the above findings.

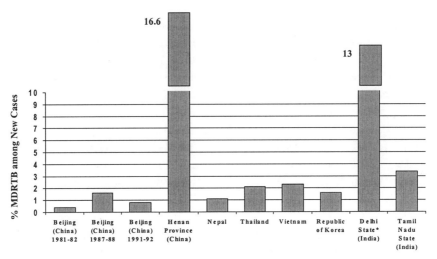

* Data refer to combined prevalence (new and retreatment cases)

Figure 3. Prevalence of MDRTB among new cases in Asia

Data from Nepal, Vietnam, and Thailand suggest that MDR among new TB cases is not a major public health problem (Figure 3) [40]. However, no data were available regarding the extent of the problem among retreatment cases. These countries have been able to implement sound control activities for several years. Hence, the results of these studies reflect effective and well-organized NTP in these countries. On the other hand, 13.3% of all TB cases in Delhi State, India, were shown to have MDRTB [40]. During the collection of these data, however, there was misclassification of retreatment cases as new cases. As a result, only the combined prevalence was reported. Recent data from Tamil Nadu State show that MDRTB prevalence is 3.4% among new cases [58]. The number of retreatment cases tested was too small to be considered meaningful.

Despite the above studies, the true magnitude of MDRTB in Asia remains undefined. Upcoming data from the provinces of Guangdong, Zhejiang, Shandong, Liaoning, and Hubei, in China, as well as other states in India, Indonesia, Mongolia, Bangladesh, and Myanmar, will contribute to a better understanding of the epidemiology of MDRTB in this region of the world. While preliminary data are pointing to the existence of high levels of MDRTB in some Asian locations, it is also apparent that countries with sound TB control programmes have been able to keep MDRTB at very low levels.

4.4   Eastern Europe

The World Bank classifies as middle-income countries most Eastern European nations, including the Russian Federation. Several previous studies carried out in the former Socialist countries are not representative with regard to the target population [38, 59-60]. Furthermore, drug resistance levels among new and retreatment cases of TB were not adequately distinguished in many of these studies. Reliable data are available from special settings (prisons and district hospitals) showing high levels of MDRTB [61,62]. Additionally, data from the WHO/IUATLD global project on DRS from the Ivanovo Oblast in Russia, Estonia, and Latvia indicate the existence of high levels of MDRTB among new and retreatment cases (Figure 4) [40]. Indeed, the Ivanovo Oblast was classified as a "hot spot" by the WHO/IUATLD global project because MDRTB was observed in 4% of the new cases surveyed [40]. Recent data show an increasing trend with levels of 9% between 1997 and 1998, and highlight an emergency situation [63]. In other parts of Russia, MDRTB is also a problem [64]. In Latvia, the WHO/IUATLD study carried out in 1996 showed 14% MDRTB among new cases. This study might have overestimated to a certain extent the true magnitude of the problem for it did not cover the whole country. Data recently published show an increasing trend from 5.2% in 1995 to 9.0% in 1997 [65]. Regardless of the exact level of MDRTB, it is clear that Latvia is experiencing a significant public health problem. The problem in Estonia also appears to be increasing in severity.

Due to a large pool of chronic cases, the high levels of MDRTB reported in several countries of Eastern Europe are likely the result of a substantial circulation of these strains in the community. This problem is common to most Eastern European countries. Chronic cases of TB are the greatest generators of MDRTB. For many years, the implementation of outdated strategies for TB control did not reduce the number of such cases in many of these countries. Other Eastern European countries, however, are making significant efforts to control TB and prevent MDRTB. This is the case of the Czech Republic where very low levels of MDRTB (1%) among new cases were reported in 1995 [40].

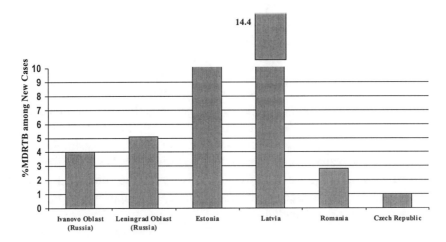

Figure 4. Prevalence of MDRTB among new cases in Eastern Europe

In summary, MDRTB in several Eastern European countries is a major public health problem and needs to be urgently addressed. If the prevalence reported from Russia, Latvia, and Estonia is not rapidly reduced, the rate of propagation of MDR cases will soon exceed their rate of removal. Thus, spread to other countries may be difficult to avoid. Feasible and cost-effective management strategies that could be implemented in the local settings must be explored in order to contain the potential spread of MDRTB. These are the objectives of the recently launched WHO DOTS-PLUS initiative [66]. However, the entire picture of drug-resistant TB in Eastern Europe is not yet defined. Azerbaijan, Bulgaria, Bosnia, Belarus, Georgia, Kazakhastan, Kyrgyzstan, Tajikistan, Ukraine, Uzbekistan, Turkmenistan, are some of the countries where reliable and representative data are needed. Many of these countries are now prioritizing surveillance of drug-resistant TB. Consequently, data should be expected in the coming years.

5.   CONCLUDING REMARKS

The epidemiology of MDRTB relies on three major factors: i) the transmissibility and virulence of MDR strains of *M. tuberculosis*; ii) the response of MDRTB to standard SSCC; and iii) the extent to which a TB control programme prevents MDRTB by curing drug-susceptible TB. Among the low- and middle-income countries, the problem of MDRTB is most critical in several Eastern European countries where urgent control measures for TB and specific management for MDRTB are needed. While the problem in other parts of the world may be limited to well-defined settings in Africa and Latin America, the true extent of the MDRTB situation in Asia is not yet known. Thus, surveillance efforts need to be urgently expanded to several areas of Asia. The vast majority of Asian countries housing the highest burden of TB are yet to generate the appropriate data.

Successes are also evident. The surveys clearly show that MDRTB has been kept at low levels in countries where DOTS is widely implemented (e.g., Benin, Botswana, Chile, Kenya, Nepal, Nicaragua, Peru, Thailand, and Vietnam). These countries, however, must continue monitoring drug-resistant TB, in order to track its course and adopt the appropriate measures, if increasing trends are detected.

ACKNOWLEDGMENTS

The author is indebted to Dr Chris Dye, Dr Catharina Lambregts-van Weezenbeek, Dr Hans Rieder, Dr Mario Raviglione, Mr. Rajesh Gupta, and Dr Thomas Frieden for their comments and contributions to this chapter.

REFERENCES

1. Crofton J, Mitchison DA. Streptomycin resistance in pulmonary tuberculosis. BMJ 1948; 2: 1009-1015.
2. Kochi A, Vareldzis B, Styblo K. Multidrug-resistant tuberculosis and its control. Res Microbiol 1993; 144: 104-110.
3. Nunn P, Felten M. Surveillance of resistance to antituberculosis drugs in developing countries. Tuberc Lung Dis 1994; 75: 163-167.
4. Alland D, Kalkut GE, Moss AR, et al. Transmission of tuberculosis in New York City - An analysis by DNA fingerprinting and conventional epidemiological methods. N Eng J Med 1994; 330: 1710-1716.
5. Small PM, Shafer RW, Hopewell PC, et al. Exogenous reinfection with multi-drug-resistant Mycobacterium tuberculosis in patients with advanced HIV infection. N Eng J Med 1993; 328: 1137-1144.

6. Monno L, Angarano G, Carbonara S, et al. Emergence of drug-resistant Mycobacterium tuberculosis in HIV-infected patients. Lancet 1991; 337: 852.

7. Bouvet E. Transmission nosocomiale de tuberculose multirésistante parmi les patients infectés par le VIH: en France, à Paris. Bulletin Epidémiologique Hebdomadaire 1991; 45: 196-197.

8. Farmer P, Kim JY. Community-based approaches to the control of multidrug-resistant tuberculosis: introducing "DOTS-PLUS". BMJ 1998; 317: 671-674.

9. Farmer P, Bayona J, Becerra M, et al. The dilemma of MDRTB in the global era. Int J Tuberc Lung Dis 1998; 2: 869-76.

10. Espinal MA, Kim SJ, Hong YP, et al. Standard short course chemotherapy for drug resistant tuberculosis. Treatment outcomes in six countries. (Manuscript submitted).

11. The World Bank. Global Economic Prospects and the Developing Countries 1998/99. The World Bank, Washington, DC, 1999.

12. Smith PG, Moss AR. Epidemiology of tuberculosis. In: Bloom BR (ed.), Tuberculosis: pathogenesis, protection, and control. AMS Press, Washington, DC, 1994.

13. Comstock GW, Livesay VT, Woolpert SF. The prognosis of a positive tuberculin reaction in childhood and adolescence. Am J Epidemiol 1974; 99: 131-138.

14. British Medical Association. BCG and vole bacillus vaccines in the prevention of tuberculosis in adolescents. First (progress) report to the medical research council by their tuberculosis vaccines clinical trials committee. BMJ 1956; 1: 1-15.

15. British Medical Association. BCG and vole bacillus vaccines in the prevention of tuberculosis in adolescents. Second report to the medical research council by their tuberculosis vaccines clinical trials committee. BMJ 1959; 2: 379-396.

16. British Medical Association. BCG and vole bacillus vaccines in the prevention of tuberculosis in adolescence and early adult life. Third report to the medical research council by their tuberculosis vaccines clinical trials committee. BM J 1963; 1: 973-978.

17. D'Arcy Hart P, Sutherland I. BCG and vole bacillus vaccines in the prevention of tuberculosis in adolescence and early adult life. Final report to the Medical Research Council. BMJ 1977; 2: 293-295.

18. Ferebee SH. Controlled chemoprophylaxis trials in tuberculosis. A general review. Adv Tuberc Res 1969; 17: 28-106.

19. Lambregts-van Weezenbeek CSB. Drug-resistant tuberculosis in the Netherlands; trifle or threat? Thesis University of Amsterdam, Amsterdam , February 1998.

20. Zhang Y, Heym B, Allen B, Young D, Cole S. The catalase-peroxidase gene and isoniazid resistance of *Mycobacterium tuberculosis*. Nature 1992; 358: 591-593.

21. Heym B, Honoré N, Truffot-Pernot C, et al. Implications of multidrug resistance for the future of short-course chemotherapy of tuberculosis: a molecular study. Lancet 1994; 344: 293-298.

22. Mitchison DA. How drug resistance emerges as a result of poor compliance during short course chemotherapy for tuberculosis. Int J Tuberc Lung Dis 1998; 2: 10-15.

23. Cohn ML, Oda U, Kovitz C, Middlebrook G. Studies on isoniazid and tubercle bacilli: the isolation of isoniazid-resistant mutants *in vitro*. Am Rev Tuberc 1954; 70: 465-475.

24. Cohn ML, Kovitz C, Oda U, Middlebrook G. Studies on isoniazid and tubercle bacilli: the growth requirements, catalase activities, and pathogenic properties of isoniazid-resistant mutants. Am Rev Tuberc 1954; 70: 641-664.

25. De Cock KM, Chaisson RE. Will DOTS do it? A reappraisal of tuberculosis control in countries with high rates of HIV infection. Int J Tuberc Lung Dis 1999; 3: 457-465.

26. Ritacco V, Di Lonardo M, Reniero A, et al. Nosocomial spread of human immunodeficiency virus-related multidrug-resistant tuberculosis in Buenos Aires. J Infect Dis 1997; 176: 637-42.

27. Edlin BR, Tokars JI, Grieco MH, et al. An outbreak of multidrug-resistant tuberculosis among hospitalized patients with the acquired immunodeficiency syndrome. N Engl J Med 1992; 326: 1514-21.

28. Marchal G. Recently transmitted tuberculosis is more frequent than reactivation of latent infections. Int J Tuberc Lung Dis 1997; 1: 192.

29. van Soolingen D, Lambregts-van Weezenbeek CSB, de Haas PEW, Veen J, van Embden JDA. Transmission of sensitive and resistant strains of *Mycobacterium tuberculosis* in The Netherlands, 1993-1995, studied by means of DNA-fingerprinting. Ned Tijdschr Geneeskd 1996; 140: 2286-2289.

30. Lambregts-van Weezenbeek CSB. Drug-resistant tuberculosis. Eur Respir Mon 1997; 4: 298-326.

31. Lambregts-van Weezenbeek CSB, Veen J. Control of drug-resistant tuberculosis. Tubercle Lung Dis 1995; 76: 455-459.

32. Mahmoudi A, Iseman MD. Pitfalls in the care of patients with tuberculosis: common errors and their association with the acquisition of drug resistance. JAMA 1993; 270: 65-68.

33. Trébucq A, Anagonou S, Gninafon M, Lambregts K, Boulahbal F. Prevalence of primary and acquired resistance of *Mycobacterium tuberculosis* to antituberculosis drugs in Benin after 12 years of short-course chemotherapy. Int J Tuberc Lung Dis 1999; 3: 466-470.

34. Valenzuela MT, Garcia P, Ponce J, Lepe R, Velasco M, Piffardi S. Drug resistance of *M. tuberculosis* in Chile: rates of initial resistance for 1986 and acquired resistance for 1985. Bull Int Union Tuberc Lung Dis 1989; 64: 13-14.

35. Chaisson RE, Coberly JS, De Cock. DOTS and drug resistance: a silver lining to a darkening cloud. Int J Tuberc Lung Dis 1999; 3: 1-3.

36. Kenyon TA, Mwasekaga MJ, Huebner R, Rumisha D, Binkin N, Maganu E. Low levels of drug resistance amidst rapidly increasing tuberculosis and human immunodeficiency virus co-epidemics in Botswana. Int J Tuberc Lung Dis 1999; 3: 4-11.

37. Uplekar MW, Rangan S. Private doctors and tuberculosis control in India. Tuberc Lung Dis 1993; 74: 332-337.

38. Cohn D, Bustreo F, Raviglione MC. Drug resistance in tuberculosis: review of the worldwide situation and WHO/IUATLD global surveillance project. Clin Infect Dis 1997; 24(Suppl. 1): S121-S130.

39. WHO/IUATLD. Anti-Tuberculosis Drug Resistance in the World. World Health Organization, Geneva, Switzerland, 1997. WHO/TB/97.229.

40. Pablos-Mendez A, Raviglione MC, Laszlo A et al. Global surveillance for antituberculosis-drug resistance, 1994-1997. New Eng J Med 1998; 338: 1641-1649.

41. Boulahbal F, Khaled S, Tazir M. The interest of follow-up of resistance of the tubercle bacillus in the evaluation of a programme. Bull IUATLD 1989; 64: 23-25.

42. Githui WA, Kwamanga D, Chakaya JM, Karimi FG, Waiyaki PG. Anti-tuberculosis initial drug resistance of *Mycobacterium tuberculosis* in Kenya: a ten-year review. East Afr Med J 1993; 70: 609-612.

43. Weyer K, Groenewald P, Zwarenstein M, Lombard CJ. Tuberculosis drug resistance in the Western Cape. S Afr Med J 1995; 85: 499-504.

44. Glynn JR, Jenkins PA, Fine PEM, et al. Patterns of initial and acquired antituberculosis drug resistance in Karonga District, Malawi. Lancet 1995; 345: 907-910.

45. National Tuberculosis/Leprosy Programme in Tanzania. Summary reports, 1991-1995. National drug resistance surveillance World Health Organization. 6106.1. Tuberculosis Programme Country Reports. WHO, Geneva, Switzerland.

46. Bretzel G, Wendl-Richter U, Adatu F, Aisu T. Drug resistance in Uganda. Proceedings of the Global Congress on Lung Health, 29th World Conference of the International Union Against Tuberculosis and Lung Disease (IUATLD/UICTMR). Abstract 11-PD. Bangkok, Thailand, 23-26 November 1998. Int J Tuberc Lung Dis 1998; 2: S324-S325.

47. Weyer K, Lancaster J, Balt E, Dürrheim D. Tuberculosis drug resistance in Mpumalanga Province, South Africa. Proceedings of the Global Congress on Lung Health, 29th World Conference of the International Union Against Tuberculosis and Lung Disease (IUATLD/UICTMR). Abstract 669-PD. Bangkok, Thailand, 23-26 November 1998. Int J Tuberc Lung Dis 1998; 2: S332-S333.

48 Laszlo A, De Kantor IN. A random sample survey of initial drug resistance among tuberculosis cases in Latin America. Bull World Health Organ 1994; 72: 603-610.

49. National Institute Microbiology, Buenos Aires. National drug resistance surveillance. World Health Organization. Global Tuberculosis Programme Country Reports. WHO, Geneva, Switzerland, 1994.

50. Farga V. The origins of DOTS. Int J Tuberc Lung Dis 1999; 3: 85-86.

51. Ministerio de Salud. Actualización de normas técnicas. Programa Nacional de Control de la Tuberculosis. Chile, 1996.

52. Espinal MA, Báez J, Soriano G. Drug-resistant tuberculosis in the Dominican Republic: results of a nationwide survey. Int J Tuberc Lung Dis 1998; 2: 490-498.

53. Centers for Disease Control and Prevention. Population-based survey for drug resistance of tuberculosis. MMWR 1998; 47: 371-75.

54. Chacón L, Cruz JR, Tardencilla A. Primary resistance and MDRTB in Nicaragua. Proceedings of the Global Congress on Lung Health, 29th World Conference of the International Union Against Tuberculosis and Lung Disease (IUATLD/UICTMR). Abstract 567-PD. Bangkok, Thailand, 23-26 November 1998. Int J Tuberc Lung Dis 1998; 2: S332.

55. Netto EM, Dye C, Raviglione MC. Progress in global tuberculosis control 1995-1996, with emphasis on 22 high-incidence countries. Int J Tuberc Lung Dis 1999; 3: 310-320.

56. Zhang LX, Kan GQ, Tu DH, Li JS, Liu XX. Trend of initial drug resistance of tubercle bacilli isolated from new patients with pulmonary tuberculosis and its correlation with the tuberculosis programme in Beijing. Tubercle Lung Dis 1995; 76: 100-103.

57. Guobin W, Yili P, Guolong Z, et al. Drug resistance surveillance (DRS). Report in Henan, China. Proceedings of the Global Congress on Lung Health, 29th World Conference of the International Union Against Tuberculosis and Lung Disease (IUATLD/UICTMR). Abstract 600-PC. Bangkok, Thailand, 23-26 November 1998. Int J Tuberc Lung Dis 1998; 2: S297-S298.

58. Paramasivan CN, Venkataraman P, Bhaskaran K, Chandrasekaran V, Narayanan PR. WHO/IUATLD sponsored surveillance of drug reistance in tuberculosis in Tamil Nadu State, India. Proceedings of the Global Congress on Lung Health, 29th World Conference of the International Union Against Tuberculosis and Lung Disease (IUATLD/UICTMR). Abstract 373-PC. Bangkok, Thailand, 23-26 November 1998. Int J Tuberc Lung Dis 1998; 2: S297.

59. Fodor T, Vadasz I. Primary resistance examination in pulmonary tuberculosis cases in Budapest. Med Thoracalis 1993; 46: 376-381.

60. Rudoy NM, Krivenko GT. Drug resistance of *Mycobacterium tuberculosis*. Vrach Delo 1987; 5: 92-95.

61. Coninx R, Mathieu C, Debacker M, et al. First-line tuberculosis therapy and drug-resistant *Mycobacterium tuberculosis* in prisons. Lancet 1999; 353: 969-73.

62. Kimerling ME, Kluge H, Vezhnina N, et al. Inadequacy of the current WHO re-treatment regimen in a central Siberian prison: treatment failure and MDRTB. Int J Tuberc Lung Dis 1999; 3: 451-453.

63. Centers for Disease Control and Prevention. Primary multidrug-resistant tuberculosis—Ivanovo Oblast, Russia, 1999. MMWR 1999; 48: 661-663.

64. Viljanen MK, Vyshnevskiy BI, Otten TF. Survey of drug-resistant tuberculosis in Northwestern Russia from 1984 through 1994. Eur J Clin Microbiol Infect Dis 1998; 17: 177-183.

65. Leimane V, Leimans J. Surveillance of multi-drug-resistant tuberculosis in Latvia. Proceedings of the Global Congress on Lung Health, 29th World Conference of the International Union Against Tuberculosis and Lung Disease (IUATLD/UICTMR). Abstract 360-PC. Bangkok, Thailand, 23-26 November 1998. Int J Tuberc Lung Dis 1998; 2: S297.

66. Communicable Diseases. Report. Multidrug resistant tuberculosis – Basis for the development of an evidence-based case-management strategy for MDR-TB within the WHO's DOTS strategy. Proceedings of 1998 Meetings and Protocol Recommendations. Edited by Espinal MA. Geneva, 1999. WHO/TB/99.260.

Chapter 4

The interaction of human immunodeficiency virus and multidrug-resistant *Mycobacterium tuberculosis*

Eugene McCray and Ida M. Onorato
Division of Tuberculosis Elimination, Centers for Disease Control and Prevention, Atlanta, GA

1.   INTRODUCTION

The association of human immunodeficiency virus infection (HIV) with increased rates of multidrug-resistant (MDR) tuberculosis (TB) in the United States (US) has been well-documented [1-4]. Furthermore, a number of studies conducted in the US have identified HIV infection as a risk factor for acquired drug resistance [5-6]. During the late 1980s and early 1990s, large outbreaks of MDRTB primarily involving HIV-infected patients occurred in hospitals, correctional facilities and other institutional settings in the US [7-12]. Similar outbreaks also occurred in other established market economies during the 1990s [13-17]. In these outbreaks, active TB developed within a few weeks or months following exposure to an infectious MDRTB patient, leading to multiple transmissions in a short period of time. Furthermore, the outbreaks were characterized by delayed diagnosis, extended infectious periods, and delays in initiation of appropriate treatment, which contributed to high mortality and morbidity. More recent data have documented a decline in new MDRTB cases and improvement in clinical outcomes for HIV-infected patients [2,18-20]. This chapter describes trends in MDRTB and HIV co-infection and key characteristics of MDRTB patients with HIV infection in the US based on national surveillance data from 1993-1997, and summarizes the key findings in published outbreaks of MDRTB involving HIV-infected persons in US and other established market economies. This

45

I. Bastian and F. Portaels (eds.), Multidrug-Resistant Tuberculosis, 45-57.
© 2000 *Kluwer Academic Publishers. Printed in the Netherlands.*

chapter will demonstrate that the association of HIV infection with drug-resistant TB is largely attributable to nosocomial outbreaks of MDRTB in various congregate settings. However, HIV-infected patients may be at some increased risk of acquired drug resistance, particularly rifampicin monoresistance, and various plausible but unproven explanations for this association are presented.

2. TRENDS IN MDRTB AND HIV CO-INFECTION, AND CHARACTERISTICS OF MDRTB PATIENTS WITH HIV INFECTION IN THE UNITED STATES, 1993-1997

During the resurgence of TB in the US from 1985 to 1992, MDRTB became a serious public health concern [21]. To monitor trends in drug-resistant TB and assess the impact of HIV on TB morbidity, the Centers for Disease Control and Prevention (CDC) added initial drug susceptibility test results and HIV information to the individual TB case report used for national surveillance beginning in 1993. In addition, cross-matching of TB and HIV/AIDS registries in state and local health departments was conducted to supplement limited reporting of HIV results in case reports to the national surveillance system. Based on information submitted to the national surveillance system combined with data from TB and HIV/AIDS registry matches, at least 33% of MDRTB cases reported during 1993-1997 were co-infected with HIV (Table 1). During this period, the number of reported MDRTB patients with HIV infection (MDRTB-AIDS) was 568; 60% (342) were reported from New York City and an additional 32% (181) were reported from 7 areas (New York excluding New York City, 45; Florida, 40; New Jersey, 31; Illinois, 30; California 13; and 11 each from Texas and the District of Columbia). The number and proportion of MDRTB-AIDS patients decreased each year from 192 or 6.5% in 1993 to 32 or 1.8% in 1997 (Table 1). The decrease in MDRTB-AIDS patients was influenced by a substantial decline in the number and proportion reported from New York City. During this period, the number of MDRTB-AIDS patients reported from New York City declined 85% from 126 in 1993 to 19 in 1997, and the proportion dropped from 66% in 1993 to 59% in 1997. The number of reported MDRTB-AIDS patients from other areas of the US outside New York City declined 80% from 66 in 1993 to 13 in 1997 and the proportion increased from 34% to 41% during the same period.

Selected demographic and clinical characteristics of patients with MDRTB-AIDS and MDRTB without documented HIV infection (MDR non-AIDS TB) are shown in Table 2. Compared to MDR non-AIDS TB,

MDRTB-AIDS patients were more likely to be persons 25-44 years old, born in the US, and have extrapulmonary disease (with or without pulmonary involvement) and less likely to have a history of previous TB (p<0.001 for all comparisons). Among MDRTB patients with pulmonary involvement (with or without extrapulmonary TB), the percentage with sputum smear positive for acid fast bacilli at the time of diagnosis was similar for those with AIDS (71%) and non-AIDS (69%). Because history of treatment for TB is not collected on the TB case report form used for national surveillance, previous history of TB is used to estimate primary and acquired anti-TB drug resistance. Previous history of treatment for TB is a known risk factor for development of MDRTB and is considered secondary or acquired resistance. The proportion of MDRTB-AIDS patients who reported a previous history of TB was only 9% (51/563) compared to 22% (250/1115) for MDRTB non-AIDS patients suggesting that primary transmission of MDRTB rather than acquired MDRTB was more common among HIV positive patients.

Table 1. Number and percentage of patients with multidrug-resistant tuberculosis, AIDS versus non-AIDS, by year, United States, 1993-1997

Year	TB-AIDS	Non-AIDS TB	Total TB
1993	192 (6.5%)	295 (2.0%)	487 (2.8%)
1994	150 (5.1%)	281 (1.9%)	431 (2.5%)
1995	131 (5.1%)	194 (1.3%)	325 (1.9%)
1996	63 (2.9%)	186 (1.3%)	249 (1.5%)
1997	32 (1.8%)	166 (1.3%)	198 (1.3%)
Total	568 (4.6%)	1122 (1.6%)	1690 (2.0%)

TB, tuberculosis; AIDS, acquired immunodeficiency syndrome. Chi-square for linear trend by year: p<0.001 for TB-AIDS, non-AIDS TB, and total TB. Chi-square comparison of TB-AIDS versus non-AIDS TB: p<0.05 for each year and overall. Non-AIDS TB includes patients with negative HIV test results and those with unknown HIV status. Patients with an indeterminate HIV test result were excluded from the analysis (n=110).

Based on follow-up data available for patients reported 1993-1996, 69% (330/475) of MDRTB-AIDS patients died during therapy compared with only 19% (153/821) of MDR non-AIDS TB patients. Among those who did not die during therapy, the percentage completing anti-TB therapy was similar for patients with MDRTB-AIDS (78%) and MDR non-AIDS TB (75%). The proportion of MDRTB-AIDS reported to the national surveillance system who died during therapy represents all-cause mortality (MDRTB may not have been the cause of death) and is slightly lower than the high mortality reported in published outbreaks of MDRTB (see below).

3.   OUTBREAKS OF MDRTB INVOLVING HIV-INFECTED PATIENTS

During the late 1980s and early 1990s, outbreaks of MDRTB primarily involving HIV-infected patients occurred in a number of institutional settings in the US and in other established market economies. In these outbreaks, most MDRTB cases appeared to be the result of nosocomial transmission on hospital wards or other locations where AIDS or HIV-infected patients were housed or received medical treatment. Table 3 summarizes information from 12 outbreaks of MDRTB published in the medical literature during 1992 to 1999. Most of the outbreaks occurred in hospitals (10) and the one outbreak reported from the New York State prison system was linked to an outbreak of MDRTB in a hospital in New York City [7-16,22]. The community outbreak of MDRTB that occurred in South Carolina involved a source patient who lived in New York City and was hospitalized in 1991 in one of the hospitals that was experiencing an MDRTB outbreak due to nosocomial transmission [23].

Table 2. Selected demographic and clinical characteristics of patients with multidrug-resistant tuberculosis, TB-AIDS versus non-AIDS TB, United States, 1993-1997

Characteristic	Number (percentage) with characteristic	
	TB-AIDS	Non-AIDS TB
Age group (years)		
0-14	3 (<1%)	22 (2%)
15-24	9 (2%)	121 (11%)
25-44	442 (78%)	464 (41%)
45-64	109 (19%)	338 (30%)
65+	5 (<1%)	177 (16%)
Birth country[a]		
United States	503 (89%)	510 (46%)
Foreign	60 (11%)	598 (54%)
Previous TB[b]		
Yes	51 (9%)	250 (22%)
No	512 (91%)	865 (78%)
Site of disease		
Pulmonary	371 (65%)	976 (87%)
Extrapulmonary	87 (15%)	92 (8%)
Both	110 (20%)	54 (5%)

TB, tuberculosis; AIDS, acquired immunodeficiency syndrome. [a]Birth country was unknown for 5 TB-AIDS and 14 non-AIDS TB patients. [b]History of previous TB unknown for 5 TB-AIDS and 7 non-AIDS TB patients. Chi-square comparison of TB-AIDS versus non-AIDS TB: p<0.001 for age group 25-44 years, born in the US, previous TB and extrapulmonary TB (with or without pulmonary TB) site of disease.

The MDRTB outbreaks primarily involved HIV-infected patients and health care workers; all studies reported documented HIV co-infection rates of at least 75% except the community outbreak in South Carolina, which had an HIV co-infection rate of 40%. In each of the published outbreaks, the authors provided both epidemiologic and laboratory evidence (i.e., anti-TB drug resistance patterns and DNA fingerprints) supporting nosocomial or community transmission of MDRTB. Results of DNA fingerprinting with restriction fragment-length polymorphism (RFLP) were also reported when available. In 11 of the published outbreaks, RFLP analysis of available isolates consistently identified an outbreak strain of MDRTB with identical or nearly identical DNA fingerprints. For example, the outbreak involving 39 inmates in the New York State prison system identified 31 inmates who were epidemiologically linked to one another, and the 29 available specimens had identical drug resistance (to isoniazid, rifampicin, streptomycin, ethambutol, ethionamide, rifabutin, and kanamycin) and RFLP patterns [11]. In a multi-institutional outbreak of MDRTB in New York City, 367 patients were identified with isolates resistant to at least isoniazid, rifampicin, ethambutol, and streptomycin (and rifabutin if tested); 267 with available isolates for analysis had identical or nearly identical RFLP patterns and epidemiologic linkages were identified for 70% [12].

Mortality in the reported outbreaks range from 78% to 100% except in a recent study from Portugal reporting an all-cause mortality of 49% among 43 MDRTB cases; 29 (77%) were infected with HIV [16]. MDRTB in HIV-infected patients was characterized by rapid progression from diagnosis to death with the median interval from diagnosis to death ranging from 28 days to 133 days. Compared to the extremely high mortality observed in the reported outbreaks of MDRTB, several recent studies have documented substantial improvement in clinical outcome of these patients [18-20]. Improved clinical outcome was associated with early identification of MDRTB patients and prompt initiation of effective anti-TB treatment. For example, in a prospective study of 34 patients with MDRTB and HIV infection, the overall response rate was 50% and the median survival was 315 days [18]. In another prospective study involving 13 patients with MDRTB and HIV infection, there was 100% bacteriologic conversion rate and 59% of the patients survived more than one year [19]. Both studies identified receipt of appropriate therapy (defined as receiving at least two drugs with *in vitro* activity against the MDRTB isolate for at least 2 weeks) as the most significant variable associated with both initial and overall response. In a retrospective study involving 90 patients with MDRTB and HIV infection, the median survival of patients appropriately treated with at least two active anti-TB medications was 14.1 months compared to less than 2 months in those not receiving appropriate therapy [20].

These published outbreaks identified several common factors contributing to tuberculosis transmission. First, delays in identifying persons

TABLE 3. Selected published outbreaks of multidrug-resistant tuberculosis in the United States and other established market economies, 1992 to 1999*

Authors	Location	Outbreak Period	No. of Patients Involved	Percent HIV Infected	Anti-TB Drug Resistance Pattern (No.)	All Cause Mortality	Median Interval from Diagnosis to Death[†]
Beck-Sagué et al., 1992	Hospital Miami, FL	5/88-1/90	25	100	H, R (18) H, R, E (7)	84%	49 days
Fischl et al., 1992	Hospital & Community Miami, FL	1/88-11/90	62	100	H, R (16) H, R, E (10) H, R, ET (10) H,E,ET (2) H, R, E, ET (21) H,R,E,S (1) H,R,E,ET,C (2)	84%	63 day
Edlin et al., 1992	Hospital NYC, NY	1/89-4/90	18	100	H,S	78%	133 days
Valway et al., 1994	State Prison NY	1/90-12/91	39	97 (38/39)	H,R (2) H,R,E (2) H,R,S,E (33) H,R,S,ET (2)	87%	105 days
Pearson et al., 1992	Hospital NYC, NY	1/90-3/91	23	91 (21/23)	at least H,R	83%	28 days
Frieden et al., 1996[¶]	41 Hospitals NYC, NY	1/90-8/93	267	86 (230/267)	at least H,R,S,E	83%	66 days

Authors	Location	Outbreak Period	No. of Patients Involved	Percent HIV Infected	Anti-TB Drug Resistance Pattern (No.)	All Cause Mortality[v]	Median Interval from Diagnosis to Death[†]
Kenyon et al., 1997	Hospital Chicago, IL	8/94-9/95	7	100	H,R	Not stated	Not stated
Agerton et al., 1997	Community SC	1/95-5/95	5	40 (2/5)	at least H,R,S	80%	Not stated
Herrera et al., 1996	Hospital Madrid, Spain	6/91-1/95	48	100	H,R,S,E	100%	78 days
Moro et al., 1998‡	Hospital A	10/91-7/95	85	98 (83/85)	H,R,S,E	95%	93 days
	Hospital B Milan, Italy	10/91-7/95	31	100	H,R,S,E	97%	79 days
Samper et al., 1997	Hospital 1 Madrid, Spain	11/93-2/95	19	100	H,R,S,E,Z	Not stated	Not stated
	Hospital 2 Malaga, Spain	1/95-2/96	20	100	H,R,S,E,Z	100%	<3 months
Portugal et al., 1999	11 Hospitals Lisbon, Portugal	1/96-12/97	43	77 (29/43)	H,R,S (33) H,R,E (7) H,R,S,E (3)	49%	Not stated

* FL indicates Florida; NYC, New York City; NY, New York; IL, Illinois; SC, South Carolina; H, isoniazid; R, rifampin; S, streptomycin sulfate; E, ethambutol hydrochloride; Z, pyrazinamide; ET, ethionamide; C, capreomycin sulfate.

† For HIV positive patients only.

¶ 357 patients identified with MDRTB but clinical and epidemiologic information presented only for 267 (75%) patients with matching DNA fingerprints.

‡ 10 patients in hospital A were lost to follow-up and information on mortality was unknown.

who were symptomatic or suspected to have TB resulted in failure to implement appropriate infection control procedures. Second, delays in recognition of drug resistance (i.e., laboratory delays in obtaining AFB smears and identifying MDRTB) resulted in failure to institute effective therapy and adequate isolation of some patients with infectious TB. Third, lapses in application of appropriate infection control procedures (including infectious TB patients leaving their rooms, and doors to TB isolation rooms being left open rendering negative pressure ventilation inoperable). Finally, performance of cough-inducing procedures such as administration of aerosolized pentamidine to TB patients in HIV clinic rooms with positive pressure relative to treatment and waiting areas also increased transmission to susceptible patients.

The factors contributing to nosocomial transmission described above show that the institutions involved in these outbreaks often did not adhere to published recommendations for preventing the transmission of TB in health care settings [24,25]. Improved diagnosis of MDRTB, prompt initiation of appropriate treatment, and implementation and adherence to appropriate infection control have since curtailed nosocomial transmission of MDRTB in many of the institutions that experienced outbreaks in the late 1980s and early 1990s [26,27]. In New York City, improved TB infection control practices in hospitals that experienced MDRTB outbreaks and expanded use of directly observed therapy (DOT) played an important role in the decline of reported MDRTB [28].

4. ASSOCIATION OF HIV AND TB CO-INFECTION WITH ACQUIRED DRUG RESISTANCE

Several published reports in the US have suggested that the presence of HIV infection favours the development of acquired drug resistance [5,29-31] and that AIDS may be an independent risk factor for acquired drug resistance [6]. Acquisition of isolated rifampicin resistance in persons with HIV infection and TB has recently been reported [5,29-34]. One report (a retrospective case control study) found that nonadherence to anti-TB therapy was correlated independently with the development of isolated rifampicin resistance among HIV-infected patients [33]. A second report confirmed nonadherence to anti-TB therapy in the medical records of six of seven HIV-positive patients who developed isolated rifampicin resistance [32]. However, nonadherence did not explain the acquisition of rifampicin resistance in all of the HIV-positive patients in these two reports. Most reports of isolated rifampicin resistance describe HIV patients who were adherent to anti-TB therapy, and do not clearly identify specific factors associated with acquired resistance [29-31,34].

In addition to nonadherence to anti-TB therapy, several other hypotheses have been proposed on the mechanism for developing isolated rifampicin resistance in HIV-infected patients. Exogenous reinfection with a new resistant strain of *M. tuberculosis*, during or after therapy for drug-susceptible TB, which has been described among patients with advanced HIV disease, may be responsible [35]. However, several of the reports found identical RFLP patterns for the first and second isolates recovered from HIV patients whose cultures became positive for isolated rifampicin-resistant TB during or after therapy for drug susceptible TB, demonstrating that reinfection did not occur [31,34]. Interactions between rifampicin and other drugs used to treat patients with AIDS may alter the therapeutic efficacy of rifampicin as well as other anti-TB medications and lead to isolated rifampicin resistance [36]. Malabsorption of drugs in HIV-infected patients perhaps caused by AIDS-associated enteropathy may result in low serum levels of rifampicin and lead to development of resistance. Several reports have suggested or shown that malabsorption of anti-TB drugs may encourage development of acquired drug resistance, especially in HIV-infected patients [37-39]. In most of the published reports of isolated rifampicin resistance, drug levels were not monitored so malabsorption could not be excluded. Exposure to rifabutin (a rifamycin antimicrobial agent related to rifampicin used for prophylaxis against infection due to *Mycobacterium avium-intracellulare* complex) may lead to isolated rifampicin resistance if AIDS patients with incubating TB concurrently receive rifabutin prophylaxis. It is probable that treatment with rifabutin led to the development of rifampicin resistance in some of the HIV-infected patients who were receiving rifabutin at the time the first specimen with the rifampicin-resistant isolate was obtained [33,40]. However, most HIV-infected patients with isolated rifampicin resistance did not receive treatment with rifabutin. Finally, assuming that drug resistance results from spontaneously occurring mutations, it is possible that a large organism burden in combination with several of the factors described above may favour the emergence of acquired resistance to rifampicin in HIV-positive patients.

The recent reports of acquired rifampicin monoresistance strongly suggest that factors other than nonadherence may contribute to the genesis of HIV-associated MDRTB during therapy for susceptible TB. Several investigators suggest that acquisition of isolated rifampicin resistance is the key step in the development of acquired MDRTB associated with HIV infection [31,32]. Factors associated with the development of isolated rifampicin resistance must be identified and studied if the public health threat of this unusual drug-resistance phenotype is to be limited.

5.   SUMMARY AND CONCLUSIONS

HIV-associated MDRTB surfaced as a serious public health problem during the resurgence of TB in the US in the late 1980s and early 1990s. The occurrence of MDRTB outbreaks among HIV/AIDS patients in institutional settings (i.e., hospitals and correctional facilities) alerted the nation to serious weaknesses in TB control efforts, especially those directed towards prevention and control of TB in health-care facilities. National guidelines for preventing TB transmission in health care settings were developed in 1990 and revised in 1994 [24-25]. During 1993-1997, the number and proportion of MDRTB-AIDS cases reported in the US markedly decreased, mostly driven by decreases in reported MDRTB-AIDS cases from New York City. Improvement in basic infection control policies and procedures in hospitals and other institutions, along with improved diagnosis and treatment (including the expanded use of DOT) curtailed the MDRTB outbreaks, and were partly responsible for the decline [12,26-28]. Additionally, aggressive contact investigation and use of alternative preventive therapy regimens for persons infected with MDRTB may have further reduced transmission.

HIV-associated MDRTB is a potential public health threat in many countries throughout the world, particularly those countries with high TB incidence and an ongoing AIDS epidemic. Several countries with a high prevalence of MDRTB (i.e., former Soviet Union, Asia, the Dominican Republic and Argentina) and an ongoing or increasing AIDS epidemic are likely to experience increases in the prevalence of HIV-associated MDRTB unless sound TB control policies are implemented [41].

Finally, while nosocomial outbreaks of MDRTB largely account for the apparent association of MDRTB and HIV infection, the recent observation of the unusual pattern of acquired isolated rifampicin resistance in patients with HIV infection raises concerns that HIV-infected patients are at increased risk of acquired drug resistance and that such resistance may not be prevented completely in HIV-infected patients by effective supervised therapy (e.g., DOT). Further studies are needed to identify and quantify the drug interactions and host factors that may predispose HIV/AIDS patients to the development of isolated rifampicin resistance.

REFERENCES

1. Freiden TR, Sterling T, Pablos-Méndez A, Kilburn JO, Cauthen GM, Dooley SW. The emergence of drug-resistant tuberculosis in New York City. N Engl J Med 1993; 328: 521-526.
2. Moore M, Onorato IM, McCray E, Castro KG. Trends in drug-resistant tuberculosis in the United States, 1993-1996. JAMA 1997; 278: 833-837.
3. Gordin FM, Nelson ET, Matts JP, Cohn DL, Ernst J, Benator D, Besch CL, Crane LR, Sampson JH, Braggs PS, El-Sadr W. The impact of human immunodeficiency virus infection on drug-resistant tuberculosis. Am J Respir Crit Care Med 1996; 154: 1478-1483.
4. Moore M, McCray E, Onorato IM. Cross-matching of TB and AIDS registries: TB patients with HIV co-infection, United States, 1993-1994. Publ Health Rep 1999; 114: 269-277.
5. Small PM, Schecter GF, Goodman PC, Sande MA, Chaisson RE, Hopewell PC. Treatment of tuberculosis in patients with advanced human immunodeficiency virus infection. N Engl J Med 1991; 324: 289-294.
6. Bradford WZ, Martin JN, Reingold AL, Schecter GF, Hopewell PC, Small PM. The changing epidemiology of acquired drug-resistant tuberculosis in San Francisco, USA. Lancet 1996; 348: 928-931.
7. Edlin BR, Tokars JI, Grieco MH, Crawford JT, Williams J, Sordillo EM, Ong KR, Kilburn JO, Dooley SW, Jarvis WR, Holmberg SD. An outbreak of multidrug-resistant tuberculosis among hospitalized patients with the acquired immunodeficiency syndrome. N Engl J Med 1992; 326: 1514-1521.
8. Pearson ML, Jereb JA, Frieden TR, Crawford JT, Davis BJ, Dooley SW, Jarvis WR. Nosocomial transmission of multidrug-resistant *Mycobacterium tuberculosis*: a risk to patient and health care workers. Ann Intern Med 1992; 117: 191-196.
9. Beck-Sague C, Dooley SW, Hutton MD, Otten J, Breeden A, Crawford JT, Pitchenfik AE, Woodley C, Cauthen GW, Jarvis WR. Hospital outbreak of multidrug-resistant *Mycobacterium tuberculosis* infections: factors in transmission to staff and HIV-infected patients. JAMA 1992; 268: 1280-1286.
10. Fischl MA, Uttamchandani RB, Daikos GL, Poblete RB, Moreno JN, Reyes RR, Boota AM, Thompson LM, Cleary TJ, Lai S. An outbreak of tuberculosis caused by multiple-drug resistant tubercle bacilli among patients with HIV Infection. Ann Intern Med 1992; 117: 177-183.
11. Valway SE, Greifinger RB, Papania M, Kilburn JO, Woodley C, Diferdinando GT, Dooley SW. Multidrug-resistant tuberculosis in the New York State Prison System, 1990-1991. J Infect Dis 1994; 170: 151-156.
12. Frieden TR, Sherman LF, May KL, Fujiwara PI, Crawford JT, Nivin B, Sharp V, Hewlett D, Brudney K, Alland D, Kreiswirth BN. A multi-institutional outbreak of highly drug-resistant tuberculosis: epidemiology and clinical outcome. JAMA 1996; 276: 1229-1235.
13. Centers for Disease Control. Multidrug-resistant tuberculosis outbreak on an HIV ward–Madrid Spain, 1991-1995. MMWR Morb Mort Wkly Rep 1996; 45: 330-333.
14. Moro ML, Gori A, Errante I, Infuso A, Franzetti F, Sodano L, Iemoli E, the Italian Multidrug-Resistant Tuberculosis Outbreak Study Group. An outbreak of multidrug-resistant tuberculosis involving HIV-infected patients from two hospitals in Milan, Italy. AIDS 1998; 12: 1095-1102.

15. Samper S, Marin C, Pinedo A, Rivero A, Blazquez J, Baquero F, van Soolingen D, van Embden J. Transmission between HIV-infected patients of multidrug-resistant tuberculosis caused by *Mycobacterium bovis*. AIDS 1997; 11: 1237-1242.

16. Portugal I, Covas MJ, Brum L, Viveiros M, Ferrinho P, Moniz-Pereira J, David H. Outbreak of multiple drug-resistant tuberculosis in Lisbon: detection by restriction fragment length polymorphism analysis. Int J Tuberc Lung Dis 1999; 3: 207-213.

17. Breathnach AS, de Ruiter A, Holdsworth GMC, Bateman NT, O'Sullivan DBM, Rees PJ, Snashall D, Milburn HJ, Peters BA, Watson J, Drobniewski FA, French GL. An outbreak of multi-drug-resistant tuberculosis in a London teaching hospital. J Hosp Infect 1998; 39: 111-117.

18. Turett GS, Telzak EE, Torian LV, Blum S, Alland D, Weisfuse I, Fazal BA. Improved outcomes for patients with multidrug-resistant tuberculosis. Clin Infect Dis 1995; 21: 1238-1244.

19. Salomon N, Perlman DC, Friedmann P, Buchstein S, Kreiswirth BN, Mildvan D. Predictors and outcome of multidrug-resistant tuberculosis. Clin Infect Dis 1995; 21: 1245-1252.

20. Park MM, Davis AL, Schluger NW, Cohen H, Rom WN. Outcome of MDR-TB patients, 1983-1993: prolonged survival with appropriate therapy. Am J Respir Crit Care Med 1996; 153: 317-324.

21. Centers for Disease Control. National action plan to combat multidrug-resistant tuberculosis. MMWR Morb Mortal Wkly Rep 1992; 41(No. RR-11): 1-45.

22. Kenyon TA, Ridzon R, Luskin-Hawk R, Schultz C, Paul WS, Valway SE, Onorato IM, Castro K. A nosocomial outbreak of multidrug-resistant tuberculosis. Ann Intern Med 1997; 127: 32-36.

23. Agerton TB, Valway SE, Gore B, Pozsik C, Plikaytis B. Woodley C, Onorato I. Transmission of a highly drug-resistant strain (Strain W1) of *Mycobacterium tuberculosis*. JAMA 1997; 278: 1073-1077.

24. Centers for Disease Control. Guidelines for preventing the transmission of tuberculosis in health-care settings, with special focus on HIV-related issues. MMWR Morb Mortal Wkly Rep 1990; 39(No.RR-17): 1-27.

25. Centers for Disease Control and Prevention. Guidelines for preventing the transmission of *Mycobacterium tuberculosis* in health-care facilities, 1994. MMWR Morb Mortal Wkly Rep 1994; 43(No.RR-13): 1-132.

26. Maloney SA, Pearson ML, Gordon MT, Del Castillo R, Boyle JF, Jarvis WR. Efficacy of control measures in preventing nosocomial transmission of multidrug-resistant tuberculosis to patients and health care workers. Ann Intern Med 1995; 122: 90-95.

27. Wenger PN, Otten J, Breeden A, Orfas D, Beck-Sague CM, Jarvis WR. Control of nosocomial transmission of multidrug-resistant *Mycobacterium tuberculosis* among health care workers and HIV infected patients. Lancet 1995; 345: 235-240.

28. Freiden TR, Fujiwara PI, Washko RM, Hamburg MA. Tuberculosis in New York City: turning the tide. N Engl J Med 1995; 333: 229-233.

29. Dylewski J. Thibert L. Failure of tuberculosis chemotherapy in a human immunodeficiency virus-infected patient. J Infect Dis 1990; 162: 778-779.

30. Godfrey-Fausset P, Stoker NG, Scott JAG, Pasvol G, Kelly P, Clancy L. DNA fingerprints of *Mycobacterium tuberculosis* do not change during the development of rifampin resistance. Tuber Lung Dis 1993; 74:240-243.

31. Nolan CM, Williams DL, Cave D, Eisenach KD, El-Hajj, Hooton TM, Thompson RL, Goldberg SV. Evolution of rifampin resistance in human immunodeficiency virus-associated tuberculosis. Am J Respir Crit Care Med 1995; 152: 1067-1071.

32. Lutfey M, Della-Latta P, Kapur V, Palumbo LA, Gurner D, Stotzky G, Brudney K, Dobkin J, Moss A, Musser JM, Kreiswirth BN. Independent origin of mono-rifampin-resistant *Mycobacterium tuberculosis* in patients with AIDS. Am J Respir Crit Care Med 1996; 153: 837-840.

33. Munsiff SS, Joseph S, Ebrahimzadeh A, Frieden TR. Rifampin-monoresistant tuberculosis in New York City, 1993-1994. Clin Infect Dis 1997; 25: 1465-1467.

34. March F, Garriga X, Rodríguez P, Moreno C, Garrigó M, Coll P, Prats G. Acquired drug resistance in *Mycobacterium tuberculosis* isolates recovered from compliant patients with human immunodeficiency virus-associated tuberculosis. Clin Infect Dis 1997; 25: 1044-1047.

35. Small P, Sharer RW, Hopewell PC, et al. Exogenous reinfection with multidrug-resistant *Mycobacterium tuberculosis* in patients with advanced HIV infection. N Engl J Med 1993; 328: 1137-1144.

36. Lee BL, Safrin S. Interactions and toxicities of drugs used in patients with AIDS. Clin Infect Dis 1992; 14:773-779.

37. Peloquin CA, MacPhee AA, Berning SE. Malabsorption of antimycobacterial medications. N Engl J Med 1993; 329: 1122-1123.

38. Patel KB, Belmonte R, Crowe HM. Drug malabsorption and resistant tuberculosis in HIV-infected patients. N Engl J Med 1995; 2: 336-337.

39. Peloquin CA, Nitta A, BurmanW. et al. Low antituberculosis drug concentrations in patients with AIDS. Ann Pharmacother 1996; 30: 919-925.

40. Ridzon R, Whitney CG, McKenna MT, et al. Risk factors for mono-resistant tuberculosis. Am J Respir Crit Care Med 1998; 157: 1881-1884.

41. Pablos-Méndez A, Raviglione MC, Laszlo A, et al. Global surveillance for antituberculosis-drug resistance, 1994-1997. N Engl J Med 1998; 338: 1641-1649.

Chapter 5

Clinical mismanagement and other factors producing antituberculosis drug resistance

Ariel Pablos-Méndez[1] and Klaus Lessnau[2]
[1]*Divisions of General Medicine and Epidemiology, Columbia University, New York*
[2]*Division of Pulmonary and Critical Care Medicine, The Brooklyn Hospital Center, New York*

1. THE GENESIS OF ANTI-TUBERCULOSIS DRUG RESISTANCE

Antimicrobial resistance in previously susceptible organisms readily emerges when antimicrobials are used in human and veterinary medicine. Although soil bacteria normally produce small amounts of antibiotics, our ecosystem has very recently been loaded with tons of man-made antibiotics, creating a sudden, unprecedented evolutionary stress for all susceptible microorganisms. Naturally resistant strains are then selected, creating a virtual arms race between our technology and microbial evolution. These increasing levels of resistance pose new challenges for both clinical management and control programmes [1].

Drug-resistant tuberculosis is a significant threat to tuberculosis control because only a few effective drugs are available against *Mycobacterium tuberculosis* [2,3]. In particular, the spread of strains resistant to the two most important drugs, rifampin (RIF) and isoniazid (INH), could have serious repercussions on the epidemiology and control of tuberculosis. Not only are patients infected with strains resistant to multiple drugs less likely to be cured [4,5], but second- or third-line treatment is much more toxic and expensive than treatment of patients with susceptible organisms [5,6].

Resistance of *M. tuberculosis* to anti-tuberculosis drugs is a man-made amplification of a natural phenomenon. Unlike most bacteria, *M.*

59

I. Bastian and F. Portaels (eds.), Multidrug-Resistant Tuberculosis, 59-76.
© 2000 *Kluwer Academic Publishers. Printed in the Netherlands.*

tuberculosis does not seem to share resistance horizontally through plasmids. Wild strains of *M. tuberculosis* that have never been exposed to anti-tuberculosis drugs are almost never drug-resistant, though natural resistance to specific drugs has been documented for *M. bovis* (pyrazinamide, PZA). However, through a random process, spontaneous genetic mutations can produce a resistant mutant. Mutations resulting in resistance of *M. tuberculosis* to RIF occur at a rate of 10^{-10} per cell division and lead to an estimated prevalence of 1 in 10^8 bacilli in drug-free environments; the rate for INH is approximately 10^{-7} to 10^{-9}, resulting in resistance in 1 out of 10^6 bacilli [2].

Since bacillary populations larger than 10^7 are common in cavitary TB [7], *genetic resistance* emerges even in the absence of anti-microbial exposure, although diluted by the majority of drug-susceptible microorganisms. However, exposure to a single drug, due to irregular drug supply, inappropriate prescription or poor adherence to treatment, provides drug-resistant strains a survival advantage. In a matter of weeks, these bacilli become predominant [8,9]. This phenomenon is called *acquired or secondary resistance* [10]. Subsequent transmission of such organisms to other persons may lead to disease which is drug-resistant from the outset, without previous treatment, a phenomenon known as *initial or primary resistance* (see Figure 1)[11]. Every active drug against *M. tuberculosis* is bound to induce resistance, and the more active a drug is, and the longer it is used, the more likely it is to induce clinical resistance [7].

Multidrug resistance due to spontaneous mutations is virtually impossible, since there is no single gene for MDR and mutations resulting in resistance to various drugs are genetically unlinked [13]. However, in a bacterial population with baseline resistance to INH, spontaneous mutation may result in resistance to RIF in some bacilli. In such situations, treatment with INH and RIF alone will select strains resistant to both antimicrobials. A similar sequence of events may lead to resistance to additional drugs, and eventually to all first-line anti-tuberculosis medications [14,15]. Prevention of this train of events is the rationale for multidrug regimens and fixed dose combination (FDC) tablets in the treatment of tuberculosis [16,17].

Population geneticists claim that burdening an organism with a large number of mutations carries a fitness cost. In other words, the selective advantage of resisting the actions of a specific drug is accompanied by a survival disadvantage in the absence of the drug [18]. Soon after the introduction of INH, laboratory studies made it clear that drug resistant strains are less viable in vitro [19], and less likely to cause disease in experimental animals [19-21]. While MDRTB strains are clearly contagious [22-24], the controversy has not been resolved and the answer will impact modelled predictions of the behaviour of MDRTB in the community [25]. In summary, drug-resistance is generated by spontaneous mutations and selected by monotherapy, and then spreads to other people much the same as drug-susceptible organisms.

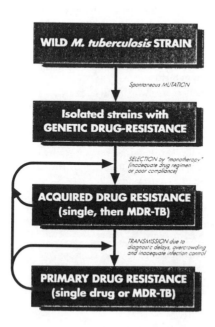

Figure 1. Development of antituberculosis drug resistance. Reproduced from reference 12 with permission.

2.   CLINICAL MISMANAGEMENT PRODUCING DRUG RESISTANCE

The prevalence of MDRTB increases ten-fold after unsuccessful treatment of new TB cases [10]. Thus, the highest priority in fighting MDRTB is its prevention by appropriate treatment of new cases [26]. Clinicians and other health providers play crucial roles in MDRTB prevention, and lack of training or caring on their part may actually fan the problem of MDRTB. The errors in the treatment of TB that can lead to the development or dissemination of MDRTB are reviewed below (Table 1).

Preventing MDRTB in the first place is more feasible and effective than treating it once it develops. Ideally, a physician who is an expert on TB should be consulted about any unusual problems during therapy; it is also useful to have expert consultants audit the charts of "active" TB patients.

The treating physician should be accountable and his/her adherence to established guidelines should be reviewed periodically [27-30]. Although resources may be constrained in some settings, district officials and national programme managers should address settings where less than 85% of patients are being cured. Private practitioners should be included if any organized effort is to be successful [31].

Table 1. Clinical mismanagement and other factors producing antituberculosis drug resistance

Examples of clinical mismanagement
Delayed diagnosis and isolation of smear-positive cases
Inadequate initial drug regimens (eg. < 4 drugs where INH resistance exists)
Failure to recognise pre-existing drug resistance
    Failure to ascertain previous treatment
    Inadequate history of contact with index cases of MDRTB
    Failure to submit baseline samples for culture and drug susceptibility testing
        (where such facilities exist)
Adding a single first-line or two weak second-line drugs to a failing regimen
Ignoring and promoting poor adherence with treatment
    Insufficient patient education
    Use of unsupervised intermittent therapy
    Not monitoring treatment adherence (by pill counting, etc)
    Relying on friends or relatives for DOT
    Not mandating DOT once poor adherence is detected
Inadequate treatment duration

Programmatic factors associated with drug resistance
Weak political commitment and irregular drug supply
Lack of standardized SCC regimens and the mechanisms to implement them
"Sloppy" or no DOTS in settings with cure rates under 85% (in HIV-negative cases)
Unrestricted availability of anti-tuberculosis drugs over the counter
Limited use of FDC tablets in settings without DOT
Lack of surveillance data to inform programme priorities

2.1   Delayed diagnosis and isolation

Delayed identification of patients with TB does not generate drug resistance. However, patients with smear-positive sputum may infect several other people [32]. While this will occur regardless of the drug-susceptibility pattern, undiagnosed MDRTB-infected patients will contribute to the spread of drug resistance. Explosive MDRTB outbreaks among HIV infected patients could be prevented by appropriate isolation practices in hospitals and similar settings [33]. In addition, delayed diagnosis and treatment of TB lead to unnecessary mortality, especially among HIV-infected patients [34,35]. The essential first step is for physicians to "Think TB" and act accordingly in patients with pneumonia or febrile wasting [36].

The optimal methods for early identification of MDRTB remain undefined. Clinical signs of MDRTB are limited and non-specific. Weight loss or fever after 2 weeks of intensive treatment is rare in patients with pan-susceptible TB [37]. Chest radiographs should not worsen after the first month of appropriate therapy, and the number of bacilli in serial sputum smears should decrease [36]. While not specific, combinations of such events should alert clinicians to the possibility of MDRTB [38]. However, WHO defines treatment failure as the persistence of positive sputum smears after 5 months of treatment, and recommends re-treatment regimens only after a second course of DOT fails [17]. The timeliness of such policies and cost-effective alternatives require further investigation.

MDRTB can be ascertained with drug-susceptibility testing (DST). However, in most TB endemic countries, routine DST is not available. Furthermore, routine DST in these settings may distract from smear microscopy, and the results may not be accurate in laboratories with a low volume of tests (eg. <300/year)[39]. In addition, DST results may cause confusion and lead to inappropriate tinkering with therapeutic regimens (ie. changing standardized regimens in patients with INH or streptomycin mono-resistance). More importantly, second line drugs are not available or affordable in most settings, and their use outside expert hands or without DOT may generate resistance to those drugs as well.

Timely DST and individualized regimens administered by experts is clearly the best approach in settings with sound TB control, adequate laboratory facilities, and enough resources for second-line drugs [40]. However, as Raviglione argues in another chapter [41], there is a low prevalence of MDRTB in most areas of the world, and standard DOTS programmes should suffice in these settings. Appropriate isolation of patients suspected of having MDRTB should nonetheless be implemented. Access to DST and MDRTB treatment may be warranted in countries with a high prevalence of drug-resistance.

2.2   Inappropriate drug regimens

2.2.1   Inadequate initial therapy

WHO and the IUATLD, as well as CDC, ATS and other professional bodies recommend standardized (ie. empirical) short-course chemotherapy with 4 drugs as the initial treatment of new patients with tuberculosis [26-28,30]. There are multiple rationales for this recommendation. INH has early bactericidal activity but is inefficient in ultimately sterilizing TB lesions. RIF is both rapidly bactericidal and also kills persisting semi-dormant bacilli. RIF and PZA, which is also crucial in achieving sterilization, are responsible for shortening the duration of treatment from the up to 18 months to the current 6-month standard [42]. Six-month regimens with initial combinations of INH, RIF and EMB lead to over 10% relapse rate [43]. Six-month regimens with initial combination of INH, RIF, and PZA are adequate in patients with pan-susceptible organisms [28,36,44]. In most settings, however, a 4-drug combination allows the use of the cost-effective 6-month courses without risking the development of MDR in cases with primary INH-resistance. Other standardized regimens exist, which are based on local traditions and rely on low prevailing levels of resistance [13], but they cannot be broadly recommended.

Over-treatment at the initiation of therapy is preferred to under-treatment, as resistance can easily develop in the presence of a high number of organisms during the first weeks of therapy. If there is suspicion of initial MDRTB (eg. in an infant living with an index case), it is advisable to start with 6 drugs (including an injectable agent)[36]. The regimen can be adjusted once susceptibility results are obtained. In settings with a high prevalence of primary MDRTB, standardizing such regimens should be carefully considered, based on local epidemiology and the assured availability and administration of the additional medications. The best approach in such settings is yet to be defined, particularly when resources are constrained.

2.2.2   Premature cessation of treatment

An incomplete course of anti-tuberculosis treatment may also cause MDRTB to develop. Recommended lengths of therapy vary. In the most common scenario, 4 drugs are used for 2 months, and then INH and RIF are continued for an additional 4 months. The continuation phase needs to be increased to 7 or 10 months (with RIF and EMB) in cases of INH resistance or intolerance [28,45,46]; alternatively the 4-month continuation phase should include RIF/EMB/PZA [28]. In cases of PZA intolerance (or if PZA is avoided in pregnancy), the maintenance phase should be prolonged to 7 months. RIF mono-resistance requires streptomycin (SM) in the initial phase, and a 16-month continuation phase on INH and EMB [46]. Rifabutin is the preferred rifamycin for use in HIV-infected patients on protease inhibitors [47,48]. This drug may also be used if susceptibility to rifabutin is demonstrated in patients with RIF mono-resistance [49]. However, caution is required because some experts doubt that the *in vitro* demonstration of rifabutin susceptibility in RIF-resistant isolates accurately predicts a therapeutic *in vivo* response [45]. Detailed regimens for treating MDRTB with/without additional drug resistances are provided in an accompanying chapter [50].

2.2.3   Inappropriate treatment modifications when complications arise

Inappropriate changes to treatment regimens are another common clinical error. General physicians should limit themselves to prescribing a well-recognised, standardized regimen. Departures from standard therapy should be well justified and discussed with a local expert. Patients who experience gastric discomfort or minor adverse effects need not switch drugs. Patients could split the daily dose (or take their medication twice weekly), take it with light meals, or even use a lower dose for a few days until tolerance is achieved.   Medications must be discontinued in patients who develop hepatitis. After liver enzymes decrease to below 3-5 times normal, reintroduce ethambutol, which causes the least hepatic dysfunction, then RIF, and finally INH. RIF should be reintroduced within 1 or 2 weeks to avoid MDR in cases of INH-resistance; otherwise an aminoglycoside and levofloxacin can be considered [36]. Monitoring serum drug-levels, even in patients with AIDS, is of little utility in guiding therapy [51].

2.2.4   Adding a single drug to a failing regimen

Adding a single first line drug (or two oral second line drugs) in the setting of therapeutic failure increases the risk of losing an additional medication to drug resistance without significantly improving the chances of treatment success [5]. DST should be obtained prior to changing a failing drug regimen. If DST is not available, it is then preferable to add at least two or three drugs not previously used by that patient. Commonly used drugs against MDRTB include the injectable agents, such as streptomycin, amikacin, or capreomycin; oral drugs such as para-aminosalicylic acid (PAS), cycloserine, ethionamide, and levofloxacin are used to prevent the acquisition of resistance to the "basic" injectable [30,36]. A general physician treating a patient with MDRTB is strongly recommended to seek expert advice.

2.2.5   Failure to adjust preventive therapy

INH chemoprophylaxis is not known to cause drug-resistance if the patient truly has a dormant infection [28]. However, the use of isoniazid "prophylaxis" in the setting of active TB disease (inadvertent monotherapy) can induce INH-resistant TB [5]. Moreover, prophylaxis with INH cannot be expected to be effective in cases infected with INH-resistant organisms. Recently introduced regimens with RIF and PZA over two months may be a reasonable chemoprophylactic substitute when INH-resistance is suspected

[52]. For PPD-positive contacts of MDRTB cases, guidelines have been developed that take into account the probability of infection from the index case (high for close exposure with PPD conversion) and the risk of progression to active disease (high in HIV infection and infancy)[36]. Alternative interventions include an appropriate multidrug regimen, careful follow-up and treatment only if active disease occurs, or simple INH chemoprophylaxis if otherwise indicated. We believe these chemoprophylaxis policies contribute little to the control of MDRTB.

2.3   Poor treatment adherence and incomplete follow-up

Patients who disregard treatment recommendations were problematic even in Hippocrates' time [53], and the problem of "irregularity" in the ambulatory treatment of tuberculosis was noted soon after the introduction of effective drug therapy [54]. During the 1970s, when tuberculosis rates were declining, the problem was rarely discussed. With the recent resurgence of tuberculosis and the emergence of drug resistance [55,56], non-adherence has again reached center stage and is considered a serious problem in TB control [57]. Reported correlates of non-adherence to antituberculosis therapy include homelessness, alcoholism, injection drug use, unemployment, and other sociomedical characteristics [58]. Treatment default has been linked to increased rates of relapse [59], and it contributes to many of the chronic cases with acquired drug-resistance.

Before the tuberculosis control programme in New York City was revamped, a cohort of 184 new patients with tuberculosis was studied [60]. Half of the patients defaulted treatment for two months or longer but only 12% of patients received directly observed therapy (DOT), usually after non-adherence was noted. Although more common among the homeless and injection drug users, non-adherence occurred frequently and unpredictably in other patients. Non-adherent patients remained infectious longer and, despite longer regimens, were half as likely to complete therapy. Not surprisingly, non-adherent subjects returning to the system were more likely to have newly acquired drug-resistance (RR 5.6 [95% CI, 0.7 to 44.2]); among the non-adherent returning patients were three cases of newly acquired MDRTB [60]. Protracted tuberculosis among non-adherent patients thus contributes to the emergence and spread of drug-resistant tuberculosis.

The reasons for non-adherence include clinical improvement, medication side-effect, forgetfulness, and concomitant illness [61,62]. While the failure to keep physicians' appointments is a worrisome sign, the best predictor of non-adherence is a previous history of non-adherence [63]. However, the clinical recognition of non-adherence is unreliable [5,60], and generalised prevention of non-adherence is therefore most important.

Hence, the responsibility of physicians and pharmacists does not end with writing or filling the correct prescription [64]. While not legally mandated, health providers should ensure treatment completion or refer patients to the appropriate TB control programme. The health provider plays a crucial role in promoting adherence, detecting poor compliance, and acting in a timely manner when default occurs. Such responsibility should be upheld whether in public clinics or in private offices. Good communication and ongoing education are important in promoting adherence, as are flexible appointments, short waiting times, accessibility, appropriate incentives and enablers, acceptability of health workers, and privacy protection [36]. Patient convenience and well-being must always be considered. For example, drug regimens can often be changed to twice weekly dosing after the first two weeks of daily treatment [65]. Injecting drug users require higher maintenance doses of methadone while on RIF, which decreases the efficacy of opium derivatives. Such consideration of the patient improves adherence and makes involuntary detention a last resort that is rarely required [66,67].

While successful treatment completion may be achieved without DOT, this approach is necessary when a programme cannot reach a cure rate of 85%. DOT is the ideal mode of treatment for all patients with active tuberculosis. Treatment should be observed, preferably by a TB professional and not by a friend or a family member. This is particularly true when injectable agents are used, as there is a tendency to skip doses. DOT should be mandatory when treating MDRTB [30,36].

Health care providers should not only report the diagnosis of every case of TB to coordinating authorities but also the treatment outcomes. A central TB registry, accessible to clinicians, is quite helpful when managing a previously treated case. Communication between providers and TB control programmes aids treatment continuity when patients transfer to other districts. A completion letter can be given to the patient at the end of treatment, specifying length of therapy, drugs used, and percent adherence [36].

3.   PROGRAMMATIC FACTORS ASSOCIATED WITH DRUG RESISTANCE

Drug resistance will inevitably develop wherever antimicrobial agents are introduced. However, the speed with which resistance emerges (or disappears) can be influenced by changes in the quality of the local TB control programme [68,69]. Examples of accelerated resistance development are New York during the 1980s [70], Djibouti and Thailand. Examples of suppression of drug resistance include Algeria [71], Korea [69], Texas, and New York (after

1992)[40]. While treatment for TB in most areas of the US is available to all individuals regardless of insurance status or ability to pay for medical care, geographic or financial access is limited in many parts of the world [72]. Political commitment to a national programme is even more important in such settings. Erratic drug supply in the context of a poorly-run TB programme is harmful and has the same adverse effect as inadequate drug regimens or low adherence. In addition, variability in the bioavailability of antituberculosis drugs manufactured in developing countries could theoretically promote drug resistance. Programmatic strategies therefore influence the development of drug resistance and periodic surveillance is essential to provide feedback and identify hot zones or populations to be targeted by special efforts [12].

3.1   Use of treatment regimens other than Standardized Short-Course Chemotherapy (SCC)

A crucial component of the strategy for control of tuberculosis adopted by WHO and IUATLD is the provision of standardized SCC to all smear-positive cases under DOT [73]. This recommendation is based on the principle that capricious variations in patient management are a source of MDRTB [74]. In most countries, the uncontrolled multiplication of regimens also prevents the rational distribution of drugs, and the cost of non-standard regimens may be higher than that of the recommended regimens.

Well-managed standardized SCC works in poor or rich countries. In Algeria, the introduction of a standardized 12-month regimen after 1967 produced a rapid decrease in the prevalence of both acquired (from 82% to 61.5%) and primary (from 15% to 10%) drug resistance. With the introduction of standard SCC in the mid 1980s, the prevalence of drug resistance was further reduced to 21% (acquired) and 5.2% (primary) in the late 1980s [71]. The impact of sound treatment policies has been demonstrated in places like New York [75,76]. Nineteen per cent of all culture-proven TB cases in New York in April 1991 were found to be resistant to both INH and RIF [14]. A major reorganization of the TB control programme followed, together with an influx of necessary resources. The number of MDRTB cases fell by 92% between 1992 and 1998 [77]. This reduction in just a few years suggests programme improvements can have a major impact on the epidemiology of MDRTB.

3.2   Failure to employ direct observation of treatment

The problem of non-compliance, as that of drug-resistance, was noted soon after the introduction of effective anti-tuberculosis therapy [8,78]. DOT has proven effective against the resurgence of tuberculosis [79], and the emergence of drug resistance [68], and is cost-effective [80-83]. Yet DOT may be deemed unnecessary where cure rates exceed 90% with self-administered protocols. The recent success of US efforts was not due solely to DOT but to a comprehensive restoration of control programmes, intensive educational campaigns, hospital isolation policies, and individualized management. Even with DOT, full adherence is not guaranteed [84], especially if applied incorrectly (ie. "sloppy DOTS"). Furthermore, there must be a threshold of MDR prevalence above which standardized SCC regimens, regardless of DOT, will not work and may even fan additional drug-resistance [41,85].

3.3   Availability of antituberculosis drugs over the counter and in fixed dose combinations

The over-the-counter (OTC) availability of antituberculosis drugs in local pharmacies runs counter to all the above principles. In the Philippines, as an example, there are dozens of commercial products combining isoniazid with vitamins which people seek for unspecified respiratory ailments. The black market for RIF exists in many countries and is even more worrisome. While the phenomenon cannot be well quantified, such practices must contribute to the emergence of MDRTB in many communities around the world. In Brazil, where all antituberculosis drugs are dispensed through the national programme, the prevalence of primary MDRTB was under 1% despite no DOT [10]. While political and economic pressures cannot be ignored, open access to antituberculosis drugs should be restricted.

Fixed dose combination tablets (eg. Rifamate™ and Rifater™) preclude monotherapy and may prevent drug resistance. The use of FDC tablets, recommended by both WHO and IUATLD since 1988 [86], is based on the rationale that FDC preparations ensure polychemotherapy and enhance adherence [87,88]. When used appropriately, FDC tablets should decrease the risk that MDRTB will develop [89]. In the WHO/IUATLD Global Surveillance Project, most countries that provided anti-tuberculosis drugs as FDC tablets in over 95% of cases (eg. Brazil, Lesotho, New Zealand, Scotland and Swaziland) reported very low levels of drug resistance and MDR [12]. On the other hand, some countries that did not use FDC tablets (eg. Botswana, Cuba, Nepal, Korea, Zimbabwe) also had low MDR levels. FDC preparations do not guarantee patient adherence, and low-quality preparations or sub-therapeutic doses could still lead to drug resistance [90]. Furthermore, FDC preparations need to be administered daily and may be more expensive overall than individual drugs given in twice-weekly regimens under direct observation. While not a substitute for DOT, FDC tablets should be considered as a safety net where DOT is not feasible [89,91].

3.4   Failure to isolate MDRTB patients

Although priority should be given to preventing the emergence of MDRTB by appropriate treatment of all new TB cases, a second line of containment is the isolation of patients to diminish the spread of the disease [22]. Patient isolation may be the only feasible strategy to curtail transmission of MDRTB where individualized treatment with second-line drugs is not available or affordable. Isolation in a household setting, after the index case is diagnosed, is unlikely to protect close contacts. However, the isolation of any TB patient suspected of harbouring MDR strains is appropriate in congregate settings [92,93], especially in hospitals and prisons with immunologically vulnerable patients [92]. Healthcare and maintenance workers are indeed at risk of infection and deserve appropriate protection [93]. The wisdom of this control strategy is particularly relevant to the management of patients whose therapy has failed or who have documented MDRTB. The heightened suspicion of TB by physicians and the rigorous application of isolation policies by hospital epidemiologists have been important components in the victory over MDRTB in New York [40,77]. Hospital isolation policies need to be tailored to regional conditions and resources.

Detention and forced isolation should be considered when all other efforts to promote adherence to therapy have failed. Such tactics protect contacts from developing MDRTB infection, even if the patient refuses treatment. In New York City, where a fifth of patients are intravenous drug users, only 139 of more than 8,000 TB patients (<2%) required detention [66]. It is possible that the legislation acted as a deterrent to treatment default. Due process and civil rights protection need to be carefully considered. Together with enablers and incentives, detention should be part of the public health measures to improve treatment completion and prevent the generation and spread of MDRTB.

4.   CONCLUSIONS

The emergence of MDRTB has been associated with clinical mismanagement, patient-related factors, and a variety of programmatic weaknesses (Table 1). In many countries, programme deficiencies may include the lack of a standardized therapeutic regimen, or poor implementation compounded by shortages of drugs. Use of anti-tuberculosis drugs of unproven quality is an additional concern, as is the sale of these medications over the counter and in the black market. Appropriate precautions and isolation policies are also important to stop transmission of MDRTB, especially in settings with immunocompromised patients.

The emergence of drug resistance is often caused by departures by health providers from the recommended guidelines. Problems may occur in selecting the appropriate chemotherapy regimen, sometimes due to lack of recognition of prior treatment, errors such as addition of a single drug to a failing regimen, and poor oversight of patient adherence. Referral to or close consultation with a specialized center is advisable when departures from standard regimens are deemed necessary on clinical rounds.

Patients' non-adherence to prescribed treatment also contributes to the development of drug resistance. Non-adherence is difficult to predict based on demographic or social characteristics but is less likely to occur under directly observed therapy [68]. Another patient factor that has been associated with MDRTB is HIV infection [94], but the results of various studies have been inconsistent. Exposure in congregate settings and rapid progression to active disease could explain the higher prevalence of MDRTB among HIV-positive patients in communities with increasing rates of MDRTB.

In the end, a poorly functioning National Tuberculosis Programme, not individual patients, is responsible for the emergence of drug resistance [95]. As a communicable disease, tuberculosis is a public health problem and needs to be addressed using appropriate control measures. On balance, the best approach with limited resources is to cure the largest number of patients and prevent MDR by adhering to standardized SCC regimens [17]. Countries that have secured the basic strategies of sound TB control may then devote additional resources to fight MDRTB and other specific problems.

REFERENCES

1. Neu HC. The crisis of antibiotic resistance. Science 1992; 257: 1064-73.
2. Kochi A, Vareldzis B, Styblo K. Multidrug resistant tuberculosis and its control. Res Microbiol 1993; 144: 104-10.
3. Grange JM. Drug resistance and tuberculosis elimination. Bull Int Union Tuberc Lung Dis 1990; 65: 57-79.
4. Mitchison DA, Nunn AJ. Influence of initial drug resistance on the response to short-course chemotherapy of pulmonary tuberculosis. Am Rev Respir Dis 1986; 133: 423-30.
5. Mahmoudi A, Iseman MD. Pitfalls in the care of patients with tuberculosis. JAMA 1993; 270: 65-8.
6. Geerligs WA, van Altena R, van der Werf TS. Antituberculosis-drug resistance. N Engl J Med 1998; 339: 1079-80.
7. Canetti G. Present aspects of bacterial resistance in tuberculosis. Am Rev Respir Dis 1965; 92: 687-703.

8. Crofton J, Mitchison DA. Streptomycin resistance in pulmonary tuberculosis. BMJ 1948; 2: 1009-15.
9. Mitchison DA. Development of streptomycin resistant strains of tubercle bacilli in pulmonary tuberculosis. Thorax 1950; 4: 144.
10. Pablos-Méndez A, Raviglione MC, Laszlo A, Bustreo F, Binkin N, Rieder H, Cohn D, Lambregts C, Kim SJ, Chaulet P, and Nunn P, for The WHO/IUATLD Global Working Group on Anti-tuberculosis Drug Resistance Surveillance. Global surveillance for antituberculosis drug resistance, 1994-1997. New Engl J Med 1998; 338: 164149.
11. Bustreo F, Pablos-Mendez A, Raviglione M, Murray J, Trébucq A, Rieder H. WHO/IUATLD Global Working Group on Antimicrobial Drug Resistance Surveillance. Guidelines for surveillance of drug resistance in tuberculosis, 1997 (WHO/TB/96.216). World Health Organization, Geneva 1996.
12. Pablos-Méndez A, Laszlo A, Bustreo F, Binkin N, Cohn DL, Lambregts-van Weezembeek C, Kim SJ, Chaulet P, Nunn P, Raviglione MC and the members of the WHO/IUATLD Global Project on Anti-tuberculosis Drug Resistance Surveillance. Anti-tuberculosis drug resistance in the world (WHO/TB/97.229). World Health Organization, Geneva, 1997.
13. Iseman MD, Madsen LA. Drug-resistant tuberculosis. Clin Chest Med 1989; 10: 341-53.
14. Frieden T, Sterling T, Pablos-Méndez A, et al. The emergence of drug-resistant tuberculosis in New York City. N Engl J Med 1993; 328: 521-26.
15. Plikaytis BB, Marden JL, Crawford JT, et al. Multiplex PCR assay specific for the multidrug-resistant strain W of Mycobacterium tuberculosis. J Clin Microbiol 1994; 32: 1542-6.
16. Cohn ML, Middlebrook G, Russell WF Jr. Combined drug treatment of tuberculosis: Prevention of emergence of mutant populations of tubercle bacilli resistant to both streptomycin and isoniazid in vitro. J Clin Invest 1959; 38: 1349.
17. World Health Organization. Treatment of tuberculosis: Guidelines for National Programs (WHO/TB/96.199). World Health Organization, Geneva 1996.
18. Friedman LN, Williams MT, Singh TP, Frieden TR. Tuberculosis, AIDS, and death among substance abusers on welfare in New York City. N Engl J Med 1996; 334: 828-33.
19. Cohn ML, Oda U, Kovitz C, Middlebrook G. Studies on isoniazid and tubercle bacilli: the isolation of isoniazid-resistant mutants in vitro. Am Rev Tuberc 1954; 70: 465-75.
20. Schmidt LH, Grover AA, Hoffmann R, Rehm J, Sullivan R. The emergence of isoniazid-sensitive bacilli in monkeys inoculated with isoniazid-resistant strains, p. 264. In: Trans 17th Conference on Chemotherapy of Tuberculosis, VA-Armed Forces. 1958.
21. Cohn ML, Kovitz C, Oda U, Middlebrook G. Studies on isoniazid and tubercle bacilli: the growth requirements, catalase activities, and pathogenic properties of isoniazid-resistant mutants. Am Rev Tuberc 1954; 70: 641-64.
22. Edlin BR, Tokars JL, Grieco MH, et al. An outbreak of multi-drug resistant tuberculosis among hospitalized patients with the acquired immunodeficiency syndrome. N Eng J Med 1992; 326: 1514-21.
23. Centers for Disease Control. Nosocomial transmission of multidrug-resistant tuberculosis among HIV-infected persons - Florida and New York, 1988-1991. MMWR 1991; 40: 585-91.
24. Monno L, Angarano G, Carbonara S, et al. Emergence of drug resistant Mycobacterium tuberculosis in HIV-infected patients. Lancet 1991; 337: 852.
25. Bastian I, Portaels F. Introduction: past, present, and future, Chapter 1, 1-15. In: Bastian I, Portaels F (eds.), Multidrug-resistant tuberculosis. Kluwer Academic Publications, The Netherlands 2000.

26. Crofton J. The prevention and management of drug resistant tuberculosis. Bull Intern Union Tuberc 1987; 62: 6-11.
27. Centers for Disease Control. Treatment of tuberculosis and tuberculosis infection in adults and children. Amer Rev Resp Dis 1994; 149: 1359-74.
28. American Thoracic Society. Treatment of tuberculosis and tuberculosis infection in adults and children. Am J Resp Crit Care Med 1994; 149: 1359-74.
29. Joint Tuberculosis Committee of the British Thoracic Society. Chemotherapy and management of tuberculosis in the United Kingdom: recommendations 1998. Thorax 1998; 53: 536-48.
30. Crofton J, Chaulet P, Maher D. Guidelines for the management of drug-resistant tuberculosis. Global Tuberculosis Program. World Health Organization, Geneva, 1997.
31. Sbarbaro JA. 'Multidrug'-resistant tuberculosis: it is time to focus on the private sector of medicine. Chest 1997; 111: 1149-51.
32. Styblo K. Epidemiology of Tuberculosis. Royal Netherlands Tuberculosis Association, The Hague, Netherland, 1984.
33. Coronado VG, Beck-Sague CM, Hutton MD, Davis BJ, Nicholas P, Villareal C, Woodley CL, Kilburn JO, Crawford JT, Frieden TR, et al. Transmission of multidrug-resistant Mycobacterium tuberculosis among persons with human immunodeficiency virus infection in an urban hospital: epidemiologic and restriction fragment length polymorphism analysis. J Infect Dis 1993; 168: 1052-5.
34. Pablos-Méndez A, Sterling TR, Frieden TR. The relationship between delayed or incomplete treatment and all-cause mortality in patients with tuberculosis. JAMA 1996; 276:1223-8.
35. Busillo CP, Lessnau KD, Sanjana V, Soumakis S, Davidson M, Mullen MP, Talavera W. Multidrug resistant *Mycobacterium tuberculosis* in patients with human immunodeficiency virus infection. Chest 1992; 102: 797-801.
36. Clinical Policies and Protocols, Bureau of Tuberculosis Control, New York City Department of Health, 1998. At http://www.ci.nyc.ny.us/health, accessed 5/99.
37. Barnes PF, Chan LS, Wong SF. The course of fever during treatment of pulmonary tuberculosis. Tubercle 1987; 68: 255-60.
38. Lessnau KD, Gorla M, Talavera W. Radiographic presentation and course in sensitive and multi-drug resistant *M. tuberculosis*. Chest 1994; 106: 687-9.
39. Nitta AT, Davidson PT, de Koning ML, Kilman RJ. Misdiagnosis of multidrug-resistant tuberculosis possibly due to laboratory-related errors. JAMA 1996; 276: 1980-3.
40. Frieden TR, Fujiwara PI, Washko RM, Hamburg MA. Tuberculosis in New York City - turning the tide. N Engl J Med 1995; 333: 229-33.
41. Raviglione MC. DOTS and multidrug-resistant tuberculosis, Chapter 7, 115-131. In: Bastian I, Portaels F (eds.), Multidrug-resistant tuberculosis. Kluwer Academic Publications, The Netherlands 2000.
42. Mitchison DA. The Garrod Lecture. Understanding the chemotherapy of tuberculosis – current problems. J Antimicrob Chemother 1992;29: 477-93.
43. Zierski M, Bek E, Long MW, et al. Short-course (6 month) cooperative tuberculosis study in Poland: results 18 months after completion of treatment. Am Rev Respir Dis 1980; 122: 879-89.
44. Singapore Tuberculosis Service/British Medical Research Council. Clinical Trial of six-month and four-month regimens of chemotherapy in the treatment of pulmonary tuberculosis. Am Rev Respir Dis 1979; 119: 579-85.
45. Iseman MD. Treatment of multidrug-resistant tuberculosis. N Engl J Med 1993; 329: 784-91.

46. Raviglione M, O'Brien RJ. Tuberculosis. In: Harrison's Principles of Internal Medicine, 14th Edition in CD-ROM. McGraw-Hill, New York, 1998.
47. Eagling VA, Back DJ, Barry MG. Differential inhibition of cytochrome P450 isoforms by protease inhibitors, ritonavir, squinavir and indinavir. Br J Clin Pharmacol 1997; 44: 190-4.
48. Centers for Disease Control and Prevention. Prevention and treatment of tuberculosis among patients infected with the human immunodeficiency virus: principles of therapy and revised recommendations. MMWR 1998; 47 (RR-20).
49. McGregor MM, Olliaro P, Wolmarans L, et al. Efficacy and safety of rifabutin in the treatment of patients with newly diagnosed pulmonary tuberculosis. Am J Respir Crit Care Med 1996; 154: 1462-7.
50. Iseman MD, Huitt G. Treatment of multidrug-resistant tuberculosis, Chapter 11, 175-190. In: Bastian I, Portaels F (eds.), Multidrug-resistant tuberculosis. Kluwer Academic Publications, The Netherlands 2000.
51. Choudhri SH, Hawken M, Gathua S, Minyiri GO, Watkins W, Sahai J, Sitar DS, Aoki FY, Long R. Pharmacokinetics of antimycobacterial drugs in patients with tuberculosis, AIDS, and diarrhea. Clin Infect Dis 1997; 25: 104-11.
52. Halsey NA, Coberly JS, Desormameaux J, et al. Randomised trial of isoniazid versus rifampicin and pyrazinamide for prevention of tuberculosis in HIV-1 infection. Lancet 1998; 351: 786-92.
53. Haynes RB, Taylor DW, Sackett DL (eds.), Compliance in Health Care. Johns Hopkins University Press, Baltimore, MD 1979.
54. Fox W. Adherence of patience and physicians: experience and lessons from tuberculosis-II. BMJ 1983; 287: 101-5.
55. Bloch AB, Cauthen GM, Onorato IM, et al. Nationwide survey of drug-resistant tuberculosis in the United States. JAMA 1994; 271: 665-71.
56. Bifani PJ, Plikaytis BB, Kapur V, et al. Origin and interstate spread of a New York City multidrug-resistant Mycobacterium tuberculosis clone family. JAMA 1996;275:452-457.
57. Addington WW. Patient adherence: the most serious remaining problem in control of tuberculosis in the US. Chest 1979; 76(suppl.): 741-3.
58. Sumartojo E. When tuberculosis treatment fails. A social behavioral account of patient adherence. Am Rev Respir Dis 1993; 147: 1311-20.
59. Ormerod LP, Prescott RJ. Inter-relations between relapses, drug regimens and compliance with treatment in tuberculosis. Respiratory Medicine 1991; 85: 239-42.
60. Pablos-Méndez A, Knirsch CA, Barr RG, Lerner BH, Frieden TR. Nonadherence in anti-tuberculosis treatment: predictors and consequences in New York City. Am J Med 1997; 102: 164-70.
61. Fox W. The problem of self-administration of drugs; with particular reference to pulmonary tuberculosis. Tubercle 1958; 39: 269-74.
62. Moodie AS. Mass ambulatory chemotherapy in the treatment of tuberculosis in a predominantly urban community. Am Rev Respir Dis 1967; 95: 384-97.
63. Tuberculosis Chemotherapy Centre, Madras. A concurrent comparison of intermittent (twice weekly) isoniazid plus streptomycin and daily isoniazid plus PAS in the domiciliary treatment of pulmonary tuberculosis. Bull WHO 1964; 31: 247-71.
64. Arif K, Ali SA, Amanullah S, Siddiqui I, Khan JA, Nayani P. Physician compliance with national tuberculosis treatment guidelines: a university hospital study. Int J Tuberc Lung Dis 1998; 2: 225-30.
65. Cohn DL, Catlin BJ, Peterson KL, Judson FN, Sbarbaro JA. A 62-dose, 6-month therapy for pulmonary and extrapulmonary tuberculosis. Ann Int Med 1990; 112: 407-15.
66. Gasner MR, Maw Kl, Feldman GE, Fujiwara PI, Frieden TR. The use of legal action in New York City to ensure treatment of tuberculosis. N Engl J Med 1999; 340: 359-66.

67. Oscherwitz T, Tulsky JP, Roger S, Sciortino S, Alpers A, Royce S, Lo B. Detention of persistently nonadherent patients with tuberculosis. JAMA 1997 Sep 10;278(10):843-6.

68. Chaulk CP, Moore-Rice K, Rizzo R, Chaisson RE. Eleven years of community-based directly observed therapy for tuberculosis. JAMA 1995; 274: 945-51.

69. Kim SJ, Hong YP. Drug resistance of Mycobacterium tuberculosis in Korea. Tuberc Lung Dis 1992; 73: 219-24.

70. Sepkowitz KA, Telzak EE, Recalde S, Armstrong D, the New York City Area Tuberculosis Working Group. Trends in the susceptibility of tuberculosis in New York City, 1987 1991. Clin Infect Dis 1994; 18: 755 9.

71. Chaulet P. Tuberculose et transition épidemiologique: le cas de l'Algerie. Ann Inst Pasteur 1993; 4: 181-7.

72. Murray CJ, Styblo K, Rouillon A. Tuberculosis in developing countries: burden, intervention and cost. Bull IUATLD 1990; 65: 6-64.

73. WHO Tuberculosis Programme. Framework for effective tuberculosis control (WHO/TB/94.179). World Health Organization, Geneva 1994.

74. Chaulet P, Raviglione M, Bustreo F. Epidemiology, control and treatment of multidrug-resistant tuberculosis. Drugs 1996; 52(suppl 2): 103-8.

75. Landesman SH. Commentary: tuberculosis in New York City--the consequences and lessons of failure. Am J Public Health 1993; 83: 766-8.

76. Fujiwara PI, Larkin C, Frieden TR. Directly observed therapy in New York City: history, implementation, results, and challenges. Clin Chest Med 1997; 18: 135-48.

77. Fujiwara PI, Cook SV, Rutherford CM , Crawford JT , Glickman SE , Kreiswirth BN, Sachdev PS , Osahan SS , Ebrahimzadeh A , Frieden TR. A continuing survey of drug-resistant tuberculosis, New York City, April 1994. Arch Intern Med 1997; 157: 531-6.

78. Fox W. Adherence of patients and physicians: experience and lessons from tuberculosis-II. BMJ 1983; 287: 101-5.

79. Weis SE, Slocum PC, Blais FX, et al. The effect of directly observed therapy on the rates of drug resistance and relapse in tuberculosis. N Engl J Med 1994; 330: 1179-84.

80. Bayer R, Wilkinson D. Directly observed therapy: history of an idea. Lancet 1995; 345: 1545-8.

81. Wilkinson D. High-compliance tuberculosis treatment program in a rural community. Lancet 1994; 343: 647-8.

82. Iseman MD, Cohn DL, Sbarbaro JA. Directly observed treatment of tuberculosis. We can't afford not to do it. N Engl J Med 1993; 328: 576-8.

83. Moore RD, Chaulk CP, Griffiths R, Cavalcante S, Chaisson RE. Cost-effectiveness of directly observed versus self-administered therapy for tuberculosis. Am J Respir Crit Care Med 1996; 154: 1013-9.

84. Burman WJ, Cohn DL, Rietmeijer CA, et al. Nonadherence with directly observed therapy for tuberculosis: epidemiology and effect on the outcome of treatment. Chest 1997; 111: 1168-73.

85. Farmer P, Bayona J, Becerra M, Furin J, Henry C, Hiatt H et al. The dilemma of MDR-TB in the global era. Int J Tuberc Lung Dis 1998; 2: 869-76.

86. Anonymous. The promise and reality of fixed dose combinations with rifampicin. A joint statement of the International Union against Tuberculosis and Lung Disease and the Tuberculosis Program of the World Health Organization. Tuberc Lung Dis 1994; 75: 180-1.

87. Combs DL, Geiter LJ, O'Brien RJ. The UHPS tuberculosis short-course chemotherapy trial 21: effectiveness, toxicity, and acceptability. The report of final results. Ann Intern Med 1990; 112: 397-406.

88. Singapore Tuberculosis Service/British Medical Research Council. Assessment of a daily combined preparation of isoniazid, rifampin, and pyrazinamide in a controlled trial of three 6-month regimens for smear-positive pulmonary tuberculosis. Am Rev Respir Dis 1991; 143: 707-712.

89. Moulding T, Dutt AK, Reichman LB. Fixed-dose combinations of antituberculous medications to prevent drug resistance. Ann Intern Med 1995; 122: 951-4.

90. Acocella G. Human bioavailability studies. Bull Int Union Tuberc Lung Dis 1989; 64: 38-40.

91. Reichman LB. How to ensure the continued resurgence of tuberculosis. Lancet 1996; 347: 175-7.

92. Dupon M, Texier-Maugein J, Leroy V, et al. Tuberculosis and HIV infection: a cohort study of incidence and susceptibility to antituberculosis drugs, Bordeaux, 1985-1993. AIDS 1995; 9: 577-83.

93. Pearson ML, Jereb JA, Frieden TR, et al. Nosocomial transmission of multidrug-resistant *Mycobacterium tuberculosis*: a risk to patients and health care workers. Ann Intern Med 1992; 117: 191-6.

94. Gordin FM, Nelson ET, Matts JP, et al. The impact of human immunodeficiency virus infection on drug resistant tuberculosis. Am J Resp Crit Care Med 1996; 154: 1478-83.

95. Reichman LB. Tuberculosis elimination - what's to stop us? Int J Tuberc Lung Dis 1997; 1: 3-11.

Chapter 6

The molecular mechanisms of drug resistance in *Mycobacterium tuberculosis*

Howard E. Takiff
Laboratorio de Genética Molecular, Centro de Microbiología y Biología Celular, Instituto Venezolano de Investigaciones Científicas, Caracas,Venezuela

1.   INTRODUCTION

In the early 1990's, when patients with acquired immunodeficiency syndrome (AIDS) in several large cities began dying with multidrug-resistant (MDR) strains of *Mycobacterium tuberculosis*, there was considerable alarm and uncertainty [1,2]. The sudden and seemingly simultaneous appearance of many MDR strains raised the terrifying possibility that there was a single mechanism or mutation, perhaps carried on a plasmid or transposable element, that could confer resistance to several drugs and be transferred horizontally from strain to strain, as occurs in other bacteria [3,4]. Fears of "Andromeda-strain" scenarios receded after studies of MDR strains demonstrated that no single resistance mechanism was responsible. Rather, MDR strains were found to develop through the sequential occurrence of separate mutations, each conferring resistance to a single drug or class of drugs [5,6]. Finding the mutations that cause resistance to each of the antituberculosis drugs was a major focus of research in the 1990's. The task was fairly straightforward for drugs that are also used against other pathogens, such as rifampicin (RIF), streptomycin (SM) and the fluoroquinolones (FQs), because the mechanisms were similar to those

I. Bastian and F. Portaels (eds.), Multidrug-Resistant Tuberculosis, 77-114.
© 2000 *Kluwer Academic Publishers. Printed in the Netherlands.*

described in other bacteria. The real challenge was discovering the mutations that confer resistance to drugs that are specific for mycobacteria—isoniazid (INH), pyrazinamide (PZA) and ethambutol (EMB)—whose mechanisms of action were poorly understood. The study of the genes and mutations that cause resistance has not only unravelled the mechanisms of action of these antibiotics, but has also expanded our knowledge of the basic biology of the mycobacteria.

There are several ways through which a mutation can cause drug resistance [3,7,8]. The classic mechanism is a mutation in the gene encoding the drug target, generally an enzyme, whose inhibition accounts for the toxic effects of the drug. Typically these mutations decrease the ability of the drug to bind the target, and therefore define the region on the protein that interacts with the drug. Another type of mutation doesn't alter the drug target, but merely increases its expression, so that there is simply more target than the available drug can inhibit. Some drugs, such as INH and PZA, enter the bacterium as prodrugs, and require an activation step catalyzed by a bacterial enzyme in order to become effective. Hence, any mutation in the activator that stops production of the active form of the drug will be an effective mechanism of resistance. Mutations that decrease drug accumulation within the bacterium can also lead to resistance. This can occur either by decreasing the entry of a drug into the bacterium, or increasing the rate at which the drug is removed from the cell. Finally, resistance can occur by chemical modification and inactivation of the drug. All of these mechanisms will be presented as recurrent themes in mycobacterial drug resistance.

When searching for mutations that cause drug resistance, the Holy Grail is a molecular technique for detecting these mutations that is so sensitive, specific, rapid and facile, that it can replace the laborious task of traditional bacteriologic sensitivity testing. However, technical considerations aside, for this test to be truly useful, it must be able to identify mutations in > 90% of resistant isolates. Unfortunately, at the current state of our knowledge, it is only with RIF resistance and high-level FQ resistance that causative mutations can be identified in > 90% of resistant strains. In at least 15-20% of *M. tuberculosis* isolates resistant to each of the other antituberculosis drugs, no mutation can currently be found to explain their resistance.

Several other reviews of antibiotic resistance in mycobacteria have appeared in recent years [9-12]. This summary will provide an overview of the mechanisms of resistance to the first and second-line anti-tuberculosis agents, and highlight how the mechanisms of resistance have elucidated the mode of action of the various drugs and provided insights into the biology of *M. tuberculosis*. For more details on the specific mutations reported in the many published studies, the reader is referred to the comprehensive review by Ramaswamy and Musser [13].

2. ISONIAZID RESISTANCE

After nicotinamide, a precursor of vitamin B_3, was shown to have a weak antibacterial effect on *M. tuberculosis* [14], many different analogues were tested. In 1952, three pharmaceutical companies simultaneously reported the efficacy of INH. Ethionamide and PZA were also discovered during the same search (Figure 1). Although isoniazid is extremely effective against *M. tuberculosis* (MIC 0.01-0.25 μg/ml), other bacteria, even most other mycobacteria, are innately resistant to it. This specificity has made INH an intriguing antibiotic, and INH has been the subject of more recent studies than any other agent used against *M. tuberculosis*. These studies have focused not only on how *M. tuberculosis* becomes resistant to INH, but also on the characteristics that make this mycobacterium exquisitely sensitive to this simple compound [15]. Attempts to answer these two overlapping questions have advanced our understanding of several aspects of *M. tuberculosis* biology, including its synthesis of mycolic acids [16], oxidative stress response [17], and virulence[18].

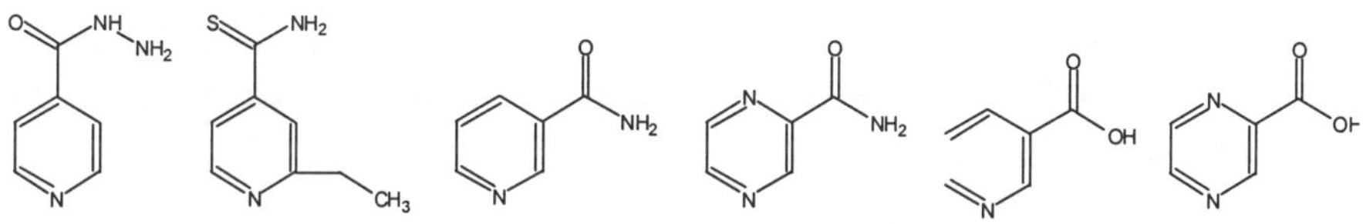

Isoniazid INH | Ethionamide ETH | Nicotinamide | Pyrazinamide PZA | Nicotinic Acid | Pyrazinoic Acid POA

Figure 1. Isoniazid, ethionamide and pyrazinamide are analogues of nicotinamide. PncA, the nicotinamidase/pyrazinamidase, converts nicotinamide to nicotinic acid and pyrazinamide to pyrazinoic acid, the active form of the drug [19]

2.1 The catalase/peroxidase, KatG

Early reports of INH-resistant (INH^R) *M. tuberculosis* noted that several of these resistant strains lacked catalase-peroxidase activity [20], and appeared to have reduced virulence [21]. Forty years later, Zhang et al showed that INH sensitivity and full virulence could be restored to catalase-minus strains by introducing an intact copy of the *katG* gene [22,23]. INH enters the bacterium as a prodrug that is not active until oxidized by KatG, a bi-functional catalase/peroxidase. Any mutation that compromises the ability of KatG to activate INH will result in INH^R. About half of all INH^R isolates of *M. tuberculosis* have mutations in *katG* [24-35], and a variety of amino acid substitutions have been described that either reduce the activity of the enzyme, or lead to rapid proteolysis [36]. Occasionally, the entire gene has been deleted. However, the loss of KatG activity comes at a cost to the bacterium; strains without catalase/peroxidase activity are less virulent [37]. Exactly how KatG contributes to virulence is not certain, but it could promote intracellular survival by protecting against macrophage killing mechanisms, detoxifying reactive oxygen intermediates, or perhaps detoxifying nitric oxide [38]. Therefore, the TB bacillus really wants to accomplish a slight alteration to KatG that no longer activates INH, yet still retains catalase/peroxidase activity. The mutation Ser315Thr does exactly that, and accounts for about half of all *katG* mutations [36,39]. INH^R strains with this mutation retain full virulence and are perhaps those with the most potential to become widely disseminated MDR isolates [40] (D. van Soolingen, personal communication).

When INH reacts with KatG, none of the stable products are very toxic for the bacterium [41](Figure 2), and it is thought that the active form of the drug must be a transient reactive intermediate. Additional toxicity could also be caused by reactive oxygen species produced during the reaction [42]. In vitro chemistry suggested that the active intermediate was likely an acyl cation or radical [43], but the exact target with which it reacted remained a mystery. However, it was recently shown that oxidation of INH in the presence of NAD$^+$ produces a stable NAD/INH complex that may be the inhibitory form of the drug [44].

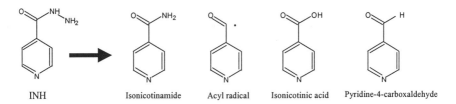

| INH | Isonicotinamide | Acyl radical | Isonicotinic acid | Pyridine-4-carboxaldehyde |

Figure 2. Oxidation of isoniazid in vitro produces the stable products isonicotinic acid, isonicotinamide, and pyridine-4-carboxaldehyde. The acyl radical may be a reactive intermediate in the formation of isonicotinic acid, pyridine-4-carboxaldehyde and the NAD$^+$/INH adduct (see text) [41].

2.2   InhA, KasA, and AcpM

Many studies had shown that INH inhibits the synthesis of mycolic acids in *M. tuberculosis* [45-47]. Hence, it was not surprising that a genetic selection in the rapid-growing model species, *Mycobacterium smegmatis*, identified a protein involved in mycolic acid synthesis that confers INH resistance when mutated or over-expressed [48]. This protein, InhA, is an enoyl acyl carrier protein (ACP) reductase that uses NADH as a cofactor

[49]. Some 20% of INH^R clinical isolates of *M. tuberculosis* have mutations in the *inhA* gene, almost all occurring in the promoter region, apparently increasing its expression (Figure 3). Rarely, INH^R mutations result in amino acid substitutions, and all of these decrease the affinity of the InhA protein for the NADH cofactor [50]. X-ray crystallographic studies with INH showed that the NADH binding pocket of InhA was occupied by the NAD$^+$/INH complex [51], whose affinity for InhA is 200 fold greater than that of NADH[44]. Thus this complex is a very effective inhibitor.

The mutations in *inhA* also confer resistance to ethionamide (ETH), and InhA also appears to be the target for this infrequently-used second-line agent. This would explain reports that ETH resistance was sometimes acquired with resistance to INH [52,53], and suggestions that ETH also acted by inhibiting mycolic acid biosynthesis [54,55]. ETH is also likely to be a prodrug that requires activation by an enzyme that has not yet been identified [43]. Additionally, InhA is the drug target for triclosan, a topical antimicrobial agent commonly used in soaps and toothpaste [56]. Triclosan-resistant mutants of *M. smegmatis* are completely cross-resistant to INH, but triclosan-resistant mutants of *M. tuberculosis* show only weak cross-resistance to INH [57].

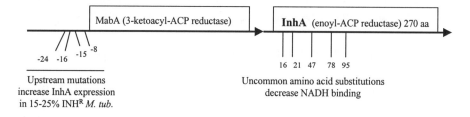

Figure 3. Location of mutations in inhA associated with resistance to INH. The genes encoding the proteins MabA and InhA are expressed together from a promoter upstream of *mabA* [48]. Sequence changes that increase promoter activity are found in 15-20% of INH^R isolates of *M. tuberculosis* [11,13]. Mutations in the coding region for the protein InhA are much less common in INH^R stains [58], and all appear to reduce NADH binding affinity.

While the InhA enzyme is clearly the target for INH in the rapid-growing *M. smegmatis* [59], its relevance for INH resistance in *M. tuberculosis* has been questioned. If InhA functions as an acyl carrier protein (ACP) reductase [49], then InhA inhibition should produce an accumulation of unsaturated fatty acids, but when *M. tuberculosis* is treated with INH, saturated fatty acids accumulate [58]. An alternative *M. tuberculosis* target for INH, KasA, has been proposed as being more consistent with the biochemical data. KasA is a ketoacyl ACP synthase, which was isolated in a covalent complex with INH and another protein, AcpM. AcpM is an acyl carrier protein specific for long chain fatty acids that are mycolic acid precursors. In the presence of INH, saturated C26 precursors accumulated on AcpM, and there was an increase in the presence of both KasA and AcpM proteins, reflecting some mechanism for up-regulation. One study found *kasA* mutations in 4 of 28 INH-resistant clinical isolates [59], supporting its role as an INH drug target, but other studies identified some of the same mutations in INH-sensitive strains [60,61]. Also, as neither KasA nor AcpM appear to bind either NADH or NAD^+, inhibition by an INH/NAD^+ complex would seem unlikely. However, it is possible that other reactive INH intermediates could be toxic for protein targets without the need to combine with NAD^+.

One unifying possibility is that InhA, KasA, AcpM and the other enzymes encoded by adjacent genes are all components of the same Type II Fatty Acid Synthetase (FAS) system [62], interacting as part of a multi-enzyme complex involved in the biosynthesis of mycolic acids [57]. The direct effect of INH on any one component of this system could cause indirect effects on other enzymes in the complex, and the saturated fatty acids that accumulate in *M. tuberculosis* in the presence of INH could be products of a Type I FAS system (W.R Jacobs, Jr. personal communication). To explain the precise mechanism of INH toxicity will probably require a better understanding of the biochemistry of mycolic acid synthesis.

2.3   OxyR and regulators of the peroxide response

Several studies have tried to explain why the drug is especially toxic for *M. tuberculosis* [15,17,63,64]. The *katG* homologue in *E. coli* is one of several genes under the control of OxyR, the central regulator of the peroxide stress response in enteric bacteria [65,66]. *E. coli* strains lacking OxyR are hypersensitive to INH, and the *M. tuberculosis* oxyR gene contains so many mutations, deletions, and stop codons that it must be a non-functional pseudogene (Figure 4)[67, 68]. Nevertheless, INH sensitivity cannot be attributed simply to the absence of OxyR, because M. smegmatis has no OxyR [69] and yet is intrinsically INH resistant (MIC 5 µg/ml). Even without an OxyR gene, when M. smegmatis is exposed to hydrogen peroxide, there is an increase in the expression of nine proteins [67]. When *M. tuberculosis* is treated with peroxide, only the expression of KatG is induced, but it is still much more resistant to peroxides than maximally induced *M. smegmatis*, perhaps owing to the cyclopropanes present in the mycolic acids of *M. tuberculosis* [70,71]. In the absence of OxyR, the regulators of the peroxide response in *M. smegmatis* and *M. tuberculosis* remain unclear, but strong contenders are the iron responsive elements FurA, located 471 bp upstream of *katG* and IdeR [72].

Adjacent to the *oxyR* pseudogene in *M. tuberculosis,* and transcribed in the opposite direction, is the *ahpC* gene [72,73] (Figure 4). This gene encodes an alkyhydroperoxidase whose homologue in *E.coli* is also regulated by OxyR [65,66]. Although the AhpC protein is undetectable in wild type *M. tuberculosis*, its expression is increased and its presence detectable in some KatG minus strains. [73-75]. Promoter mutations responsible for this up-regulation of *ahpC* have been found in perhaps 10% of INH[R] strains. The increased AhpC expression is thought to compensate for the loss of KatG activity by providing increased protection from peroxides [75], but it does not, by itself, confer INH resistance, nor does it restore virulence to KatG deficient strains [74]. However, an intact AhpC seems to be necessary for full virulence [37,76]. Mutations causing increased AhpC expression are less common in INH[R] strains with the Ser315Thr *katG* mutation [77,78], presumably because the KatG activity is not seriously compromised, and thus no compensatory increase in AhpC activity is required [36,39].

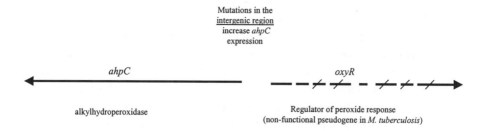

Figure 4. The *M. tuberculosis ahpC* and *oxyR* genes. The M. tuberculosis OxyR gene appears to be a non-functional pseudogene because it contains several deletions and stop codons [67, 68], The expression of AhpC is increased in some INH[R] KatG-minus isolates of M. tuberculosis, and some of these strains have mutations in the intergenic region, between ahpC and the pseudogene oxyR, that increase the strength of the ahpC promoter [73-75].

Although these studies have provided valuable information on the response of *M. tuberculosis* to peroxides and its importance in virulence, the peculiar sensitivity of *M. tuberculosis* for INH remains unexplained. One intriguing possibility is that the amount of free NAD[+] in the bacterium may be important. Only the NAD[+] form will react with activated INH, so if more free NAD[+] is present in the bacterium, more of the inhibitory NAD[+]/INH adduct can be produced. This idea is supported by mutations in the *M. smegmatis* NADH dehydrogenase that result in lower NAD[+]/NADH ratio and also confer INH resistance. No studies are yet available on the NAD[+]/NADH ratio of *M. tuberculosis* [79].

About 15-25% of INH^R strains have no mutations in *inhA, kasA, katG,* or *ahpC,* and hence no recognised mechanism of drug resistance. One possibility is an enzyme found in both *M. smegmatis* and *M. tuberculosis* that can acetylate INH and prevent its activation [80]. Over-expression of the acetylase in *M. smegmatis* causes a three-fold higher resistance to INH, and a promoter mutation in *M. tuberculosis* could have the same effect. Another possibility could be increases in the expression INH exporting efflux pumps, such as those recently shown to export INH from *M. smegmatis* [81].

3.   PYRAZINAMIDE

Pyrazinamide is an important first-line drug for short-course tuberculosis therapy. It was shown to be an active agent in 1952, but was not used extensively as a first-line agent until the 1980's. Unlike INH, RIF, SM, and EMB, which are only effective against actively metabolizing bacteria, PZA kills semi-dormant bacteria in acidic environments, such as within the macrophage [82]. PZA is similar to INH in several respects:

1. PZA is an analogue of nicotinamide;
2. PZA is specific for *M. tuberculosis*—other mycobacteria are intrinsically PZA-resistant;
3. PZA, like INH, is a prodrug that must be converted by a pyrazinamidase (PZase) to the active bactericidal form—pyrazinoic acid (POA); and
4. strains of *M. tuberculosis* without PZase activity are resistant to PZA [83, 84], just as strains without KatG activity are resistant to INH.

The active form, POA, is not an effective drug in animal models, presumably due to poor gastrointestinal absorption and good binding to serum proteins. The enzyme that converts PZA to POA was thought to be a nicotinamidase, so the sequence of the *E. coli* nicotinamidase was used as a guide to amplify the gene, *pncA,* that encodes the *M. tuberculosis* nicotinamidase/PZase [19]. The function of PncA, a protein of 186 amino acids, is to degrade nicotinamide to nicotinic acid in order to be recycled into NAD [85]. As PZA is an analogue of nicotinamide, PncA also converts PZA to POA, but its activity as a PZase is about 100 fold less than as a nicotinamidase [86](Figure 5).

Several studies have sequenced the *pncA* gene in PZA^R, PZase-deficient strains of *M. tuberculosis,* and all have found that at least 70% contain mutations in *pncA*. The proof that the *pncA* mutations were responsible for the drug resistance was provided by introducing a wild-type plasmid copy of the *pncA* gene into resistant strains and showing that PZase activity and PZA sensitivity were restored. One study [87] found *pncA* mutations in only 48 (72%) of 67 PZA^R clinical *M. tuberculosis* isolates, but no mutations in 51

PZA sensitive strains. Other studies of PZA^R *M. tuberculosis* isolates have found *pncA* mutations in 31 of 36 (86%) [88], 33 of 38, (87%) [89] 16 of 23 (70%) [90] and 32 of 33 (97%) [91] strains. The mutations don't cluster in a particular region, but instead are found in diverse sites distributed over most of the *pncA* gene. Single amino acid substitutions, often with a proline, were most common, but stop codons, small deletions and insertions were also found, and two mutations were located just upstream of the coding region, perhaps reducing *pncA* expression.

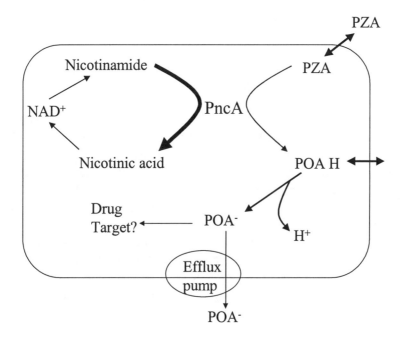

Figure 5. The fate of pyrazinamide (PZA) in mycobacteria (see text for details).

PZA susceptibility testing is notoriously difficult and unreliable, principally because the drug is only active at acidic pH [92,93]. Detecting mutations in the *pncA* gene could be a more reliable method for determining PZA resistance, but the diversity of mutations would require that the entire *pncA* gene be examined—some 600 bases [94]. In addition, the utility of such a test would depend upon the true percentage of PZA^R *M. tuberculosis* strains with *pncA* mutations, which has varied from 70% or 97%, depending on the study.

Although *M. bovis* is closely related to *M. tuberculosis*, it is innately resistance to PZA [95], and the lack of PZase activity of *M. bovis* has been used to distinguish it from *M. tuberculosis* [96]. In most *M. bovis* strains examined [87], this intrinsic PZA^R is due to a C→G change at nucleotide 169 of *pncA,* changing the histidine at position 57 in wild-type *M. tuberculosis* to an aspartic acid [97].

The mechanisms of intrinsic PZA resistance in other mycobacteria are different. *M. kansasii* may be less sensitive to PZA (MIC 125 µg/ml) than *M. tuberculosis* (MIC 16-50 µg/ml)[86], because its PZase is 5-fold less active. *M. smegmatis* has a very active PZase yet is highly resistant to PZA (MIC >2000 µg/ml) [98], probably because it has an efflux pump that transports POA out of the bacteria [99]. A POA efflux pump is also present in *M. tuberculosis*, but is about 100-fold less active than the *M. smegmatis* pump.

Recent accumulation studies using [^{14}C]-labelled PZA and POA have provided a plausible explanation for the increased activity of PZA in acidic conditions (Figure 5). PZA, a neutral amide, diffuses freely across the *M. tuberculosis* cell membrane, and inside the bacteria is converted by PncA to POA, a weak lipophilic acid that can also freely diffuse. However, at the neutral pH within the bacteria, most of the POA will dissociate the proton to leave a negative charge that does not diffuse across the membrane. In an extracellular environment with a low pH, much more of the POA will be in the weak acid form, which will diffuse across the membrane, dissociate its proton in the higher intracellular pH, and be trapped within the bacteria [99]. Thus, PZA is more effective in acidic environments because higher concentrations of POA accumulate within the bacteria.

What could be the mechanism of drug resistance in the 3%-30% of PZA^R strains with no *pncA* mutations—presuming the bacteriologic determination of PZA^R was accurate? Neither the mode of action of POA nor its target are known, but this drug target could be a site for resistance mutations. Mutations that increase the expression or activity of the weak *M. tuberculosis* efflux pump might also confer resistance.

4.   ETHAMBUTOL

Ethambutol is another first-line drug useful only against mycobacteria. It was discovered in 1961 in a screen of randomly selected compounds for antituberculosis activity [100]. Studies of the effects of EMB on mycobacteria suggested that it inhibited the transfer of D-arabinose into cell wall arabinogalactams [101]. The arabinogalactams are arabinose-containing, complex branched polysaccharides that connect the mycolic acids to the inner peptidoglycan of the cell wall [102]. Resistance mutations were then found to map in a group of genes encoding arabinosyl transferases [103], termed the *emb* operon. In *M. tuberculosis* this operon is composed of three arabinosyl transferases *embC*, *embA*, and *embB*, that are about 60% identical, and must have arisen by gene duplication [104]. These proteins each contain more than 1000 amino acids, and predictions of protein topology suggest that they are integral membrane proteins with 12 transmembrane domains and a globular C-terminal region of 400 amino acids residing in the periplasm [104]. However, almost all EMB^R mutations described replace the single methionine in EmbB at position 306, usually with a leucine or isoleucine. This region of the EmbB protein has been termed the EMB-resistance determining region (ERDR), and protein structure predictions place it in a loop that extends into the cytoplasm between the third and fourth transmembrane segments.

In two studies of EMB^R *M. tuberculosis* clinical isolates, 13/28 (47%)[104] and 8/16 (50%) [105] had mutations in amino acid 306 of *embB*. The mutation was never found in the many EMB-sensitive strains examined. A larger study of 69 EMB^R isolates found *embB* mutations in 69%, and 89% of these were replacements of Met306. Less common amino acid substitutions were found in amino acids 285, 330, and 630 [13].

The paucity of amino acids positions in which EMB^R mutations are found suggests that these may be the only mutations that can preserve the EmbB arabinosyl transferase activity while altering its interaction with EMB. It has been proposed that EMB is an analog of D-arabinose and only the dextro isomer of the drug is active, so the interaction must be quite specific. Very similar Emb genes were found in 13 other mycobacterial species, including three species with innate EMB resistance, *M. abscessus, M. chelonae,* and *M. leprae*. These three strains were found to have a variant amino acid motif in their ERDR region that might reduce the affinity of the proteins for EMB and thus explain their intrinsic resistance [106]. Most *M. tuberculosis* isolates containing ERDR mutations have higher levels of resistance ($\geq$ 20 μg/ml) than strains lacking these mutations (MIC~10 μg/ml) [106], and the mechanism of resistance in these wild-type *embB* strains is speculative. Selection of high level EMB^R mutants of *M. smegmatis* required three successive steps [104]. While only the highly resistant had *embB* mutations, some of the low and intermediately resistant *M. smegmatis* mutants showed increased EmbB protein on Western blotting. The site of the mutations causing up-regulation of EmbB expression, perhaps the first step in developing resistance, has not been identified.

5.   RIFAMPICIN

The rifamycins are a family of antibiotics originally isolated from *Streptomyces mediterranei* [100]. Although the naturally occurring compounds had some antibacterial activity, they required chemical modification to be clinically useful. Rifampicin (or rifampin) is a semi-synthetic antibiotic that was derived from rifamycin S and has become a valuable first line drug for treatment of tuberculosis [107]. Extensive studies in *E. coli* have shown that the target of RIF is the RNA polymerase, and mutations that confer resistance impede the binding of the drug to the enzyme [108]. In the presence of RIF, the RNA polymerase is unable to extend nascent RNA transcripts beyond the first few ribonucleotides, and only very short RNA oligomers (dimers or trimers) are produced [109]. Equivalent effects of RIF have been observed in *M. smegmatis* [110].

The RNA polymerase core enzyme is composed of four polypeptides, two α-subunits, one β-subunit, and one β′-subunit, which are the products of the *rpoA*, *rpoB*, and *rpoC* genes, respectively. The σ-subunit is added to this core to form the holoenzyme for transcription initiation. The basic structure of RNA polymerase has been well conserved throughout evolution, and the amino acid sequences of the sub-units are similar in all prokaryotes [108]. As in *E.coli*, the mutations that confer RIF resistance in *M. tuberculosis* are located in the *rpoB* gene [111]. Although the protein is quite large—1172 amino acids in *M. tuberculosis* [112]—almost all mutations occur in an 81 bp segment of the *rpoB* gene that encodes amino acids 507-533 (Figure 6) [5,113-117]. The clustering of RIF resistance mutations in this segment, termed the Rifampicin Resistance Determining Region (RRDR), simplifies their detection by molecular methods, and several techniques for this have been described.

Ramaswamy and Musser [13] reviewed several studies from different geographic areas and collated the mutations found in 478 RIF^R strains. Mutations in the RRDR were found in 96% of these strains. In 86%, a substitution was found in one of three amino acids: 531 (41%), 526 (36%) or 516 (9%) (Figure 6). Mutations causing substitutions in 11 other amino acids within the RRDR were present in 11% of the RIF^R isolates. In-frame deletions were found in eight strains, insertions in five, and one RIF^R isolate only had a mutation causing a substitution at amino acid 381. Most mutations in codons 516, 526 and 531 conferred high level RIF resistance (MIC>32 μg/ml), but some substitutions were associated with lower MICs: Asp516Tyr (2 μg/ml), His526Leu (8 μg/ml), and His526Asn (8 μg/ml).

Several new rifamycin derivatives—rifapentine, rifabutin and KRM-1648—have been developed and some have been found to be effective against a subgroup of *M. tuberculosis* isolates resistant to RIF. These RIF^R strains were then analyzed to determine whether particular mutations were still sensitive to these new agents. All mutations that conferred resistance to RIF (MIC > 8 μg/ml) conferred equal resistance to rifapentine, but some were still moderately sensitive to rifabutin or KRM-1648. MICs of <1 μg/ml for either KRM-1648, rifabutin or both drugs, were found in strains with substitutions Leu511Pro [118,119], Asp516Tyr [120], Asp516Val, Asn519Lys, Ser522Leu, and some, but not all with the His526Leu substitution.

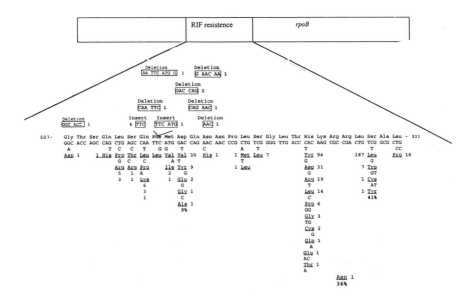

Figure 6. In 93-98% of RIF^R isolates of *M. tuberculosis*, mutations are found in an 81-bp region of *rpoB*, the gene for the β subunit of RNA polymerase. Mutations have been described in 14 of the 27 amino acids encoded by this region (amino acid's 507-533), but they most commonly affect three positions. In a compilation of 478 RIF^R isolates, 41% had substitutions at Leu531, 36% had substitutions at His526, and 9% at Asp516 [13]. The nucleotide replacements appear above the amino acid substitutions, and the number of RIF^R isolates containing this mutation are indicated. The small in-frame deletions and insertions that have been described are also depicted. This figure is a modification of one previously published [13].

In most studies, 2%-7% of the RIF^R *M. tuberculosis* isolates have no detectable *rpoB* mutations [115-117]. In *M. smegmatis*, which is innately more resistant to RIF than *M. tuberculosis* (MIC 4 µg/ml) [121], a gene has been described that inactivates RIF by ribosylation [122]. Other mechanisms for inactivating RIF have been described in other species [123], but none have been shown to play a role in RIF resistance in *M. tuberculosis*. Most strains of the *M. avium-intracellulare* complex (MAC) don't contain *rpoB* mutations [124,125], yet are intrinsically resistant to RIF (MIC > 4 µg/ml) presumably because the MAC cell wall acts as a permeability barrier to prevent drug entry [126]. *M. leprae* is similar to *M. tuberculosis*, and most RIF^R strains contain *rpoB* mutations [127].

6.   STREPTOMYCIN

Streptomycin is an aminoglycoside that was isolated from *Streptomyces griseus* in 1944. It was the first antibiotic found to be active against *M. tuberculosis* [1] but initial use of SM as monotherapy was accompanied by a significant incidence of drug resistance. The drug's mechanism of action and the development of resistance to SM have been studied extensively in *E. coli* [128] and other organisms [129]. In the presence of SM, there is a reduction in translation initiation and a decrease in ribosomal proof-reading capacity that results in more incorrect amino acids being incorporated into the nascent polypeptide chains [130]. The most common site for mutations conferring SM^R is *rpsL*, the gene encoding the S12 protein of the small ribosomal subunit [131,132]. These *rpsL* mutations increase the accuracy of the ribosomal proof-reading, thereby counteracting the effect of SM. There is also a class of less frequent mutations that produce such a marked increase in the proof reading accuracy that the ribosomes become hyper-accurate, and translational efficiency is seriously impaired. These mutants are termed SM dependent because they grow very poorly unless the proof-reading stringency is relaxed by the presence of SM [133].

Several studies have found that one-third to one-half of SM^R *M. tuberculosis* isolates have mis-sense mutations in *rpsL*. The mutations usually affect amino acids 43 or 88, which are equivalent to amino acids substituted in SM^R isolates of other bacterial species. The most frequent mutation results in a Lys43Arg substitution, but the Lys88Arg replacement is also fairly common, and Lys43Thr and Lys88Gln are occasionally observed [134-136].

SM binds to the ribosome, one drug molecule per ribosome [137], and SM^R ribosomes bind less drug [138]. SM doesn't bind to S12 [139], as might have been expected, but rather binds two regions on the 16S rRNA that should lie close to each other in the molecule's tertiary structure. Even though SM doesn't appear to bind to proteins, the ribosomal proteins S3 and S5 are needed to maintain the proper rRNA configuration for SM binding [140, 141].

One of the two sites of SM binding, determined using the *E.coli* 16S rRNA, is in the region of nucleotides 912-915 (Figure 7)[130,142]. The other is in a highly conserved segment of the 16S rRNA, termed the 530 loop. It has been proposed that in the 16S rRNA tertiary structure there is base pairing in this loop between residues 507 and 524, and between 506 and

525 [143,144], which leads to the formation of a pseudoknot. S12 appears to bind to the 912 region, and may also interact with the 530 loop to facilitate the rRNA folding [145,146]. The mutations in S12 may alter the complex rRNA structure slightly so that the SM binding sites are less accessible to the drug, and perhaps also less tolerant of codon anti-codon mismatches.

Because *E. coli* contains seven genes for ribosomal rRNA, and SM sensitivity is dominant over resistance [147], SM[R] mutations in the *E. coli* 16S RNA are not found naturally, and can only be studied by expressing them on multi-copy plasmids or in mutant strains [148]. However, in organisms with only one copy of the rRNA gene *(rrs)*[149-151], such as *M. tuberculosis* [152], 16S rRNA mutations that cause SM resistance are fairly common. Mutations in *rrs*, the gene encoding the rRNA, have been found in 5% to 33% of SM[R] *M. tuberculosis* strains. In the 912 region, mutations occur in nucleotides 903 and 904, that correspond to the *E. coli* positions 912 and 913. The most common changes reported are A→G at position 904, and C→A or C→G at position 903.

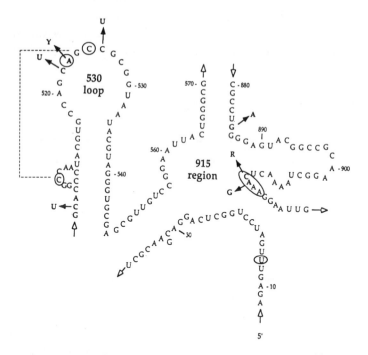

Figure 7. Secondary-structure model of the 16S rRNA of *M. tuberculosis* with sites of mutations associated with SM[R], based on a model structure of *E. coli* 16S rRNA. For actual numbers of *M. tuberculosis* positions subtract 10 from the 530 loop, and 8 from the 915 region. Mutations associated with SM resistance in *M. tuberculosis* are indicated with arrows, Y = U or C; R = A or G. Sites of SM[R] mutations in *E. coli* are circled. Dotted lines indicate regions of base pairing to form a pseudoknot. This figure is a modification of two figures previously published [11,142].

In the 530 loop, mutations are found at nucleotides 491, 512, 513, and 516, which are equivalent to *E. coli* positions 501, 522, 523, and 526 [153,154]. C→T replacements are seen at positions 491, 512, and 516, and A→C or A→T changes have been observed at position 513. Novel mutations have also been reported at positions 798, 877, and 906 [155]. One SM dependent strain of *M. tuberculosis* was found to have an extra cytosine inserted between 16S rRNA positions 512 and 513 [154]. In 25 to 35% of the SM^R isolates, no mutations are found in either *rpsL* or *rrs*.

Mitchison observed that SM^R *M. tuberculosis* strains could be segregated into three groups by their level of resistance [156]. These groups can now be tentatively correlated with specific mutations. Strains with amino acid substitutions in S12 demonstrate high level resistance, with MICs of 250 - 1000 µg/ml, strains with *rrs* mutations have moderate levels of resistance (MIC 50-500 µg/ml), and those strains wild type for both *rpsL* and *rrs* exhibit only low-level resistance (10-50 µg/ml)[157]. Some sort of permeability barrier could be at work in strains without *rrs* or *rpsL* mutations, as their resistance decreases in the presence of the detergent Tween [157]. Aminoglycoside-modifying enzymes confer resistance to SM in other bacteria [158,159], but these have not been found in *M. tuberculosis*, and SM^R strains are not cross-resistant to other aminoglycosides [157].

7.   FLUOROQUINOLONES

The appearance of *M. tuberculosis* isolates resistant to several of the traditional antimycobacterial agents prompted consideration of other antibiotics as second- or third-line therapeutic options. One class of antibiotics that is commonly used against a broad spectrum of bacteria is the FQs [160], which have moderate activity against mycobacteria [161]. The FQs are among the most prescribed antibiotics worldwide, but their efficacy has been seriously compromised by the frequent appearance of drug-resistant strains [162]. FQ^R isolates of *M. tuberculosis* appeared soon after ciprofloxacin (CIP) and ofloxacin (OFL) (Figure 8) began to be used against strains resistant to first-line agents [163]. The mechanisms of FQ resistance are basically similar in the many bacteria that have been studied, including the mycobacteria [164]. Resistance develops progressively by the sequential addition of mutations in several sites. [165]. It has been proposed that FQ resistance mutations appear at an increased frequency as a result of adaptive mutations in specific genes that allow inhibited bacteria to resume growth in the presence of the drug [166].

The FQs act by inhibiting type II topoisomerases [169,170]. These complex enzymes introduce a double-stranded cut into the DNA chromosome, covalently bind the two ends, pass another section of double-stranded DNA through the break, and then re-ligate the cut ends. The FQs bind to these topoisomerases in a complex with DNA, inhibiting their activity and leaving the breaks in the chromosome un-ligated. The topoisomerase-FQ complex is frozen on the chromosome, blocking both DNA replication and RNA transcription [170,171].

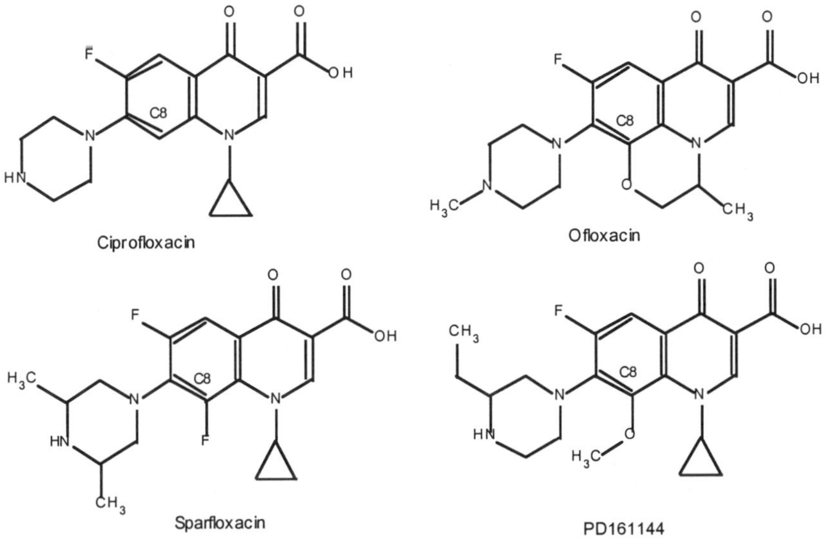

Figure 8. Structure of some fluoroquinolones (FQ) active against *M. tuberculosis.* Ciprofloxacin and ofloxacin were the first FQs used against MDR strains of *M. tuberculosis.* Levofloxacin (not shown), which is also used to treat *M. tuberculosis*, is the levo form of ofloxacin. Sparfloxacin is hydrophobic, and may be the most active FQ against *M. tuberculosis* [167]. The C8 position appears to be important for activity against mycobacteria, and structures with a methoxy group at this position, such as PD161144, may be particularly effective [168].

Most bacteria contain two type II topoisomerases which are similar in structure: DNA gyrase [172] introduces negative supercoils into the chromosome to maintain its topological state, while topo IV [173,174], separates newly replicated DNA chromosomes, which are interlinked, or concatenated after replication. The amino acid sequences of these enzymes are well conserved among bacteria [175], especially in the regions that interact with DNA, which are also close to the sites where most FQ resistance mutations are found [176]. Both gyrase and topo IV are composed of two A and two B sub-units. For gyrase these are encoded by the *gyrA* and *gyrB* genes, and for topo IV they are encoded by *parC* and *parE* (or *grlA* and *grlB*)[177]. The first site identified with FQ^R mutations was a short segment of *gyrA* termed the Quinolone Resistance Determining Region (QRDR)[178]. A few FQ^R mutations have also been described in *gyrB*, usually in a region of the protein thought to interact with the QRDR to form the FQ binding pocket [179,180]. Topoisomerase IV was discovered in *E. coli,* and found to be present in most bacteria. Mutations conferring FQ resistance map in analogous regions of its A and B sub-units[181,182]. In mycobacteria, FQ^R mutations were found in the QRDR of *gyrA* [183], and it was assumed that mutations would also occur in the mycobacterial topo IV, which, for some reason, could not be identified. When the sequence of the *M. tuberculosis* chromosome was completed [184], surprisingly, no topo IV was found, and presumably gyrase performs its function, decatenating the newly replicated sister chromosomes.

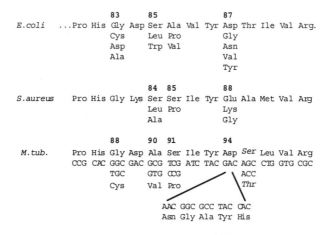

MUTATIONS in the FQ RESISTANCE DETERMINING REGION of GyrA

Figure 9. Mutations in the Quinolone Resistance Determining Region (QRDR) of *gyrA.* Isolates of *M. tuberculosis* that are resistant to >3 μg/ml of ciprofloxacin, levofloxacin, or ofloxacin generally contain a mutation in a small segment of *gyrA* termed the QRDR. The QRDR is near the tyrosine that becomes covalently bound to the cut DNA strand (position 130 in *M. tuberculosis,* 122 in *E. coli* [185]). The most common mutations cause substitutions for Ala90 and Asp94, but replacements of Ser91 and Gly88 have also been described [183]. Equivalent amino acids are commonly substituted in FQ^R isolates of *E. coli* and *S. aureus* [186]. A naturally occurring Ser/Thr polymorphism, that is unrelated to FQ^R [183], occurs in *M. tuberculosis* at amino acid 95.

The *gyrA* mutations that cause FQ^R in mycobacteria occur in the amino acids that are equivalent to those associated with FQ^R in other bacteria (Figure 9) [163,183,186-192]. The three most frequently mutated amino acids of *M. tuberculosis*, 90, 91, and 94, are equivalent to the commonly mutated amino acids in *E. coli*, 83, 84 and 87 [178,193], and in *S. aureus*, 84, 85, and 88 [194]. Presumably the mutant amino acids alter the protein structure so as to reduce FQ binding [172]. In *E. coli*, the most common FQ^R mutation replaces the serine at position 83, which seems to be a key site for the gyrase/drug interaction. Species of mycobacteria with a serine at this position, such as *M. fortuitum* and *M. aurum* are more sensitive to the FQs than those with an alanine, such as *M. tuberculosis* [188,195].

Mutations in *gyrA* can be selected in the laboratory in one step, at a frequency of 10^{-7} to 10^{-9}, and generally have MICs for CIP and OFL of at least 2-3 µg/ml [183,187]. More resistant isolates (MICs for CIP and OFL > 8 µg/ml) arise at frequencies less than 10^{-9} and result from the step-wise occurrence of additional mutations. Second-step mutations in *gyrB* were obtained from a laboratory strain of *M. tuberculosis* containing a *gyrA* mutation [196], but *gyrB* mutations have not been found in FQ^R clinical isolates of *M. tuberculosis* (D. Williams and S. Sreevatsan, personal communications).

Although the QRDR region of the gyrase A subunit is the most important site for mutations conferring FQ^R, mutations in other sites must be responsible for the low-level resistance seen in strains without gyrase mutations [191], and for the varying levels of resistance found in different isolates with identical *gyrA* mutations [188]. In other bacteria, FQ-transporting efflux pumps [197], such as NorA in *S. aureus* [198] or MecCD in *Ps. aeruginosa*, have been implicated in drug resistance [199], usually as a result of regulatory mutations that increase their expression [200]. Genes coding for transcriptional regulators of the AraC/XylS/TetR family are often found adjacent to the genes encoding the efflux pumps. For example, the gene for regulator NfxB [199] is located next to the genes for the MecCD pump that it regulates. In some cases the expression of the pumps can be induced by the presence of some of the transported compounds [201].

An efflux pump, LfrA, was identified in *M. smegmatis* [202-204], and found to confer low-level resistance (ie. 10-fold increase in MIC) to CIP, OFL, and other hydrophilic FQs, but not to the hydrophobic sparfloxacin (SPAR). Upstream of *lfrA* is a gene for a putative regulator with similarity to NfxB. Although the *M. tuberculosis* genome contains at least 15 putative efflux pumps [184], none of them closely resembles *lfrA*, and it is not known if any play a role in the development of FQ^R.

Many different FQ structures have been tested, and several are currently marketed, but none qualify as first-line agents, even ignoring their high cost, because resistant strains of *M. tuberculosis* appear too readily at non-toxic concentrations. The affinity of the FQ for the gyrase is likely the principal determinant of the MIC, and the C8 position appears to play a critical role.

Some FQ analogues with a bromine or methoxy group at the C8 position (Figure 8) have sufficient affinity for the gyrase that they are still active, at achievable drug levels (0.6-1.2 µg/ml), against *M. tuberculosis* isolates containing a *gyrA* mutation [168,205]. This would mean that the appearance of a *gyrA* mutation would not necessarily result in treatment failure. However, once *M. tuberculosis* has two *gyrA* mutations, even these agents are no longer effective.

The ideal FQ should be so effective that the concentration at which virtually no resistant mutants appear (termed the mutant prevention concentration-MPC [206]) is well below the achievable, non-toxic, serum drug level. For a FQ to be a real anti-TB champion, resistant *M. tuberculosis* colonies should appear at a frequency of less than 10^{-10} at a drug concentration of 0.05-0.1 µg/ml, with an achievable serum level of 2 - 4 µg/ml. This dream drug should also penetrate infected tissues well, be non-toxic, and affordable [207]. With CIP, resistant colonies of *M. tuberculosis* arise at a frequency of 10^{-7} to 10^{-8} in a drug concentration of 2.0 µg/ml, which is about the achievable serum drug level, and these isolates do not even contain *gyrA* mutations [183]. The rapid appearance of CIP-resistant clinical isolates was predictable.

At present, sparfloxacin (SPAR) appears to be the most useful FQ for treating tuberculosis [167], perhaps owing to the pharmacologic characteristics of the drug. Most of the FQs are hydrophilic and subject to transport by efflux pumps such as NorA and LfrA. In contrast, SPAR is hydrophobic, and not a substrate for most of the FQ pumps that have been described. In addition, the order of occurrence of resistance mutations in some bacteria (in gyrase or in topo IV first) is different for SPAR than for the hydrophilic FQs [208], suggesting that SPAR's affinity for the topoisomerase targets could be distinct. In strains of *M. bovis* BCG with a *gyrA* mutation, SPAR has an MIC of 1.0 µg/ml (unpublished results from the author's laboratory) similar to that seen with the C8 methoxy FQs. However, SPAR has not been carefully compared to the most effective C8 methoxy FQs, and SPAR's clinical use is limited by side-effects, principally photo-sensitivity [209].

8.   KANAMYCIN AND AMIKACIN, VIOMYCIN AND CAPREOMYCIN

Viomycin (VIO) and Capreomycin (CAP) are peptide antibiotics [210], Kanamycin (KAN) and Amikacin (AMK) are aminoglycosides [211]. All are second- or third-line drugs that are used against *M. tuberculosis* strains resistant to the first-line agents [212], or against infections with other mycobacteria [213]. These drugs appear to exert their effects on the ribosome by blocking the translocation from the A to the P sites [214, 215]. Cross-resistance between VIO and CAP has been complete in some studies [216], and variable in others [217], while cross-resistance between CAP and KAN is generally variable and low-level. Between KAN and AMK, cross-resistance is standard, as the same mutations are found in resistant isolates selected by either drug [218]. None of these drugs engender cross-resistance to streptomycin [219].

Two studies of human *M. tuberculosis* isolates resistant to KAN and AMK found that all those with high-level resistance (>200 µg/ml) contained an A→G change at position 1400 of the 16S rRNA, which is encoded by the *rrs* gene. This mutation was absent in strains with low-level resistance and all KAN-sensitive strains [218,220]. Of 43 *M. tuberculosis* isolates from Japan that were resistant to > 200 µg/ml KAN, 26 (60%) had an A→G change at nucleotide 1400, one had a C→T change at 1401, and one had both a C→A change at 1401 and a G→T change at 1483. No 16S rRNA mutations were found in 14 (33%) KAN^R strains nor in 71 KAN-sensitive strains [221]. Finally, the *rrs* and *rpsL* genes were sequenced from 10 clinical isolates of *M. tuberculosis* resistant to SM, KAN and VIO. Of four strains with high level KAN^R (>200 µg/ml), three had the same A→G mutation at nucleotide 1400, and one strain had a mutation at position 705 and a Lys43Arg mutation in RpsL, the latter causing the SM resistance. Five strains with low level KAN or VIO resistance (MIC<50 µg/ml) lacked mutations in either the *rpsL* and *rrs* genes [222].

Almost all clinical and *in vitro* isolates of *M. abscessus* and *M. chelonae* resistant to KAN, AMK, tobramycin and neomycin had mutations at nucleotide 1408 of their 16S rRNAs, which is equivalent to 1400 of *M. tuberculosis* [223]. Most *M. smegmatis* strains resistant to high levels of KAN and AMK had an A→G mutation at position 1389, also equivalent to 1400 of *M. tuberculosis* [220, 222]. Two strains had mutations at nucleotide 1387. *M. smegmatis* contains two copies of the rRNA genes, so 16S rRNA mutations causing antibiotic resistance are difficult to obtain.

Low-level aminoglycoside resistance in *M. tuberculosis* is unexplained, but there are a few possibilities. Aminoglycoside resistance in other bacteria [224] is often associated with aminoglycoside-modifying enzymes [225], and one of these, aminoglycoside 2'-N-acetyltransferase, is present in the chromosomes of all mycobacteria examined, including *M. tuberculosis* [226]. Increased enzyme expression confers aminoglycoside resistance in *M. smegmatis*, but the enzyme has yet to be implicated in drug resistance in *M. tuberculosis*. An efflux pump from *M. fortuitum* confers low-level aminoglycoside and tetracycline resistance when present on a plasmid in *M. smegmatis*. A similar gene exists in the *M. tuberculosis* genome, but it is not known whether it is involved in clinical drug resistance [227]. Aminoglycoside-producing organisms, such as Streptomyces, protect themselves from the drug by methylating an adenine at the drug target site in the 16S rRNA to prevent drug binding [228], but this mechanism has not been described in mycobacteria.

Few studies have looked at VIO resistance in mycobacteria. Two different classes of mutations have been identified genetically in VIO^R *M. smegmatis*, *vicA* and *vicB* [215]. No rRNA mutations were identified in the vicA mutants, but the vicB group had either G→A or G→T changes at position 1473 of 16S rRNA [222], with the G→T change causing a higher level of cross-resistance to KAN. Based on the secondary structure of *E. coli* 16S rRNA, nucleotide 1473 of the *M. smegmatis* 16S rRNA lies very close to nucleotide 1389, where mutations are found in high-level aminoglycoside resistant strains [229]. The 1473 mutation might engender cross-resistance to kanamycin by altering the conformation of the aminoglycoside-binding site adjacent to nucleotide 1389. There are no available studies of mutations found in isolates resistant to CAP.

9.   CYCLOSERINE

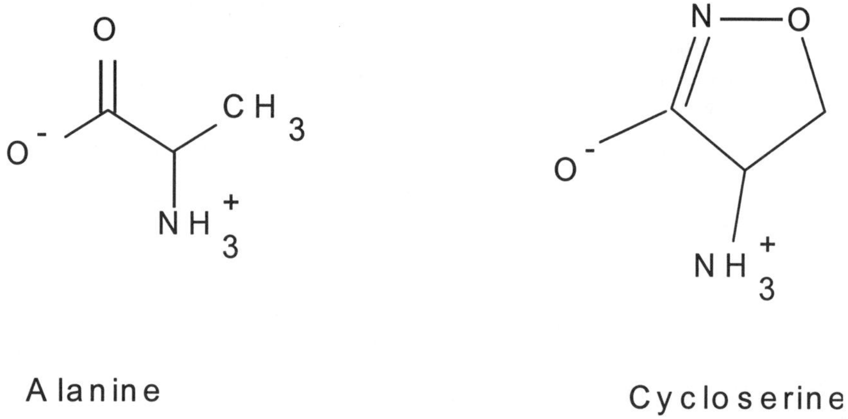

A la n in e   C y c lo s e rin e

Figure 10. D-cycloserine (DCS) is an analog of D-alanine. Cycloserine enters the bacteria via the D-alanine transporter and targets the alanine racemase and the D-alanine ligase [230].

D-Cycloserine (DCS) is an analog of D-alanine (Figure 10) that inhibits cell wall synthesis [230]. Because of neurotoxicity ("psychoserine"), DCS is not commonly prescribed except in MDR strains resistant to most other agents. The mechanisms of resistance in *M. tuberculosis* have not been well documented, but from older studies in both mycobacteria and other bacteria, and one recent study in *M. smegmatis* [231], some likely mechanisms of resistance can be inferred. DCS inhibits two enzymes critical in cell wall synthesis, D-alanine racemase, which converts L-alanine to D-alanine, and D-alanine ligase, which forms D-alanine dipeptides [232]. Excess D-alanine reverses growth inhibition by DCS [233]. Studies of DCS-resistant streptococci found one mutant with higher than normal levels of both the ligase and racemase enzymes, but most mutants appeared to be defective in D-alanine uptake. [230]. It appears that there is a single transport system for accumulating L- and D-alanine and also glycine, D-serine and DCS [234]. Therefore, decreased D-alanine accumulation will also result in decreased DCS accumulation and hence drug resistance.

A recent study in *M. smegmatis* identified a gene, *alrA*, which encodes a D-alanine racemase. Over-expression of this enzyme conferred DCS resistance in *M. smegmatis, M. intracellulare,* and *M. bovis* BCG [231]. In addition, one of four spontaneous DCS-resistant mutants of *M. smegmatis* had a promoter mutation resulting in high expression of the AlrA racemase. The mutations causing resistance in the other DCS^R *M. smegmatis* strains were not found, but there are three other possible sites:

1. promoter mutations increasing the expression of the D-alanine ligase, as yet unidentified;
2. mutations in an alanine transporter that would decrease both alanine and DCS accumulation; or
3. mutations in a dipeptide transporter that would selectively increase alanine, but not DCS uptake [235].

10. CONCLUSION

This chapter has reviewed the most recent information on the molecular mechanisms of resistance to the first- and second-line drugs used against *M. tuberculosis*. It was hoped that improved understanding of the resistance mechanisms would foster better methods for detecting drug resistance and also lead to the rational design of new antituberculosis agents. Although gaps remain in our understanding of the actions of INH and PZA, most the important resistance mechanisms have now been defined, but this knowledge has yet to have an impact on the fight against MDR tuberculosis. It is proving much more difficult to outwit the bacillus than to learn how it has outfoxed our therapy.

ACKNOWLEDGMENTS

The author thanks to D. Alland, C. Barry, S. Cole, V. Deretic, K. Drlica, M. Gonzatti, W. Jacobs, J. Musser, D. van Soolingen, D. Williams, and Y. Zhang, for advice, critical readings, and helpful discussions during the preparation of this chapter. Studies from the author's laboratory were supported by grants from CONICIT (S1-96-1322), ICGEB (VEN 96/02), and the Venezuelan Program for Operational Research in Endemic Diseases (Ven/96/002 021-37).

REFERENCES

1.   Bloom BR, Murray CJ. Tuberculosis: commentary on a reemergent killer. Science 1992; 257: 1055-1064.
2.   Centers for Disease Control. Transmission of multidrug- resistant tuberculosis among immunocompromised persons, correctional system--New York, 1991. JAMA 1992; 268: 855-856.
3.   Neu HC. The crisis in antibiotic resistance. Science 1992; 257: 1064-1073.
4.   Poole K, Krebes K, McNally C, Neshat S. Multiple antibiotic resistance in *Pseudomonas aeruginosa*: evidence for involvement of an efflux operon. J Bacteriol 1993; 175: 7363-7372.
5.   Heym B, Honore N, Truffot-Pernot C, et al. Implications of multidrug resistance for the future of short-course chemotherapy of tuberculosis: a molecular study. Lancet 1994; 344: 293-298.
6.   Morris S, Bai GH, Suffys P, Portillo-Gomez L, Fairchok M, Rouse D. Molecular mechanisms of multiple drug resistance in clinical isolates of *Mycobacterium tuberculosis*. J Infect Dis 1995; 171: 954-960.
7.   Maiden MC. Horizontal genetic exchange, evolution, and spread of antibiotic resistance in bacteria. Clin Infect Dis 1998; 27 Suppl 1: S12-S20.
8.   Spratt BG. Resistance to antibiotics mediated by target alterations. Science 1994; 264: 388-393.
9.   Blanchard JS. Molecular mechanisms of drug resistance in *Mycobacterium tuberculosis*. Annu Rev Biochem 1996; 65: 215-239.
10.   Cole ST, Telenti A. Drug resistance in *Mycobacterium tuberculosis*. Eur Respir J Suppl 1995; 20:701s-713s.
11.   Musser JM. Antimicrobial agent resistance in mycobacteria: molecular genetic insights. Clin Microbiol Rev 1995; 8: 496-514.
12.   Davies J. Antibiotic resistance in mycobacteria. Novartis Found Symp 1998; 217: 195-205.

13. Ramaswamy S, Musser JM. Molecular genetic basis of antimicrobial agent resistance in *Mycobacterium tuberculosis:* 1998 update. Tuberc Lung Dis 1998; 79: 2-29.

14. McKenzie D, Malone L, Kushner S, Oleson J, Subbarow J. The effect of nicotinic acid amide on experimental tuberculosis of white mice. Lab Clin Med 1948; 33: 1249-1253.

15. Zhang Y, Dhandayuthapani S, Deretic V. Molecular basis for the exquisite sensitivity of *Mycobacterium tuberculosis* to isoniazid. Proc Natl Acad Sci U S A 1996; 93: 13212-13216.

16. Yuan Y, Mead D, Schroeder BG, Zhu Y, Barry CE, 3rd. The biosynthesis of mycolic acids in *Mycobacterium tuberculosis*. Enzymatic methyl(ene) transfer to acyl carrier protein bound meromycolic acid in vitro. J Biol Chem 1998; 273: 21282-21290.

17. Deretic V, Song J, Pagan-Ramos E. Loss of oxyR in *Mycobacterium tuberculosis*. Trends Microbiol 1997; 5: 367-372.

18. Manca C, Paul S, Barry CE, 3rd, Freedman VH, Kaplan G. *Mycobacterium tuberculosis* catalase and peroxidase activities and resistance to oxidative killing in human monocytes in vitro. Infect Immun 1999; 67: 74-79.

19. Scorpio A, Zhang Y. Mutations in pncA, a gene encoding pyrazinamidase/nicotinamidase, cause resistance to the antituberculous drug pyrazinamide in tubercle bacillus. Nat Med 1996; 2: 662-667.

20. Middlebrook G. Isoniazid-resistance and catalase activity of tubercle bacilli. Am Rev Tuberc 1954; 69: 471-472.

21. Middlebrook G, and Cohn, M.L. Some observations on the pathogenicity of isoniazid-resistant variants of tubercle bacilli. Science 1953; 118: 297-299.

22. Zhang Y, Heym B, Allen B, Young D, Cole S. The catalase-peroxidase gene and isoniazid resistance of *Mycobacterium tuberculosis*. Nature 1992; 358: 591-593.

23. Zhang Y, Garbe T, Young D. Transformation with *katG* restores isoniazid-sensitivity in *Mycobacterium tuberculosis* isolates resistant to a range of drug concentrations. Mol Microbiol 1993; 8: 521-524.

24. Stoeckle MY, Guan L, Riegler N, et al. Catalase-peroxidase gene sequences in isoniazid-sensitive and - resistant strains of *Mycobacterium tuberculosis* from New York City. J Infect Dis 1993; 168: 1063-1065.

25. Altamirano M, Marostenmaki J, Wong A, FitzGerald M, Black WA, Smith JA. Mutations in the catalase-peroxidase gene from isoniazid-resistant *Mycobacterium tuberculosis* isolates. J Infect Dis 1994; 169: 1162-1165.

26. Goto M, Oka S, Tachikawa N, et al. KatG sequence deletion is not the major cause of isoniazid resistance in Japanese and Yemeni *Mycobacterium tuberculosis* isolates. Mol Cell Probes 1995; 9:433-439.

27. Cockerill FR, 3rd, Uhl JR, Temesgen Z, et al. Rapid identification of a point mutation of the *Mycobacterium tuberculosis* catalase-peroxidase (*katG*) gene associated with isoniazid resistance. J Infect Dis 1995; 171: 240-245.

28. Heym B, Alzari PM, Honore N, Cole ST. Missense mutations in the catalase-peroxidase gene, *katG*, are associated with isoniazid resistance in *Mycobacterium tuberculosis*. Mol Microbiol 1995; 15: 235-245.

29. Musser JM, Kapur V, Williams DL, Kreiswirth BN, van Soolingen D, van Embden JD. Characterization of the catalase-peroxidase gene (*katG*) and *inhA* locus in isoniazid-resistant and -susceptible strains of *Mycobacterium tuberculosis* by automated DNA sequencing: restricted array of mutations associated with drug resistance. J Infect Dis 1996; 173: 196-202.

30. Dobner P, Rusch-Gerdes S, Bretzel G, et al. Usefulness of *Mycobacterium tuberculosis* genomic mutations in the genes *katG* and *inhA* for the prediction of isoniazid resistance. Int J Tuberc Lung Dis 1997; 1: 365-369.

31. Pretorius GS, van Helden PD, Sirgél F, Eisenach KD, Victor TC. Mutations in *katG* gene sequences in isoniazid-resistant clinical isolates of *Mycobacterium tuberculosis* are rare. Antimicrob Agents Chemother 1995; 39: 2276-2281.

32. Victor TC, Pretorius GS, Felix JV, Jordaan AM, van Helden PD, Eisenach KD. *katG* mutations in isoniazid-resistant strains of *Mycobacterium tuberculosis* are not infrequent. Antimicrob Agents Chemother 1996; 40: 1572.

33. Marttila HJ, Soini H, Huovinen P, Viljanen MK. *katG* mutations in isoniazid-resistant *Mycobacterium tuberculosis* isolates recovered from Finnish patients. Antimicrob Agents Chemother 1996; 40: 2187-2189.

34. Rouse DA, Li Z, Bai GH, Morris SL. Characterization of the *katG* and *inhA* genes of isoniazid-resistant clinical isolates of *Mycobacterium tuberculosis*. Antimicrob Agents Chemother 1995; 39: 2472-2477.

35. Ferrazoli L, Palaci M, Telles MA, et al. Catalase expression, *katG*, and MIC of isoniazid for *Mycobacterium tuberculosis* isolates from Sao Paulo, Brazil. J Infect Dis 1995; 171: 237-240.

36. Saint-Joanis B, Souchon H, Wilming M, Johnsson K, Alzari PM, Cole ST. Use of site-directed mutagenesis to probe the structure, function and isoniazid activation of the catalase/peroxidase, KatG, from *Mycobacterium tuberculosis*. Biochem J 1999; 338: 753-760.

37. Wilson TM, de Lisle GW, Collins DM. Effect of *inhA* and *katG* on isoniazid resistance and virulence of *Mycobacterium bovis*. Mol Microbiol 1995; 15: 1009-1015.

38. Wengenack NL, Jensen MP, Rusnak F, Stern MK. *Mycobacterium tuberculosis* KatG is a peroxynitritase. Biochem Biophys Res Commun 1999; 256: 485-487.

39. Wengenack NL, Uhl JR, St. Amand AL, et al. Recombinant *Mycobacterium tuberculosis* KatG(S315T) is a competent catalase-peroxidase with reduced activity toward isoniazid. J Infect Dis 1997; 176: 722-727.

40. Marttila HJ, Soini H, Eerola E, et al. A Ser315Thr substitution in KatG is predominant in genetically heterogeneous multidrug-resistant *Mycobacterium tuberculosis* isolates originating from the St. Petersburg area in Russia. Antimicrob Agents Chemother 1998; 42: 2443-2445.

41.   Johnsson K, Schultz PG. Mechanistic studies of the oxidation of isoniazid by the catalase peroxidase from *Mycobacterium tuberculosis*. J Am Chem Soc 1994; 116: 7425-7426.

42.   Shoeb HA, Bowman BU, Ottolenghi AC, Merola AJ. Enzymatic and nonenzymatic superoxide-generating reactions of isoniazid. Antimicrob Agents Chemother 1985; 27: 408-412.

43.   Johnsson K, King DS, Schultz PG. Studies on the mechanism of action of isoniazid and ethionamide in the chemotherapy of tuberculosis. J Am Chem Soc 1995; 117:5009-5010.

44.   Wilming M, Johnsson K. Spontaneous formation of the bioactive form of the tuberculosis drug isoniazid. Angew Chem Int Ed 1999; 38: 2588-2590.

45.   Winder FG, Collins PB. Inhibition by isoniazid of synthesis of mycolic acids in *Mycobacterium tuberculosis*. J Gen Microbiol 1970; 63: 41-48.

46.   Quemard A, Lacave C, Laneelle G. Isoniazid inhibition of mycolic acid synthesis by cell extracts of sensitive and resistant strains of *Mycobacterium aurum*. Antimicrob Agents Chemother 1991; 35: 1035-1039.

47.   Winder FG. Mode of action of the antimycobacterial agents and associated aspects of the molecular biology of the Mycobacteria, p.354-438. In: Ratledge C, Stanford J (eds.), The Biology of the Mycobacteria. Academic Press, San Diego, 1982.

48.   Banerjee A, Dubnau E, Quemard A, et al. *inhA*, a gene encoding a target for isoniazid and ethionamide in *Mycobacterium tuberculosis*. Science 1994; 263: 227-230.

49.   Quemard A, Sacchettini JC, Dessen A, et al. Enzymatic characterization of the target for isoniazid in *Mycobacterium tuberculosis*. Biochemistry 1995; 34: 8235-8241.

50.   Basso LA, Zheng R, Musser JM, Jacobs WR, Jr., Blanchard JS. Mechanisms of isoniazid resistance in *Mycobacterium tuberculosis*: enzymatic characterization of enoyl reductase mutants identified in isoniazid-resistant clinical isolates. J Infect Dis 1998; 178: 769-775.

51.   Rozwarski DA, Grant GA, Barton DHR, Jacobs WR, Jr., Sacchettini JC. Modification of the NADH of the isoniazid target (InhA) from *Mycobacterium tuberculosis*. Science 1998; 279: 98-102.

52.   Canetti G. Present aspects of bacterial resistance in tuberculosis. Am Rev Respir Dis 1965; 92: 687-703.

53.   Lefford MJ. The ethionamide sensitivity of British pre-treatment strains of *Mycobacterium tuberculosis*. Tubercle 1966; 47: 198-206.

54.   Winder FG, Collins PB, Whelan D. Effects of ethionamide and isoxyl on mycolic acid synthesis in *Mycobacterium tuberculosis* BCG. J Gen Microbiol 1971; 66: 379-80.

55.   Quemard A, Laneelle G, Lacave C. Mycolic acid synthesis: a target for
       ethionamide in mycobacteria? Antimicrob Agents Chemother 1992; 36: 1316-
       1321.

56.   McMurry LM, McDermott PF, Levy SB. Genetic evidence that InhA of
       Mycobacterium smegmatis is a target for triclosan. Antimicrob Agents Chemother
       1999; 43: 711-713.

57.   Slayden RA, Barry CEI. The Genetics and Biochemistry of Isoniazid Resistance
       in *Mycobacterium tuberculosis*. Microbes and Infection (in press).

58.   Mdluli K, Sherman DR, Hickey MJ, et al. Biochemical and genetic data suggest
       that InhA is not the primary target for activated isoniazid in *Mycobacterium*
       tuberculosis. J Infect Dis 1996; 174: 1085-1090.

59.   Mdluli K, Slayden RA, Zhu Y, et al. Inhibition of a *Mycobacterium tuberculosis*
       beta-ketoacyl ACP synthase by isoniazid. Science 1998; 280: 1607-1610.

60.   60.   Piatek AS, Telenti A, Murray MR, et al. Genotypic analysis of
       Mycobacterium tuberculosis in two distinct populations using molecular beacons:
       implications for rapid susceptibility testing. Manuscript submitted.

61.   Lee AS, Lim IH, Tang LL, Telenti A, Wong SY. Contribution of kasA analysis to
       detection of isoniazid-resistant *Mycobacterium tuberculosis* in Singapore.
       Antimicrob Agents Chemother 1999; 43: 2087-2089.

62.   Bloch K. Fatty acid synthases from *Mycobacterium phlei*. Methods Enzymol
       1975; 35: 84-90.

63.   Zhang Y. Life without KatG. Trends Microbiol 1996; 4: 415-416.

64.   Deretic V, Pagan-Ramos E, Zhang Y, Dhandayuthapani S, Via LE. The extreme
       sensitivity of *Mycobacterium tuberculosis* to the front-line antituberculosis drug
       isoniazid. Nat Biotechnol 1996; 14: 1557-1561.

65.   Rosner JL. Susceptibilities of oxyR regulon mutants of *Escherichia coli* and
       Salmonella typhimurium to isoniazid. Antimicrob Agents Chemother 1993; 37:
       2251-2253.

66.   Rosner JL, Storz G. Effects of peroxides on susceptibilities of *Escherichia coli*
       and *Mycobacterium smegmatis* to isoniazid. Antimicrob Agents Chemother 1994;
       38: 1829-1833.

67.   Sherman DR, Sabo PJ, Hickey MJ, et al. Disparate responses to oxidative stress
       in saprophytic and pathogenic mycobacteria. Proc Natl Acad Sci U S A 1995; 92:
       6625-6629.

68.   Deretic V, Philipp W, Dhandayuthapani S, et al. *Mycobacterium tuberculosis* is a
       natural mutant with an inactivated oxidative-stress regulatory gene: implications
       for sensitivity to isoniazid. Mol Microbiol 1995; 17: 889-900.

69.   Dhandayuthapani S, Zhang Y, Mudd MH, Deretic V. Oxidative stress response
       and its role in sensitivity to isoniazid in mycobacteria: characterization and
       inducibility of *ahpC* by peroxides in *Mycobacterium smegmatis* and lack of
       expression in *M. aurum* and *M. tuberculosis*. J Bacteriol 1996; 178: 3641-3649.

70. Yuan Y, Lee RE, Besra GS, Belisle JT, Barry CE, 3rd. Identification of a gene involved in the biosynthesis of cyclopropanated mycolic acids in *Mycobacterium tuberculosis*. Proc Natl Acad Sci U S A 1995; 92: 6630-6634.

71. Chan J, Fujiwara T, Brennan P, et al. Microbial glycolipids: possible virulence factors that scavenge oxygen radicals. Proc Natl Acad Sci USA1989; 86: 2453-2457.

72. Pagan-Ramos E, Song J, McFalone M, Mudd MH, Deretic V. Oxidative stress response and characterization of the oxyR-*ahpC* and furA-*katG* loci in *Mycobacterium marinum*. J Bacteriol 1998; 180: 4856-4864.

73. Wilson TM, Collins DM. *ahpC*, a gene involved in isoniazid resistance of the *Mycobacterium tuberculosis* complex. Mol Microbiol 1996; 19: 1025-1034.

74. Heym B, Stavropoulos E, Honore N, et al. Effects of overexpression of the alkyl hydroperoxide reductase AhpC on the virulence and isoniazid resistance of *Mycobacterium tuberculosis*. Infect Immun 1997; 65: 1395-1401.

75. Sherman DR, Mdluli K, Hickey MJ, et al. Compensatory *ahpC* gene expression in isoniazid-resistant *Mycobacterium tuberculosis*. Science 1996; 272: 1641-1643.

76. Wilson T, de Lisle GW, Marcinkeviciene JA, Blanchard JS, Collins DM. Antisense RNA to *ahpC*, an oxidative stress defence gene involved in isoniazid resistance, indicates that AhpC of *Mycobacterium bovis* has virulence properties. Microbiology 1998; 144: 2687-2695.

77. Kelley CL, Rouse DA, Morris SL. Analysis of *ahpC* gene mutations in isoniazid-resistant clinical isolates of *Mycobacterium tuberculosis*. Antimicrob Agents Chemother 1997; 41: 2057-2058.

78. Sreevatsan S, Pan X, Zhang Y, Deretic V, Musser JM. Analysis of the oxyR-*ahpC* region in isoniazid-resistant and -susceptible *Mycobacterium tuberculosis* complex organisms recovered from diseased humans and animals in diverse localities. Antimicrob Agents Chemother 1997; 41: 600-606.

79. Miesel L, Weisbrod TR, Marcinkeviciene JA, et al. NADH dehydrogenase defects confer isoniaazid resistance and conditional lethality in *Mycobacterium smegmatis*. J Bacteriol 1998; 180: 2459-2467.

80. Payton M, Auty R, Delgoda R, Everett M, Sim E. Cloning and characterization of arylamine N-acetyltransferase genes from *Mycobacterium smegmatis* and *Mycobacterium tuberculosis*: increased expression results in isoniazid resistance. J Bacteriol 1999; 181: 1343-1347.

81. Choudhuri BS, Sen S, Chakrabarti P. Isoniazid accumulation in *Mycobacterium smegmatis* is modulated by proton motive force-driven and ATP-dependent extrusion systems. Biochem Biophys Res Commun 1999; 256: 682-684.

82. Heifets L, Lindholm-Levy P. Pyrazinamide sterilizing activity in vitro against semidormant *Mycobacterium tuberculosis* bacterial populations. Am Rev Respir Dis 1992; 145: 1223-1225.

83. McClatchy JK, Tsang AY, Cernich MS. Use of pyrazinamidase activity on *Mycobacterium tuberculosis* as a rapid method for determination of pyrazinamide susceptibility. Antimicrob Agents Chemother 1981; 20:556-557.

84. Konno K, Feldmann FM, McDermott W. Pyrazinamide susceptibility and amidase activity of tubercle bacilli. Am Rev Respir Dis 1967; 95: 461-469.

85. Foster JW, Moat AG. Nicotinamide adenine dinucleotide biosynthesis and pyridine nucleotide cycle metabolism in microbial systems. Microbiol Rev 1980; 44: 83-105.

86. Sun Z, Zhang Y. Reduced pyrazinamidase activity and the natural resistance of *Mycobacterium kansasii* to the antituberculosis drug pyrazinamide. Antimicrob Agents Chemother 1999; 43: 537-542.

87. Sreevatsan S, Pan X, Zhang Y, Kreiswirth BN, Musser JM. Mutations associated with pyrazinamide resistance in pncA of *Mycobacterium tuberculosis* complex organisms. Antimicrob Agents Chemother 1997; 41: 636-640.

88. Marttila HJ, Marjamaki M, Vyshnevskaya E, et al. pncA mutations in pyrazinamide-resistant *Mycobacterium tuberculosis* isolates from northwestern Russia. Antimicrob Agents Chemother 1999; 43: 1764-1766.

89. Scorpio A, Lindholm-Levy P, Heifets L, et al. Characterization of pncA mutations in pyrazinamide-resistant *Mycobacterium tuberculosis*. Antimicrob Agents Chemother 1997; 41: 540-543.

90. Mestdagh M, Fonteyne PA, Realini L, et al. Relationship between pyrazinamide resistance, loss of pyrazinamidase activity, and mutations in the pncA locus in multidrug-resistant clinical isolates of *Mycobacterium tuberculosis*. Antimicrob Agents Chemother 1999; 43: 2317-2319.

91. Hirano K, Takahashi M, Kazumi Y, Fukasawa Y, Abe C. Mutation in *pncA* is a major mechanism of pyrazinamide resistance in *Mycobacterium tuberculosis*. Tuberc Lung Dis 1998; 78: 117-122.

92. Salfinger M, Heifets LB. Determination of pyrazinamide MICs for *Mycobacterium tuberculosis* at different pHs by the radiometric method. Antimicrob Agents Chemother 1988; 32: 1002-1004.

93. Cutler RR, Wilson P, Villarroel J, Clarke FV. Evaluating current methods for determination of the susceptibility of mycobacteria to pyrazinamide, conventional, radiometric Bactec and two methods of pyrazinamidase testing. Lett Appl Microbiol 1997; 24: 127-32.

94. Lemaitre N, Sougakoff W, Truffot-Pernot C, Jarlier V. Characterization of new mutations in pyrazinamide-resistant strains of *Mycobacterium tuberculosis* and identification of conserved regions important for the catalytic activity of the pyrazinamidase PncA. Antimicrob Agents Chemother 1999; 43: 1761-1763.

95. Konno K, Feldman FM, McDermott W. Nicotinamidase in mycobacteria: A method for distinguishing bovine type tubercle bacilli from other mycobacteria. Nature 1959; 184.

96. Wayne LG. Simple pyrazinamidase and urease tests for routine identification of mycobacteria. Am Rev Respir Dis 1974; 109: 147-151.

97. Scorpio A, Collins D, Whipple D, Cave D, Bates J, Zhang Y. Rapid differentiation of bovine and human tubercle bacilli based on a characteristic mutation in the bovine pyrazinamidase gene. J Clin Microbiol 1997; 35: 106-110.

98. Boshoff HI, Mizrahi V. Purification, gene cloning, targeted knockout, overexpression, and biochemical characterization of the major pyrazinamidase from *Mycobacterium smegmatis*. J Bacteriol 1998; 180: 5809-5814.

99. Zhang Y, Scorpio A, Nikaido H, Sun Z. Role of acid pH and deficient efflux of pyrazinoic acid in unique susceptibility of *Mycobacterium tuberculosis* to pyrazinamide. J Bacteriol 1999; 181: 2044-2049.

100. Kucers A, Bennett NM. The Use of Antibiotics. William Heinemann Medical Books Ltd, London, 1979.

101. Mikusova K, Slayden RA, Besra GS, Brennan PJ. Biogenesis of the mycobacterial cell wall and the site′ of action of ethambutol. Antimicrob Agents Chemother 1995; 39: 2484-2489.

102. Brennan PJ, Nikaido H. The envelope of mycobacteria. Annu Rev Biochem 1995; 64: 29-63. transport. J Bacteriol 1998;180:6773-5.

103. Belanger AE, Besra GS, Ford ME, et al. The embAB genes of *Mycobacterium avium* encode an arabinosyl transferase involved in cell wall arabinan biosynthesis that is the target for the antimycobacterial drug ethambutol. Proc Natl Acad Sci U S A 1996; 93: 11919-11924.

104. Telenti A, Philipp WJ, Sreevatsan S, et al. The emb operon, a gene cluster of *Mycobacterium tuberculosis* involved in resistance to ethambutol. Nat Med 1997; 3: 567-570.

105. Sreevatsan S, Stockbauer KE, Pan X, et al. Ethambutol resistance in *Mycobacterium tuberculosis*: critical role of *embB* mutations. Antimicrob Agents Chemother 1997; 41: 1677-1681.

106. Alcaide F, Pfyffer GE, Telenti A. Role of *embB* in natural and acquired resistance to ethambutol in mycobacteria. Antimicrob Agents Chemother 1997; 41: 2270-2273.

107. Sensi P, Maggi N, Furesz S, Maffii G. Chemical modifications and biological properties of rifamycins. Antimicrob Agents Chemother 1966; 6: 699-714.

108. Jin DJ, Zhou YN. Mutational analysis of structure-function relationship of RNA polymerase in *Escherichia coli*. Methods Enzymol 1996; 273: 300-319.

109. McClure WR, Cech CL, Johnston DE. A steady state assay for the RNA polymerase initiation reaction. J Biol Chem 1978; 253: 8941-8948.

110. Levin ME, Hatfull GF. *Mycobacterium smegmatis* RNA polymerase: DNA supercoiling, action of rifampicin and mechanism of rifampicin resistance. Mol Microbiol 1993; 8: 277-285.

111. Jin DJ, Gross CA. Mapping and sequencing of mutations in the *Escherichia coli rpoB* gene that lead to rifampicin resistance. J Mol Biol 1988; 202: 45-58.

112. Cole ST, Barrell BG. Analysis of the genome of *Mycobacterium tuberculosis* H37Rv. Novartis Found Symp 1998; 217: 160-172.

113. Miller LP, Crawford JT, Shinnick TM. The *rpoB* gene of *Mycobacterium tuberculosis*. Antimicrob Agents Chemother 1994; 38: 805-811.

114. Taniguchi H, Aramaki H, Nikaido Y, et al. Rifampicin resistance and mutation of the *rpoB* gene in *Mycobacterium tuberculosis*. FEMS Microbiol Lett 1996; 144: 103-108.

115. Kapur V, Li LL, Iordanescu S, et al. Characterization by automated DNA sequencing of mutations in the gene (*rpoB*) encoding the RNA polymerase beta subunit in rifampin-resistant *Mycobacterium tuberculosis* strains from New York City and Texas. J Clin Microbiol 1994; 32: 1095-1098.

116. Telenti A, Imboden P, Marchesi F, et al. Detection of rifampicin-resistance mutations in *Mycobacterium tuberculosis*. Lancet 1993; 341: 647-650.

117. Williams DL, Waguespack C, Eisenach K, et al. Characterization of rifampin-resistance in pathogenic mycobacteria. Antimicrob Agents Chemother 1994; 38: 2380-2386.

118. Williams DL, Spring L, Collins L, et al. Contribution of *rpoB* mutations to development of rifamycin cross- resistance in *Mycobacterium tuberculosis*. Antimicrob Agents Chemother 1998; 42: 1853-1857.

119. Moghazeh SL, Pan X, Arain T, Stover CK, Musser JM, Kreiswirth BN. Comparative antimycobacterial activities of rifampin, rifapentine, and KRM-1648 against a collection of rifampin-resistant *Mycobacterium tuberculosis* isolates with known *rpoB* mutations. Antimicrob Agents Chemother 1996; 40: 2655-2657.

120. Bodmer T, Zurcher G, Imboden P, Telenti A. Mutation position and type of substitution in the beta-subunit of the RNA polymerase influence in-vitro activity of rifamycins in rifampicin- resistant *Mycobacterium tuberculosis*. J Antimicrob Chemother 1995; 35: 345-348.

121. Hetherington SV, Watson AS, Patrick CC. Sequence and analysis of the *rpoB* gene of *Mycobacterium smegmatis*. Antimicrob Agents Chemother 1995; 39: 2164-2166.

122. Quan S, Venter H, Dabbs ER. Ribosylative inactivation of rifampin by *Mycobacterium smegmatis* is a principal contributor to its low susceptibility to this antibiotic. Antimicrob Agents Chemother 1997; 41: 2456-2460.

123. Andersen SJ, Quan S, Gowan B, Dabbs ER. Monooxygenase-like sequence of a *Rhodococcus equi* gene conferring increased resistance to rifampin by inactivating this antibiotic. Antimicrob Agents Chemother 1997; 41: 218-221.

124. Portillo-Gomez L, Nair J, Rouse DA, Morris SL. The absence of genetic markers for streptomycin and rifampicin resistance in *Mycobacterium avium* complex strains. J Antimicrob Chemother 1995; 36: 1049-1053.

125. Guerrero C, Stockman L, Marchesi F, Bodmer T, Roberts GD, Telenti A. Evaluation of the *rpoB* gene in rifampicin-susceptible and -resistant *Mycobacterium avium* and Mycobacterium intracellulare. J Antimicrob Chemother 1994; 33: 661-663.

126. Hui J, Gordon N, Kajioka R. Permeability barrier to rifampin in mycobacteria. Antimicrob Agents Chemother 1977; 11: 773-779.

127. Honore N, Cole ST. Molecular basis of rifampin resistance in Mycobacterium leprae. Antimicrob Agents Chemother 1993; 37: 414-418.

128. Breckenridge L, Gorini L. Genetic analysis of streptomycin resistance in *Escherichia coli*. Genetics 1970; 65: 9-25.

129. Allen PN, Noller HF. Mutations in ribosomal proteins S4 and S12 influence the higher order structure of 16 S ribosomal RNA. J Mol Biol 1989; 208: 457-468.

130. Moazed D, Noller HF. Interaction of antibiotics with functional sites in 16S ribosomal RNA. Nature 1987; 327: 389-394.

131. Funatsu G, Wittmann HG. Ribosomal proteins. 33. Location of amino-acid replacements in protein S12 isolated from *Escherichia coli* mutants resistant to streptomycin. J Mol Biol 1972; 68: 547-50.

132. Liu XQ, Gillham NW, Boynton JE. Chloroplast ribosomal protein gene rps12 of Chlamydomonas reinhardtii. Wild-type sequence, mutation to streptomycin resistance

and dependence, and function in *Escherichia coli*. J Biol Chem 1989; 264: 16100-16108.

133. Ruusala T, Andersson D, Ehrenberg M, Kurland CG. Hyper-accurate ribosomes inhibit growth. Embo J 1984; 3: 2575-2580.

134. Katsukawa C, Tamaru A, Miyata Y, Abe C, Makino M, Suzuki Y. Characterization of the *rpsL* and *rrs* genes of streptomycin-resistant clinical isolates of *Mycobacterium tuberculosis* in Japan. J Appl Microbiol 1997; 83: 6346-40.

135. Honore N, Cole ST. Streptomycin resistance in mycobacteria. Antimicrob Agents Chemother 1994; 38: 238-242.

136. Cooksey RC, Morlock GP, McQueen A, Glickman SE, Crawford JT. Characterization of streptomycin resistance mechanisms among *Mycobacterium tuberculosis* isolates from patients in New York City. Antimicrob Agents Chemother 1996; 40: 1186-1188.

137. Bock A, Petzet A, Piepersberg W. Ribosomal ambiguity (ram) mutations facilitate diyhydrostreptomycin binding to ribosomes. FEBS Lett 1979; 104: 317-321.

138. Kaji H, Tanaka Y. Binding of dihydrostreptomycin to ribosomal subunits. J Mol Biol 1968; 32: 221-230.

139. Schreiner G, Nierhaus KH. Protein involved in the binding of dihydrostreptomycin to ribosomes of *Escherichia coli*. J Mol Biol 1973; 81: 71-82.

140. Stern S, Weiser B, Noller HF. Model for the three-dimensional folding of 16 S ribosomal RNA. J Mol Biol 1988; 204: 447-481.

141. Stern S, Powers T, Changchien LM, Noller HF. Interaction of ribosomal proteins S5, S6, S11, S12, S18 and S21 with 16 S rRNA. J Mol Biol 1988; 201: 683-695.

142. Bottger EC. Resistance to drugs targeting protein synthesis in mycobacteria. Trends Microbiol 1994; 2: 416-421.

143. Powers T, Noller HF. A functional pseudoknot in 16S ribosomal RNA. Embo J 1991; 10: 2203-2214.

144. Woese CR, Gutell RR. Evidence for several higher order structural elements in ribosomal RNA. Proc Natl Acad Sci U S A 1989; 86: 3119-3122.

145. Powers T, Noller HF. Evidence for functional interaction between elongation factor Tu and 16S ribosomal RNA. Proc Natl Acad Sci U S A 1993; 90: 1364-1368.

146. Van Ryk DI, Dahlberg AE. Structural changes in the 530 loop of *Escherichia coli* 16S rRNA in mutants with impaired translational fidelity. Nucleic Acids Res 1995; 23: 3563-3570.

147. Sander P, Meier A, Bottger EC. *rpsL+*: a dominant selectable marker for gene replacement in mycobacteria. Mol Microbiol 1995; 16: 991-1000.

148. Melancon P, Lemieux C, Brakier-Gingras L. A mutation in the 530 loop of *Escherichia coli* 16S ribosomal RNA causes resistance to streptomycin. Nucleic Acids Res 1988; 16: 9631-9639.

149. Harris EH, Burkhart BD, Gillham NW, Boynton JE. Antibiotic resistance mutations in the chloroplast 16S and 23S rRNA genes of *Chlamydomonas reinhardtii*: correlation of genetic and physical maps of the chloroplast genome. Genetics 1989; 123: 281-292.

150. Montandon PE, Nicolas P, Schurmann P, Stutz E. Streptomycin-resistance of Euglena gracilis chloroplasts: identification of a point mutation in the 16S rRNA gene in an invariant position. Nucleic Acids Res 1985; 13: 4299-4310.

151. Gauthier A, Turmel M, Lemieux C. Mapping of chloroplast mutations conferring resistance to antibiotics in Chlamydomonas: evidence for a novel site of streptomycin resistance in the small subunit rRNA. Mol Gen Genet 1988; 214: 192-197.

152. Bercovier H, Kafri O, Sela S. Mycobacteria possess a surprisingly small number of ribosomal RNA genes in relation to the size of their genome. Biochem Biophys Res Commun 1986; 136: 1136-1141.

153. Meier A, Kirschner P, Bange FC, Vogel U, Bottger EC. Genetic alterations in streptomycin-resistant *Mycobacterium tuberculosis*: mapping of mutations conferring resistance. Antimicrob Agents Chemother 1994; 38: 228-233.

154. Honore N, Marchal G, Cole ST. Novel mutation in 16S rRNA associated with streptomycin dependence in *Mycobacterium tuberculosis*. Antimicrob Agents Chemother 1995; 39: 769-770.

155. Sreevatsan S, Pan X, Stockbauer KE, Williams DL, Kreiswirth BN, Musser JM. Characterization of *rpsL* and *rrs* mutations in streptomycin-resistant *Mycobacterium tuberculosis* isolates from diverse geographic localities. Antimicrob Agents Chemother 1996; 40: 1024-1026.

156. Mitchison DA. The segregation of streptomycin-resistant variants of *Mycobacterium tuberculosis* into groups with characteristic levels of resistance. J Gen Microbiol 1951; 5: 596-604.

157. Meier A, Sander P, Schaper KJ, Scholz M, Bottger EC. Correlation of molecular resistance mechanisms and phenotypic resistance levels in streptomycin-resistant *Mycobacterium tuberculosis*. Antimicrob Agents Chemother 1996; 40: 2452-2454.

158. Benveniste R, Davies J. Mechanisms of antibiotic resistance in bacteria. Ann Rev Biochem 1973; 42: 471-506.

159. Sundin GW, Bender CL. Dissemination of the *strA-strB* streptomycin-resistance genes among commensal and pathogenic bacteria from humans, animals, and plants. Mol Ecol 1996; 5: 133-143.

160. Hooper DC, Wolfson JS. Fluoroquinolone antimicrobial agents. N Engl J Med 1991; 324: 384-394.

161. Chen CH, Shih JF, Lindholm-Levy PJ, Heifets LB. Minimal inhibitory concentrations of rifabutin, ciprofloxacin, and ofloxacin against *Mycobacterium tuberculosis* isolated before treatment of patients in Taiwan. Am Rev Respir Dis 1989; 140: 987-989.

162. Muder RR, Brennen C, Goetz AM, Wagener MM, Rihs JD. Association with prior fluoroquinolone therapy of widespread ciprofloxacin resistance among gram-negative isolates in a Veterans Affairs medical center. Antimicrob Agents Chemother 1991; 35: 256-258.

163. Sullivan EA, Kreiswirth BN, Palumbo L, et al. Emergence of fluoroquinolone-resistant tuberculosis in New York City. Lancet 1995; 345: 1148-1150.

164. Drlica K, Xu C, Wang JY, Burger RM, Malik M. Fluoroquinolone action in mycobacteria: similarity with effects in *Escherichia coli* and detection by cell lysate viscosity. Antimicrob Agents Chemother 1996; 40: 1594-1599.

165. Everett MJ, Jin YF, Ricci V, Piddock LJ. Contributions of individual mechanisms to fluoroquinolone resistance in 36 *Escherichia coli* strains isolated from humans and animals. Antimicrob Agents Chemother 1996; 40: 2380-2386.

166. Riesenfeld C, Everett M, Piddock LJ, Hall BG. Adaptive mutations produce resistance to ciprofloxacin. Antimicrob Agents Chemother 1997; 41: 2059-2060.

167. Lounis N, Ji B, Truffot-Pernot C, Grosset J. Which aminoglycoside or fluoroquinolone is more active against *Mycobacterium tuberculosis* in mice? Antimicrob Agents Chemother 1997; 41: 607-610.

168. Zhao BY, Pine R, Domagala J, Drlica K. Fluoroquinolone action against clinical isolates of *Mycobacterium tuberculosis*: effects of a C-8 methoxyl group on survival in liquid media and in human macrophages. Antimicrob Agents Chemother 1999; 43: 661-666.

169. Wang JC. DNA topoisomerases. Ann Rev Biochem 1996; 65: 635-692.

170. Drlica K. Mechanism of fluoroquinolone action. Current Opinion in Microbiology 1999; 2: 504-508.

171. Willmott CJ, Critchlow SE, Eperon IC, Maxwell A. The complex of DNA gyrase and quinolone drugs with DNA forms a barrier to transcription by RNA polymerase. J Mol Biol 1994; 242: 351-363.

172. Maxwell A. DNA gyrase as a drug target. Trends Microbiol 1997; 5: 102-109.

173. Kato J, Suzuki H, Ikeda H. Purification and characterization of DNA topoisomerase IV in *Escherichia coli*. J Biol Chem 1992; 267: 25676-25684.

174. Adams DE, Shekhtman EM, Zechiedrich EL, Schmid MB, Cozzarelli NR. The role of topoisomerase IV in partitioning bacterial replicons and the structure of catenated intermediates in DNA replication. Cell 1992; 71: 277-288.

175. Huang WM. Bacterial diversity based on type II DNA topoisomerase genes. Ann Rev Genet 1996; 30: 79-107.

176. Morais Cabral JH, Jackson AP, Smith CV, Shikotra N, Maxwell A, Liddington RC. Crystal structure of the breakage-reunion domain of DNA gyrase. Nature 1997; 388: 903-906.

177. Ferrero L, Cameron B, Manse B, et al. Cloning and primary structure of *Staphylococcus aureus* DNA topoisomerase IV: a primary target of fluoroquinolones. Mol Microbiol 1994; 13: 641-653.

178. Yoshida H, Bogaki M, Nakamura M, Nakamura S. Quinolone resistance-determining region in the DNA gyrase *gyrA* gene of *Escherichia coli*. Antimicrob Agents Chemother 1990; 34: 1271-1272.

179. Stein DC, Danaher RJ, Cook TM. Characterization of a *gyrB* mutation responsible for low-level nalidixic acid resistance in *Neisseria gonorrhoeae*. Antimicrob Agents Chemother 1991; 35: 622-626.

180. Yamagishi J, Yoshida H, Yamayoshi M, Nakamura S. Nalidixic acid-resistant mutations of the *gyrB* gene of *Escherichia coli*. Mol Gen Genet 1986; 204: 367-373.

181. Takahashi H, Kikuchi T, Shoji S, et al. Characterization of *gyrA*, *gyrB*, *grlA* and *grlB* mutations in fluoroquinolone-resistant clinical isolates of *Staphylococcus aureus*. J Antimicrob Chemother 1998; 41: 49-57.

182. Tanaka M, Onodera Y, Uchida Y, Sato K. Quinolone resistance mutations in the GrlB protein of *Staphylococcus aureus*. Antimicrob Agents Chemother 1998; 42: 3044-3046.

183. Takiff HE, Salazar L, Guerrero C, et al. Cloning and nucleotide sequence of *Mycobacterium tuberculosis gyrA* and *gyrB* genes and detection of quinolone resistance mutations. Antimicrob Agents Chemother 1994; 38: 773-780.

184. Cole ST, Brosch R, Parkhill J, et al. Deciphering the biology of *Mycobacterium tuberculosis* from the complete genome sequence. Nature 1998; 393: 537-544.

185. Horowitz DS, Wang JC. Mapping the active site tyrosine of *Escherichia coli* DNA gyrase. J Biol Chem 1987; 262: 5339-5344.

186. Nakamura S. Mechanisms of quinolone resistance. J Infect Chemother 1997; 3: 128-138.

187. Alangaden GJ, Manavathu EK, Vakulenko SB, Zvonok NM, Lerner SA. Characterization of fluoroquinolone-resistant mutant strains of *Mycobacterium tuberculosis* selected in the laboratory and isolated from patients. Antimicrob Agents Chemother 1995; 39: 1700-1703.

188. Williams KJ, Chan R, Piddock LJ. *gyrA* of ofloxacin-resistant clinical isolates of *Mycobacterium tuberculosis* from Hong Kong. J Antimicrob Chemother 1996; 37: 1032-1034.

189. Revel V, Cambau E, Jarlier V, Sougakoff W. Characterization of mutations in *Mycobacterium smegmatis* involved in resistance to fluoroquinolones. Antimicrob Agents Chemother 1994; 38: 1991-1996.

190. Cambau E, Sougakoff W, Besson M, Truffot-Pernot C, Grosset J, Jarlier V. Selection of a *gyrA* mutant of *Mycobacterium tuberculosis* resistant to fluoroquinolones during treatment with ofloxacin. J Infect Dis 1994; 170: 479-483.

191. Xu C, Kreiswirth BN, Sreevatsan S, Musser JM, Drlica K. Fluoroquinolone resistance associated with specific gyrase mutations in clinical isolates of multidrug-resistant *Mycobacterium tuberculosis.* J Infect Dis 1996; 174: 1127-1130.

192. Ito H, Yoshida H, Bogaki-Shonai M, Niga T, Hattori H, Nakamura S. Quinolone resistance mutations in the DNA gyrase *gyrA* and *gyrB* genes of *Staphylococcus aureus.* Antimicrob Agents Chemother 1994; 38: 2014-2023.

193. Conrad S, Oethinger M, Kaifel K, Klotz G, Marre R, Kern WV. *gyrA* mutations in high-level fluoroquinolone-resistant clinical isolates of *Escherichia coli.* J Antimicrob Chemother 1996; 38: 443-455.

194. Deplano A, Zekhnini A, Allali N, Couturier M, Struelens MJ. Association of mutations in *grlA* and *gyrA* topoisomerase genes with resistance to ciprofloxacin in epidemic and sporadic isolates of methicillin-resistant *Staphylococcus aureus.* Antimicrob Agents Chemother 1997; 41: 2023-2025.

195. Guillemin I, Jarlier V, Cambau E. Correlation between quinolone susceptibility patterns and sequences in the A and B subunits of DNA gyrase in mycobacteria. Antimicrob Agents Chemother 1998; 42: 2084-2088.

196. Kocagoz T, Hackbarth CJ, Unsal I, Rosenberg EY, Nikaido H, Chambers HF. Gyrase mutations in laboratory-selected, fluoroquinolone-resistant mutants of *Mycobacterium tuberculosis* H37Ra. Antimicrob Agents Chemother 1996; 40: 1768-1774.

197. Nikaido H. Multidrug efflux pumps of gram-negative bacteria. J Bacteriol 1996; 178: 5853-5859.

198. Kaatz GW, Seo SM. Mechanisms of fluoroquinolone resistance in genetically related strains of *Staphylococcus aureus.* Antimicrob Agents Chemother 1997; 41: 2733-2737.

199. Poole K, Gotoh N, Tsujimoto H, et al. Overexpression of the mexC-mexD-oprJ efflux operon in nfxB-type multidrug-resistant strains of *Pseudomonas aeruginosa.* Mol Microbiol 1996; 21: 713-724.

200. Sun L, Sreedharan S, Plummer K, Fisher LM. NorA plasmid resistance to fluoroquinolones: role of copy number and norA frameshift mutations. Antimicrob Agents Chemother 1996; 40: 1665-1669.

201. Hillen W, Schollmeier K, Gatz C. Control of expression of the Tn10-encoded tetracycline resistance operon. II. Interaction of RNA polymerase and TET repressor with the tet operon regulatory region. J Mol Biol 1984; 172: 185-201.

202. Takiff HE, Cimino M, Musso MC, et al. Efflux pump of the proton antiporter family confers low-level fluoroquinolone resistance in *Mycobacterium smegmatis.* Proc Natl Acad Sci U S A 1996; 93: 362-366.

203. Liu J, Takiff HE, Nikaido H. Active efflux of fluoroquinolones in *Mycobacterium smegmatis* mediated by LfrA, a multidrug efflux pump. J Bacteriol 1996; 178: 3791-3795.

204. Sander S, De.Rossi E, Böddinghaus B, et al. Contribution of the multidrug efflux pump LfrA to innate mycobacterial drug resistance. (manuscript submitted).

205. Dong Y, Xu C, Zhao X, Domagala J, Drlica K. Fluoroquinolone action against mycobacteria: effects of C-8 substituents on growth, survival, and resistance. Antimicrob Agents Chemother 1998; 42: 2978-2984.

206. Dong Y, Zhao X, Domagala J, Drlica K. Effect of fluoroquinolone concentration on selection of resistant mutants of *Mycobacterium bovis* BCG and *Staphylococcus aureus*. Antimicrob Agents Chemother 1999; 43: 1756-1758.

207. Piddock LJ, Johnson M, Ricci V, Hill SL. Activities of new fluoroquinolones against fluoroquinolone-resistant pathogens of the lower respiratory tract. Antimicrob Agents Chemother 1998; 42: 2956-2960.

208. Pan XS, Fisher LM. Targeting of DNA gyrase in *Streptococcus pneumoniae* by sparfloxacin: selective targeting of gyrase or topoisomerase IV by quinolones. Antimicrob Agents Chemother 1997; 41: 471-474.

209. Martin SJ, Meyer JM, Chuck SK, Jung R, Messick CR, Pendland SL. Levofloxacin and sparfloxacin: new quinolone antibiotics. Ann Pharmacother 1998; 32: 320-336.

210. Herr EB, Jr., Redstone MO. Chemical and physical characterization of capreomycin. Ann N Y Acad Sci 1966; 135: 940-946.

211. Edson RS, Terrell CL. The aminoglycosides. Mayo Clin Proc 1999; 74: 519-528.

212. Rastogi N, Labrousse V, Goh KS. In vitro activities of fourteen antimicrobial agents against drug susceptible and resistant clinical isolates of *Mycobacterium tuberculosis* and comparative intracellular activities against the virulent H37Rv strain in human macrophages. Curr Microbiol 1996; 33: 167-175.

213. Ho YI, Chan CY, Cheng AF. In-vitro activities of aminoglycoside-aminocyclitols against mycobacteria. J Antimicrob Chemother 1997; 40: 27-32.

214. Rheinberger H-J, Geigenmüeller U, Gnirke A, et al. Allosteric three-site model for the ribosomal elongation cycle. In: Hill WE, Dahlberg A, Garrett RA, Moore PB, Schlessinger D, Warner JR (eds.), The Ribosome Structure, Function & Evolution. American Society for Microbiology, Washington, D.C., 1990.

215. Yamada T, Mizugichi Y, Nierhaus KH, Wittmann HG. Resistance to viomycin conferred by RNA of either ribosomal subunit. Nature 1978; 275: 460-461.

216. Koseki Y, Okamoto S. Studies on cross-resistance between capreomycin and certain other anti-mycobacterial agents. Jap. J. M. Sc. & Biol. 1963; 16: 31-38.

217. McClatchy JK, Kanes W, Davidson PT, Moulding TS. Cross-resistance in *M. tuberculosis* to kanamycin, capreomycin and viomycin. Tubercle 1977; 58: 29-34.

218. Alangaden GJ, Kreiswirth BN, Aouad A, et al. Mechanism of resistance to amikacin and kanamycin in *Mycobacterium tuberculosis*. Antimicrob Agents Chemother 1998; 42: 1295-1297.

219. Tsukamura M, Mizuno S. Cross-resistant relationships among the aminoglucoside antibiotics in *Mycobacterium tuberculosis*. J Gen Microbiol 1975; 88: 269-274.

220. Sander P, Prammananan T, Bottger EC. Introducing mutations into a chromosomal rRNA gene using a genetically modified eubacterial host with a single rRNA operon. Mol Microbiol 1996; 22: 841-848.

221. Suzuki Y, Katsukawa C, Tamaru A, et al. Detection of kanamycin-resistant *Mycobacterium tuberculosis* by identifying mutations in the 16S rRNA gene. J Clin Microbiol 1998; 36: 1220-1225.

222. Taniguchi H, Chang B, Abe C, Nikaido Y, Mizuguchi Y, Yoshida SI. Molecular analysis of kanamycin and viomycin resistance in *Mycobacterium smegmatis* by use of the conjugation system. J Bacteriol 1997; 179: 4795-4801.

223. Prammananan T, Sander P, Brown BA, et al. A single 16S ribosomal RNA substitution is responsible for resistance to amikacin and other 2-deoxystreptamine aminoglycosides in *Mycobacterium abscessus* and *Mycobacterium chelonae*. J Infect Dis 1998; 177: 1573-1581.

224. Davies J, Wright GD. Bacterial resistance to aminoglycoside antibiotics. Trends Microbiol 1997; 5: 234-240.

225. Shaw KJ, Rather PN, Hare RS, Miller GH. Molecular genetics of aminoglycoside resistance genes and familial relationships of the aminoglycoside-modifying enzymes. Microbiol Rev 1993; 57: 138-163.

226. Ainsa JA, Perez E, Pelicic V, Berthet FX, Gicquel B, Martin C. Aminoglycoside 2'-N-acetyltransferase genes are universally present in mycobacteria: characterization of the aac(2')-Ic gene from *Mycobacterium tuberculosis* and the aac(2')-Id gene from *Mycobacterium smegmatis*. Mol Microbiol 1997; 24: 431-441.

227. Ainsa JA, Blokpoel MC, Otal I, Young DB, De Smet KA, Martin C. Molecular cloning and characterization of Tap, a putative multidrug efflux pump present in *Mycobacterium fortuitum* and *Mycobacterium tuberculosis*. J Bacteriol 1998; 180: 5836-5843.

228. Cundliffe E. How antibiotic-producing organisms avoid suicide. Annu Rev Microbiol 1989; 43: 207-233.

229. Fourmy D, Recht MI, Blanchard SC, Puglisi JD. Structure of the A site of *Escherichia coli* 16S ribosomal RNA complexed with an aminoglycoside antibiotic. Science 1996; 274: 1367-1371.

230. Reitz RH, Slade HD, Neuhaus FC. The biochemical mechanisms of resistance by streptococci to the antibiotics D-cycloserine and O-carbamyl-D-serine. Biochemistry 1967; 6: 2561-2570.

231. Caceres NE, Harris NB, Wellehan JF, Feng Z, Kapur V, Barletta RG. Overexpression of the D-alanine racemase gene confers resistance to D- cycloserine in *Mycobacterium smegmatis*. J Bacteriol 1997; 179: 5046-5055.

232. David HL, Goldman DS, Takayama K. Inhibition of the synthesis of wax D peptidoglycolipid of *Mycobacterium tuberculosis* by D-cycloserine. Infect Immun 1970; 1: 74-77.

233. Zygmunt WA. Antagonism of D-cycloserine inhibition of mycobacterial growth by D-alanine. J. Bacteriol. 1963; 85: 1217-1220.

234. David HL. Resistance to D-cycloserine in the tubercle bacilli: mutation rate and transport of alanine in parental cells and drug-resistant mutants. Appl Microbiol 1971; 21:888-892.

235. Bhatt A, Green R, Coles R, Condon M, Connell ND. A mutant of *Mycobacterium smegmatis* defective

Chapter 7

DOTS and multidrug-resistant tuberculosis

Mario C. Raviglione
Operational and Epidemiological Research Team, Communicable Diseases Prevention and Control, World Health Organization, Geneva, Switzerland

1.   INTRODUCTION

In late 1997, the World Health Organization (WHO) and the International Union against Tuberculosis and Lung Disease (IUATLD), in collaboration with a variety of institutions world-wide, published the results of studies to determine the prevalence of drug-resistant tuberculosis (TB) conducted in 35 countries and territories [1]. These studies, based on representative samples drawn from the populations under study, were undertaken using standard definitions and approaches. Proficiency testing and an overall international quality assurance programme for laboratory performance were implemented [2].   The results of these studies showed that multidrug-resistant TB (MDRTB) is more widespread than previously thought [3]. The study also allowed the identification of "hot spots" for MDRTB: these were largely in the former USSR, but also in other parts of the world.

At the same time, based on a number of considerations, the value of the WHO strategy of TB control (Directly Observed Treatment, Short-course – DOTS) to properly address the MDRTB phenomenon started to be questioned [4,5]. While recognising that the adoption of the DOTS strategy has improved the performance of TB control efforts in many settings, some challenge the traditional notion that, by introducing standardised short-

I.Bastian and F. Portaels (eds.), Multidrug-Resistant Tuberculosis, 115-131.
© 2000 *Kluwer Academic Publishers. Printed in the Netherlands.*

course chemotherapy (SCC) and halting the emergence of MDRTB, one can effectively neutralise the existing burden of MDRTB.

Novel approaches are indeed necessary where MDRTB is a major burden. WHO has recently launched a research initiative to study the feasibility of the management of MDRTB using second-line anti-tuberculosis drugs under programme conditions [6]. However, until results of large-scale feasibility assessments are available, it will not be possible to know if, in low-resource settings with a high burden of MDRTB, programmes can effectively address the issue in a sustainable manner. Thus, this chapter will look at the available evidence of the relationship of DOTS and MDRTB trying to identify appropriate solutions. It will also lay the ground for the need of a strengthened DOTS strategy, which has been named "DOTS-plus" and is the subject of another chapter in the book.

2.   DOTS: CURRENT STATUS OF TUBERCULOSIS CONTROL ACHIEVEMENTS WORLD-WIDE

DOTS is the current strategy for TB control advocated by WHO and endorsed by most institutions and agencies involved in TB control worldwide. It has been clearly defined in a number of publications [7-13]. Essentially, it consists of five elements:
1. government commitment to TB control,
2. case detection focusing on symptomatic patients self-reporting to health services, and utilising sputum smear microscopy,
3. administration of standardised (SCC) throughout the country, with direct observation of treatment during, at least, the initial phase (two months),
4. a system of regular supply of all essential anti-tuberculosis drugs, and
5. a standardised recording and reporting system allowing assessment of treatment results.

Focusing on item (iii), the recommended SCC for sputum smear-positive cases never treated previously (new cases) consists of four drugs (isoniazid, rifampicin, pyrazinamide and ethambutol or streptomycin) for 2 months, followed by isoniazid and rifampicin for 4 months or isoniazid and ethambutol for 6 months [14]. For cases who were already treated (failures, treatment interrupted, and relapses), the recommended retreatment regimen consists of the same five drugs used all together for 2 months, followed by one month of the same except streptomycin, and by 5 months of isoniazid, rifampicin and ethambutol [14].

Since 1996, the WHO global tuberculosis surveillance and monitoring project has provided information on the status of implementation of DOTS by reporting countries (Figure 1). Based on the most recent available information, of the 212 countries and territories surveyed by WHO in 1998, 102 had adopted the recommended strategy by the end of 1997 [10]. Of them, 59 had implemented DOTS in over 90% of the country. Eight countries were in the pilot phase of implementation (coverage of less than 10%) and 35 were in the expansion phase (coverage between 10% and 90%). Of the remaining 110 countries, 57 had not yet adopted DOTS, 14 were low-incidence countries (case notification rate of less than 10 per 100,000 population) not using a strategy compatible with DOTS, and 39 did not report to WHO. Overall, the number of countries using DOTS has been increasing since 1990, when only around 10 countries were using a strategy of TB control which today we would call DOTS. The increase in the number of countries was rather steady during the period 1995-1997, when the global project became operational allowing a precise evaluation of the worldwide situation.

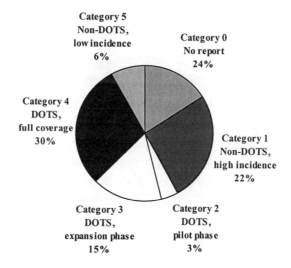

Figure 1. Proportions of countries with different levels of DOTS coverage, 1997. Data from reference 10.

Although the number of countries adopting DOTS was steadily increasing and 76% of the global population was living in countries that had adopted DOTS, in many DOTS countries adequate diagnostic and treatment services were not available in all districts. Allowing for incomplete coverage within countries, it is estimated that by the end of 1997 only 35% of the human population and an equal percentage of TB cases lived in areas where DOTS was available [10].

In 1997 nearly one million cases were notified from DOTS areas/countries, and 2.376 million from areas/countries not using DOTS. The performance of DOTS programmes has been evaluated through the use of some indicators. For instance, the percentage of new smear-positive cases out of all the new pulmonary cases is usually much higher in countries or areas using DOTS than those that do not: 65% versus 35% in 1997. This difference suggests an emphasis on sputum smear examination for diagnosis of TB. Also, documented treatment success (defined as patients completing treatment with or without bacteriological proof of smear-negativity) among the 461,149 patients treated in DOTS programmes in 1996 was 78.4%, compared with 38.6% among the 758,466 cases treated elsewhere [10]. Apart from the superiority of standardized SCC administered under direct supervision, compared to erratic and inadequate regimens used in many non-DOTS settings, one of the major reasons for this large difference is the absence of systematic evaluation of treatment results in countries or areas not using the information system recommended as part of the DOTS strategy. In summary, there is evidence that DOTS programmes are on average superior to other TB control efforts.

Prospects for further progress in TB control are encouraging, although a continued effort is necessary to achieve tangible and sustainable results. Most of the 22 countries identified by WHO as carrying some 80% of the global burden of TB are now implementing DOTS at least in pilot districts, with the aim of gradual phased expansion and, ultimately, coverage of the whole country after several years. The best examples of adequate control have been documented in Kenya, Peru, Tanzania, Viet Nam, Cambodia [10,15,16]: all of these countries reach high treatment success (above 70%) and acceptable case detection (estimated to be more than 50%). Other success stories are those of China [17], Bangladesh [18], Ethiopia and Myanmar, achieving high treatment success, although case coverage is still limited [10].

3.   THE DRUG RESISTANCE SITUATION WORLD-WIDE

As already mentioned, in 1994, WHO and IUATLD initiated the Global Project on Anti-tuberculosis Drug Resistance Surveillance [1,19]. The Global Project, based on a network of reference laboratories, aimed at measuring the prevalence of anti-tuberculosis drug resistance in countries throughout the world using comparable methodology. Cross-sectional analysis of surveys and surveillance reports allowed, for the first time, an assessment of the global situation. Participants followed guidelines that emphasized representative sampling, an accurate history of previous treatment, standardised laboratory methodology and common definitions [19,20]. A network of supranational reference laboratories provided quality assurance to country laboratories [2].

The 35 countries or regions studied during the period 1994-1997 enrolled a median of 555 tuberculosis patients (range, 59 to 14,344). A median of 9.9% (range, 2 to 41%) of the *Mycobacterium tuberculosis* strains from patients with no history of prior treatment were resistant to at least one drug ("primary" drug resistance); resistance to isoniazid (7.3%) and streptomycin (6.5%) were more common than resistance to rifampin (1.8%) or ethambutol (1.0%). The global prevalence of primary multidrug-resistance was 1.4% (range, 0 to 14.4%). Among patients with a history of prior treatment, the prevalence of any and multidrug resistance ("acquired" drug resistance) were 36% (range, 5.3 to 100%) and 13% (range, 0 to 54%), respectively. The combined prevalence (among new and retreatment cases) of any and multidrug resistance were 12.6% (range, 2.3 to 42.4%) and 2.2% (range, 0 to 22%).

Anti-tuberculosis drug resistance was found in all countries and regions surveyed. Primary multidrug resistance was identified everywhere, except in Kenya. A high prevalence of multidrug resistance was found in Latvia, Estonia and the Ivanovo Oblast, Russia (all in the former USSR), Asia (Delhi State, India), and additional "hot spots" in Latin America, particularly the Dominican Republic.

4. EVIDENCE THAT DOTS PREVENTS MDRTB

It has been claimed that SCC as part of a good TB control strategy can effectively prevent the emergence of drug- and multidrug-resistant TB [7,14]. One of the aims of the Global Project on Anti-tuberculosis Drug Resistance Surveillance was to provide evidence that this statement is true. In an attempt to correlate the levels of MDRTB with the quality of TB control programmes, the 35 participating countries were stratified into two groups:

- countries with "better" TB control which achieved coverage by DOTS of the entire country, or coverage of at least one third of the country if in a phase of expansion, or countries with a TB notification rate of less than 10 per 100,000 population;
- countries with "poorer" TB control which had not adopted DOTS, or had a coverage of less than one third of their territory if in a phase of expansion, or countries piloting DOTS.

The analysis, yet to be published, reveals that countries with "better" TB control had a lower combined prevalence of MDRTB than those with "poorer" TB control (1.6% versus 3.9%; p<0.05). In addition, they also had a lower prevalence of MDRTB among cases previously treated (7.7% versus 17%), while the prevalence of MDRTB among cases never treated was similar to that in countries with "poorer" control. Finally, the acquired MDR index (acquired MDRTB cases divided by the total number of registered patients, as an expression of the relative burden of MDRTB among cases previously treated) was significantly lower in countries with "better" control (0.6% vs 1.8%; p<0.05).

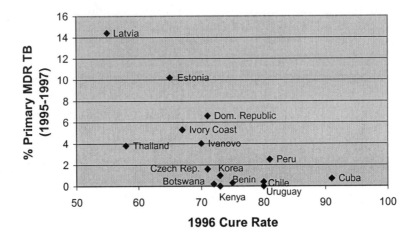

Figure 2. Relationship between primary MDR-TB prevalence and treatment success rate in selected countries worldwide, 1995-1997 (r^2 = 50%)

In addition to DOTS coverage (an "input" indicator), looking at the relationship of programme performance (an "output" indicator) and drug resistance is of great interest. The treatment success rate, as the best expression of the performance of TB control programmes, is expected to be inversely related to the prevalence of MDRTB. The situation for selected countries, for which both drug resistance and treatment result data are reliable, is shown in Figure 2. Countries achieving a high rate of treatment success have very low primary MDRTB prevalence (see bottom right section of the chart). The relationship is statistically significant (r^2=50%, p=0.003 by Pearson correlation test). This finding is stimulating and should prompt further analysis once more data on drug resistance are available. A reason for the lack of correlation in some settings where treatment success is currently high is the persistence, after implementation of revised and stronger programmes, of MDRTB created by previously weak programmes. This could explain, for instance, why some programmes which are achieving high levels of cure today (e.g., those of Peru and Viet Nam) still are working in an environment with relatively high levels of MDRTB.

These observations suggest that the proper use of standard SCC, as in many effective DOTS programmes worldwide, minimises the creation of MDRTB where it does not yet exist. African countries such as Benin, Botswana, and Kenya, which have started using rifampicin in their standard SCC regimens at the time of implementation of good TB control practices (1983, 1986, 1993, respectively) and have achieved high cure rates, have been very successful in minimizing the appearance and spread of MDRTB. Similarly, some Latin American countries, such as Chile, Cuba and Uruguay, with traditionally excellent control programmes curing most patients, have today very low levels of MDRTB. On the other hand, countries such as the Dominican Republic, Estonia, Côte d'Ivoire, Latvia, Russia and Thailand, which used rifampicin widely before introducing standard regimens countrywide and strengthening their programmes by ensuring adherence to treatment, have on average a higher prevalence of MDRTB. Therefore, effective TB control is associated with prevention of MDRTB. The situation might be different, however, in settings where MDRTB is already frequent and standard SCC including rifampicin is introduced for wide use.

5.   CAN MDRTB BE ELIMINATED AS A PUBLIC HEALTH PROBLEM BY DOTS?

Elimination of MDRTB can only occur when TB as a whole is eliminated, as resistant bacilli will always be originated by selective pressure when drugs are used. Therefore, it may be prudent to speak of "elimination as a public health problem". This is what is meant by "elimination" in this paper. The question is whether properly handled SCC based on regimens of isoniazid, rifampicin, pyrazinamide, and ethambutol (or streptomycin) [14] can effectively contain and possibly eliminate MDRTB when this is already widespread in a country. In other words, what will happen in some countries of the former USSR, for instance, upon the introduction of standard SCC as part of the DOTS strategy?

Some believe that, by adopting the standard SCC regimens endorsed by WHO and IUATLD for use countrywide, MDRTB prevalence will slowly decline until elimination. In fact, many patients will be cured even though they are infected with multidrug-resistant strains; some (25-30%) will undergo spontaneous cure, as part of the natural history of the disease [21,22]; and the rest will die quickly, thus stopping infecting others.

Beginning with case fatality, the current evidence shows that HIV-infected MDRTB patients have an extraordinarily high risk of death approaching 70-80%, with a mortality peaking between one and four months after diagnosis [23-27]. Among patients without HIV infection, the MDRTB case fatality rate was much lower: 37 of 171 patients (22%) in a study from the National Jewish Center, one of the most prestigious referral hospitals in the United States [28], and 1 of 25 in a study from various hospitals in New York City [29]. In both studies, however, second-line anti-tuberculosis drugs and surgery were used to treat patients. Even with these interventions, the median time to sputum conversion, among those who responded, appeared to be relatively long, from 2 to 705 days, with a median of 69 days in one study [29]. In summary, these data suggest that specialised and individualised treatment can cure a relatively high proportion of cases with MDRTB, thus removing them from the pool of infectious cases. At the same time, the duration of infectiousness prior to sputum conversion or death is also high. Therefore, assuming that a large number of MDRTB patients die quickly is unwarranted. However, the above assessments were made in the United States of America, where expensive individualised regimens and surgery are more clearly accessible than in most other countries.

The situation in developing countries using standard SCC as part of DOTS is globally the most important. Looking at previous published evidence and at results among cases with drug-resistant TB and MDRTB treated using standard first-line regimens in four programme settings, it appears that most cases of TB resistant to isoniazid or streptomycin alone can be cured. In the past, it was shown that the failure rate of 4-6 months' treatment, in TB resistant to isoniazid, was only 1%, though 11% relapsed [30]. Similarly, very low failure rates of 0 to 2% were observed in clinical trials when regimens of at least six months were used against strains resistant to either isoniazid or streptomycin [31]. Recent data reported to WHO from national control programmes, as distinct from controlled trials, show that cure rates of patients with strains resistant to a single drug (not including rifampicin), and given SCC, are not significantly lower than cure rates in patients with fully susceptible strains. In Peru, 90% (1029/1145) of cases with susceptible strains and 87% (105/121) of patients with resistance to a single drugs were cured (p = 0.27). In Korea, the figures were 85% (1668/1968) and 80% (104/129; p = 0.11) respectively. These data suggest that SCC may cure most cases with mono-resistance. Inevitably, however, treatment success rates of MDRTB cases are lower. In Peru and Korea, the treatment success rates of MDRTB cases have recently been measured to be 58% (14/24) and 56% (20/36), significantly lower than for susceptible cases (p < 0.001 in both studies). A multi-centre study involving four countries (Peru, Korea, the Dominican Republic and the Ivanovo Oblast in Russia) showed an average treatment success rate of 48% among new MDRTB cases, with an average failure rate of 39%. The death rate was generally below 10% [32]. Thus, some response to standard first-line drugs indeed is possible, although the failure rate is clearly unacceptable. The question remains whether achieving a treatment success rate of about 50% among new cases and a relatively low case fatality rate, but allowing a high failure rate, are sufficient to eliminate MDRTB.

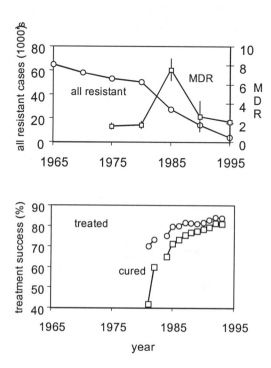

Figure 3. Trends in resistance to anti-tuberculosis drugs in Korea, in relation to treatment success rates. Top: estimated numbers of prevalent MDRTB cases (squares) and cases resistant to any drug (circles), 1965-95. Estimates were obtained by multiplying number of prevalent smear-positive cases by rates of drug resistance (95% confidence intervals are attached to numbers of MDRTB cases, which are estimated from relatively small sample sizes). Bottom: percent of sputum smear-positive patients which were cured (squares) or treated successfully (cured + completed treatment; circles), 1981-93. Data from references 33, 34, and 35.

Trends of MDRTB prevalence country-wide in good DOTS programmes could provide a direct answer to such question. Unfortunately, only very scarce data are available at the moment for developing countries. Trend data from Korea are illustrative [33,34,35]. Figure 3 (top) shows that the estimated number of all resistant cases was falling slowly in Korea from 1965 to 1980, and then more steeply from 1980-85 onwards. MDRTB cases rose between 1975 and 1985, but were lower in 1990 and 1995. The fall in all resistant cases, and in MDRTB cases, coincides with a sharp increase in cure rates in Korea, especially between 1980 and 1985 (Figure 3, bottom). This is not sufficient to prove that one can eliminate MDRTB with good programmes alone. However, these data may suggest that DOTS can influence the decline of MDRTB by preventing the emergence of new MDRTB cases.

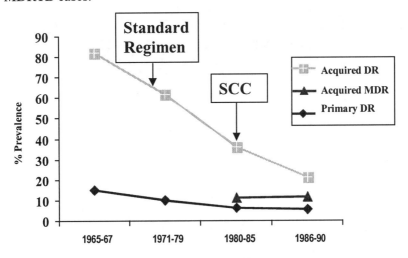

Figure 4. Drug resistance trend in Algeria between 1965 and 1990. The policy decisions that may have contributed to the trend are shown in the two boxes. Data from reference 36.

Another country where drug resistance trends have been studied is Algeria [36]. In the region of Algiers, from 1965 to 1990, drug resistance decreased from 15% to 5.2% among new cases and from 81.9% to 21% among cases for retreatment (Figure 4). This coincided with two important policy changes: the introduction of standard regimens in the late 1960s and that of rifampicin-containing SCC in 1980. However, whether the decline would have occurred regardless of these changes is not known, as previous trend data are not available. The trend of MDRTB over time has been reported among cases eligible for a retreatment regimen: there was no change in both numbers and percentages (11% and 11.5% respectively) between 1980-85 and 1986-90. Taken together, the experiences from Korea and Algeria suggest that MDRTB can be kept under control, but not substantially decreased, by introducing properly handled SCC.

In summary, the information available today on efficacy of SCC to treat TB is strongly suggesting that drug resistance will not be produced by programmes which can deliver drugs correctly to patients and cure them. On the other hand, the epidemiological information derived from the trends described above is still weak. Thus, while awaiting more conclusive data, it is fair to say that the standard SCC recommended as part of DOTS can minimise the creation of MDRTB but may not be sufficient to eliminate it, especially when it is a significant problem at the start of a revised control programme. The crucial factor fostering elimination is treatment success: at a given cure rate for both susceptible and drug- and multidrug-resistant cases, MDRTB will disappear. High cure rates of susceptible or "non-MDR drug-resistant" cases will ensure that "acquired" MDRTB is not created; as a result, "primary" MDRTB (i.e., multidrug resistant disease among new cases never treated before and therefore resulting from a primary infection with MDRTB strains) will also decline. At the same time, an increased cure rate of existing MDRTB will eliminate the sources of transmission in the community. The achievement of this cure rate remains, therefore, crucial.

6.   ELIMINATION OF MDRTB

There is evidence from the experience in New York City that MDRTB can be rapidly reduced [37]. Between 1991-1992 and 1994-1994, the total number of MDRTB cases nearly halved (44% decrease) by the implementation of effective control measures. These included proper SCC and directly observed therapy (DOT) allowing the achievement of high completion rates; infection control interventions in congregate settings, such as hospitals, shelters for the homeless, and jails; and the adoption of adequate treatment regimens for both cases with susceptible and MDR strains. The latter were treated with second-line drugs, in order to achieve high success rates [29]. Clearly, without agents such as amikacin, capreomycin, kanamycin, cycloserine, ethionamide, p-aminosalicylic acid and the fluoroquinolones, it will not be possible to substantially increase the cure rate above 50% [32]. At this level of cure, it is unlikely that MDRTB cases rapidly stop transmitting, therefore reducing the chances of elimination of MDRTB. What happened in the New York City can be summarised as follows: increased cure rates among susceptible and "non-MDR drug-resistant" cases produced a decline of "acquired" MDRTB. This, in turn, resulted in a reduction in transmission of MDRTB strains and, therefore a fall of "primary MDRTB". In addition, existing MDRTB cases were cured with second-line drugs and transmission was interrupted. Effective infection control interventions, such as isolation of infectious patients and active case finding in certain at-risk populations, also helped interrupt transmission.

As mentioned previously, standard SCC based on first-line agents (isoniazid, rifampicin, pyrazinamide, streptomycin, ethambutol, and thioacetazone) can only cure a limited proportion of MDRTB cases. This is not surprising, as the programmatic use of standard SCC regimens was conceived when MDRTB was not an issue. In addition, there is some evidence that patients, who at the start of treatment are already infected with strains resistant to isoniazid and rifampicin, risk selecting strains with additional resistance to other first-line drugs, if they are treated with standard SCC based on first-line drugs. This has been called an "amplifier effect" [4,5]. Anecdotes confirming this effect have been reported, although no published report is yet available in the scientific literature that attempts to quantify the importance of the phenomenon. Should the "amplifier effect" occur in more than a sporadic manner, the policy of providing standard regimens with first-line drugs to cases likely to be already infected with MDRTB strains will need to be revisited. Indeed, this will be particularly critical where the likelihood of (primary) MDRTB in cases never treated previously is high, as in the "hot spots" identified by the WHO/IUATLD Global Project [1].

In summary, standard SCC as recommended in DOTS programmes may not be able to achieve sufficiently high cure rates to eliminate MDRTB and carries the risk of causing additional drug resistance. Thus, one of the solutions seems to be the very cautious use of second-line drugs to treat MDRTB. Regimens based on these drugs have been shown to substantially increase the cure rate. We have already described the outcome of patients treated in New York City [29], where at least 64% were cured at the time of publication of the report, while another 28% were still on treatment and in remission (only 3 patients underwent surgery in addition to chemotherapy). Recently, a study on 107 MDRTB cases from Korea also showed treatment success in over 80% [38]. Preliminary information from a project in northern Lima, Peru, reveals that high cure rates are possible with the aggressive use of individualised regimens [5]. The National Tuberculosis Programme of Peru has also adopted new standard schemes, which include second-line drugs, for treatment of MDRTB cases. Preliminary data show relatively high (more than 70%) conversion rates at 6 and 9 months of treatment.

7. ADAPTING DOTS TO HIGH MDRTB BURDEN SETTINGS: RESEARCH ISSUES

The evidence currently available supports the necessity to adapt the DOTS strategy in settings where MDRTB is a major problem. In particular, the use of second-line line drugs in proper combinations needs to be implemented in an effective manner. The "trigger" for instituting treatment with second-line drugs needs to be re-evaluated, for instance, by introducing drug susceptibility testing earlier than the fourth month of retreatment as currently recommended [14]; and the recording and reporting system needs to be adapted to allow for longer duration of treatment and its monitoring.

A variety of research questions therefore arise. Are regimens based on second-line anti-tuberculosis drugs (also called "third-line regimens") efficacious? Are standardised regimens warranted? Is it feasible to use them under routine programme conditions, i.e., in settings, like small hospitals or even at community level [5], other than the "very specialised units" as recommended at the moment [39]?

Regarding the efficacy of third-line regimens, at best there is only empirical evidence supporting their use, due to the intrinsic difficulties of controlled clinical trials. A variety of regimens can be conceived depending upon the pattern of multidrug resistance, when this is known [39, 40]. A major issue to be faced is usefulness of standardised vs individualised regimens based on second-line drugs. The large majority of data available today and mentioned above are based on the individualised use of drugs with regimens tailored following drug susceptibility patterns. In reality, a closer look at the issue allows one to follow certain rules to design a regimen, as outlined in recent consensus recommendations [39]. By using a flexible approach, which depends on the drug susceptibility pattern, it will be possible to prescribe effective regimens in a semi-standardised manner. The use of standardised third-line regimens is indicated when the drug susceptibility pattern is not (yet) known and there is the strong suspicion of MDRTB, i.e., among chronic excretors and/or failures of standard first-line retreatment regimens [41].

The crucial question, however, is that of feasibility. Can we indeed promote the proper use of regimens based on second-line drugs at programmatic level in developing countries? A number of problems need to be solved:

1. to ensure adequate drug susceptibility testing of first-line drugs, so that MDRTB can be reliably detected;

2. to establish the best timing for performing drug susceptibility testing in order to shorten the time of detection of MDRTB and, therefore, reduce transmission;

3. to assess the possibility, using smear microscopy, to switch patients to second-line line drugs when detecting failure to convert at 2-3 months, rather than waiting until 4 months later when patients, at that point declared failures, might have infected additional contacts;
4. to ensure an uninterrupted supply of expensive and good quality second-line drugs;
5. to guarantee that these drugs are administered in proper regimens and under strict supervision, so that they are not lost for the future by the creation of additional resistance;
6. to monitor adequately the response to therapy during a 18-24-month long course of treatment; and
7. to ensure that the intervention (drug susceptibility testing, second-line drug use) is cost-effective in an era dominated by economic forces and competition with other health priorities.

In addition to these practical problems, other questions need to be answered in order to maximise our understanding of MDRTB and potentially to allow further interventions. For instance, can the duration of infectiousness be decreased in such a way that transmission is reduced, for example by conducting active case finding and rapidly detecting cases at the start? Also, is the virulence of multidrug-resistant strains of *Mycobacterium tuberculosis* somewhat lower than that of susceptible strains? If this were the case, only vulnerable fragments of the population, such as the HIV-infected, may develop disease following infection and specific interventions can be targeted effectively.

To answer some of these questions, WHO has recently established a Working Group on DOTS-plus to support pilot projects assessing the feasibility of interventions in a variety of settings prior to formulating policy recommendations on management of MDRTB [6]. For the purpose of the activities of such a Group, DOTS-plus has been preliminarily defined as a "case management strategy designed to manage MDRTB using second-line drugs within the DOTS strategy in low- and middle-income countries" [6]. Another chapter will further describe DOTS-plus.

8.   CONCLUSION

In this chapter, the current evidence on the relationship of DOTS and MDRTB both in terms of cause and effects was outlined. The main conclusion is that standard SCC as part of DOTS can prevent MDRTB from arising, but can only achieve limited success among existing MDRTB cases. On the other hand, with the careful use of second-line drugs, provided DOTS is in place to stop the production of new drug resistance, it is possible to achieve higher cure rates. These, coupled with an earlier detection of MDRTB cases, may effectively stop transmission of MDRTB in the community and eventually eliminate it as a public health problem. The confirmation of this possibility will only come from studying the trends of the prevalence of MDRTB after the implementation of DOTS-plus pilot projects. Meanwhile, modelling exercises, as described elsewhere in the book, can help predict what might happen and guide the choice of interventions.

ACKNOWLEDGEMENTS

The author would like to thank Dr H. Rieder, IUATLD, Dr C. Dye, WHO/CDS, Dr P. Nunn, WHO/CDS, and Professor J. Grosset for their comments and contributions to this paper.

REFERENCES

1. Pablos-Mendez A, Raviglione MC, Laszlo A et al. Global surveillance for antituberculosis-drug resistance, 1994-1997. N Engl J Med 1998; 338:1641-1649.
2. Laszlo A, Rahman M, Raviglione M, Bustreo F and the WHO/IUATLD Network of Supranational Reference Laboratories. Quality assurance programme for drug susceptibility testing of *Mycobacterium tuberculosis* in the WHO/IUATLD Supranational Laboratory Network: first round of proficiency testing. Int J Tuberc Lung Dis 1997; 1:231-238.
3. Cohn DL, Bustreo F, Raviglione MC. Drug resistance in tuberculosis: review of the worldwide situation and WHO/IUATLD's Global Surveillance Project. Clin Infect Dis 1997; 24(Suppl.1):S121-S130.
4. Farmer P, Bayona J, Becerra M, Furin J, Henry C, Hiatt H et al. The dilemma of MDR-TB in the global era. Int J Tuberc Lung Dis 1998; 2:869-76.
5. Farmer P, Kim JY. Community-based approaches to the control of multidrug-resistant tuberculosis: introducing "DOTS-PLUS". Br Med J 1998; 317: 671-674.
6. Communicable Diseases. Coordination of DOTS-PLUS pilot projects for the management of MDR-TB. Proceedings of a Meeting. Geneva, 29 January 1999. Edited by: Espinal MA, Raviglione MC. Geneva, 1999. WHO/TB/99.262.
7. World Health Organization. WHO Tuberculosis Programme. Framework for effective tuberculosis control. WHO/TB/94.179, Geneva, 1994.
8. World Health Organization. Global Tuberculosis Programme (Raviglione M, Schmidt S, Nunn P, Dye C, Spinaci S, Chaulet P, Grzemska M, Hanson C, Kumaresan J, Levy M, Luelmo F, Tayler E, Kochi A) Global tuberculosis control. WHO Report 1997. Geneva, Switzerland, WHO/TB/97.225.
9   World Health Organization. Global Tuberculosis Programme (Netto EM, Dye C, Schmidt S, Raviglione M). Global tuberculosis control. WHO Report 1998. Geneva, Switzerland, WHO/TB/98.237.

10 World Health Organization. Communicable Diseases (Netto EM, Dye C, Raviglione M). Global tuberculosis control. WHO Report 1999. Geneva, Switzerland, WHO/CPC/TB/99.259.

11. Raviglione MC, Dye C, Schmidt S, Kochi A for the WHO Global Surveillance and Monitoring Project. Assessment of worldwide tuberculosis control. Lancet 1997; 350:624-629.

12. Styblo K, Raviglione MC. Tuberculosis, public health aspects. In Dulbecco R., Ed. "Encyclopedia of human biology", Second Edition, Vol. 8. Academic Press, 1997.

13. Enarson DA. The International Union Against Tuberculosis and Lung Disease model National Tuberculosis Programme. Tuberc Lung Dis 1995; 76:95-99.

14. World Health Organization. Treatment of tuberculosis. Guidelines for National Programmes. Second Edition 1997. Geneva, 1997. WHO/TB/97.220.

15. Ministerio de Salud, Dirección General de Salud de Las Personas, Dirección del Programa Nacional de Control de Enfermedades Transmisibles Control de la Tuberculosis. Seminario Taller: Evaluación del Programa Nacional de Control de la Tuberculosis en el Perú-año 1997, Lima, Perú.

16. Norval P-Y, Kim San K, Bakhim T, Rith DN, Ahn DI, Blanc L. DOTS in Cambodia. Int J Tuberc Lung Dis 1998; 2:44-51.

17. China Tuberculosis Control Collaboration. Results of directly observed short-course chemotherapy in 112 842 Chinese patients with smear-positive tuberculosis. Lancet 1996; 347:358-62.

18. Kumaresan JA, Ahsan Ali AKMd, Parkkali LM. Tuberculosis control in Bangladesh: success of the DOTS strategy. Int J Tuberc Lung Dis 1998; 2:992-998.

19. Pablos-Méndez A, Laszlo A, Bustreo F, Binkin N, Cohn DL, Lambregts-van Weezembeek C, Kim SJ, Chaulet P, Nunn P, Raviglione MC and the members of the WHO/IUATLD Global Project on Anti-tuberculosis Drug Resistance Surveillance. Anti-tuberculosis drug resistance in the world. Global Tuberculosis Programme, World Health Organization, Geneva, Switzerland, 1997 (WHO/TB/97.229).

20. WHO/IUATLD Global Working Group on Antimicrobial Drug Resistance Surveillance. Guidelines for surveillance of drug resistance in tuberculosis, 1997. Edited by Bustreo F, Pablos-Mendez A, Raviglione M, Murray J, Trébucq A, Rieder H. Geneva, Switzerland, WHO/TB/96.216

21. Drolet GJ. Present trend of case fatality rates in tuberculosis. Am Rev Tuberc 1938; 37:125-151.

22. National Tuberculosis Institute, Bangalore. Tuberculosis in a rural population of India: a five-year epidemiological study. Bull World Health Organ 1974; 51:473-88.

23. Centers for Disease Control. Nosocomial transmission of multidrug-resistant tuberculosis among HIV-infected persons – Florida and New York, 1988-1991. MMWR 1991; 40: 585-591.

24. Centers for Disease Control and Prevention. Outbreak of multidrug-resistant tuberculosis at a hospital. MMWR 1993; 42: 427-434.

25. Edlin BR, Tokars JL, Brieco MH, et al. An outbreak of multi-drug resistant tuberculosis among hospitalized patients with the acquired immunodeficiency syndrome. N Engl J Med 1992; 326: 1514-1521.

26. Fischl MA, Uttamchandani RB, Daikos GL, et al. An outbreak of tuberculosis caused by multiple-drug-resistant tubercle bacilli among patients with HIV infection. Ann Intern Med 1992; 117: 177-183.

27. Busillo CP, Lessnau CD, Sanjana V et al. Multidrug resistant *Mycobacterium* tuberculosis in patients with human immunodeficiency virus infection. Chest 1992; 102:797-801

28. Goble M, Iseman MD, Madsen LA et al. Treatment of 171 patients with pulmonary tuberculosis resistant to isoniazid and rifampin. N Engl J Med 1993; 328:527-32.
29. Telzak EE, Sepkowitz K, Alpert P et al. Multidrug-resistant tuberculosis in patients without HIV infection. N Engl J Med 1995; 33:907-911.
30. Coates ARM, Mitchison DA. The role of sensitivity tests in short-course chemotherapy. Bull Int Union Tuberc Lung Dis 1983; 58:110-114.
31. Mitchison DA, Nunn AJ. Influence of initial drug resistance on the response to short-course chemotherapy of pulmonary tuberculosis. Am Rev Respir Dis 1986; 133:423-430.
32. Espinal MA, Kim SJ, Hong YP et al. Treatment outcome of multidrug resistant (MDR) tuberculosis (TB) cases under programme conditions. Proceedings of the Global Congress on Lung Health, 29th World Conference of International Union Against Tuberculosis and Lung Disease, IUATLD/UICTMR. Abstract 428-PC. Bangkok, Thailand, 23-26 November 1998. Int J Tuberc Lung Dis 1998; 2 (suppl. 2): S371.
33. Hong YP, Kim SJ, Lew WJ, Lee EK, Han YC. The seventh nationwide tuberculosis prevalence survey in Korea, 1995. Int J Tuber Lung Dis 1998; 2:27-36.
34. Kim SJ, Bai SH, Hong YP. Drug-resistant tuberculosis in Korea. Int J Tuber Lung Dis 1997; 1:302-8.
35. Espinal M, Dye C, Raviglione M, Kochi A. Rational "DOTS Plus" for the control of MDR-TB. Int J Tuber Lung Dis 1999 (in press).
36. Chaulet P. Tuberculose et transition épidémiologique: le cas de l'Algérie. Annales de l'Institut Pasteur 1993; 4:181-187.
37. Frieden TR, Fujiwara PI, Washko RM, Hamburg MA. Tuberculosis in New York City - turning the tide. N Engl J Med 1995; 333:229-33.
38. Park SK, Kim CT, Song SD. Outcome of chemotherapy in 107 patients with pulmonary tuberculosis resistant to isoniazid and rifampin. Int J Tuberc Lung Dis 1998; 2:877-884.
39. Crofton J, Chaulet P, Maher D et al. Guidelines for the management of drug-resistant tuberculosis. Geneva, 1997. WHO/TB/96.210
40. Iseman MD. Treatment of multidrug-resistant tuberculosis. N Engl J Med 1993; 329: 784-791.
41. Communicable Disease. Report. Multidrug resistant tuberculosis - Basis for the development of an evidence-based case-management strategy for MDR-TB within the WHO's DOTS strategy. Proceedings of 1998 Meetings and Protocol Recommendations. Edited by Espinal MA. Geneva, 1999. WHO/TB/99.260.

Chapter 8

Conventional methods for antimicrobial susceptibility testing of *Mycobacterium tuberculosis*

Leonid Heifets
National Jewish Medical and Research Center, Denver, Colorado

1.   INTRODUCTION

The growing prevalence of MDRTB around the world places the importance of *M. tuberculosis* drug susceptibility testing (DST), especially for initial clinical isolates, in a new perspective. An alternative to detection of MDRTB by a laboratory test is an empirical assumption based on the patient's failure to respond to the standard treatment regimen. Such an option lacks accuracy, and it can be dangerous and costly. It can be dangerous for individual patients, who may receive inappropriate treatment, and it is costly for society because of the prolonged period during which a patient with MDRTB is infectious. Management of patients with MDRTB, even if their numbers are still small, can be much more expensive than the cost of DST of the initial isolates from all new patients. The DOTS-plus strategy, which is discussed in another chapter [1], particularly administration of non-standard treatment regimens for patients with MDRTB, cannot be fully successful if such regimens are not selected on the basis of DST results.

Implementation of a system for DST in areas with increasing levels of drug resistance requires a technology that can provide a reasonable balance between the cost and turnaround time (TAT). The DST system is also most likely to be economically affordable and to provide optimal results if it is based on direct delivery of raw specimens to a central mycobacteriology laboratory that has a large operational volume, has well trained personnel,

133

I. Bastian and F. Portaels (eds.), Multidrug-Resistant Tuberculosis, 133-143.
© 2000 *Kluwer Academic Publishers. Printed in the Netherlands.*

and is properly equipped [2,3]. This chapter addresses the advantages and disadvantages of conventional methods only, and consists of the following sections: a) general principles, b) methods for egg-based solid medium, c) the proportion method for agar media, d) broth-based radiometric (BACTEC®) indirect qualitative test, and e) conclusions.

2.   GENERAL PRINCIPLES OF A DRUG SUSCEPTIBILITY TEST

The main requirement for a DST is the ability to make a distinction between susceptible and resistant *M. tuberculosis* strains. Such a distinction by a traditional phenotypic strategy based on cultivation is quite feasible because *M. tuberculosis* isolates from patients never before treated are quite uniform in the degree of their susceptibility, as evidenced by the relatively narrow ranges of the minimum inhibitory concentrations (MICs) of the conventional antituberculosis drugs [4,5]. The classical definition of a drug-resistant strain of *M. tuberculosis* is that it is significantly different by the degree of susceptibility from a wild strain that has never come into contact with the drug [6,7]. The drug concentrations to distinguish susceptible and resistant strains, so-called 'critical concentrations', should be somewhere between the highest MIC found among the wild strains and the lowest MIC found among the isolates considered resistant. Progress in molecular biology may provide a new definition of drug resistance, but also may raise new questions to be addressed, especially considering that resistance to some drugs has more than one genetic mechanism responsible for low and high levels of resistance [8]. It should also be taken into account that phenotypic differences in the degree of resistance may reflect differences in the proportions of resistant mutants in the bacterial population.

Different methods for *M. tuberculosis* drug susceptibility testing, as well as their advantages and disadvantages, have been discussed in our previous review [2]. Drug susceptibility methods based on mycobacterial cultivation on solid media, either egg- or agar-based, can be performed as a direct or indirect test. In the *direct* test a set of drug-containing and drug-free media is inoculated directly with a concentrated specimen. An *indirect* test is the inoculation of the media with a pure culture and it is classically performed with a bacterial suspension made from growth on solid media (Lowenstein-Jensen, 7H10, or 7H11 agar). A 7H9 broth culture can be used for the same purpose when it is grown up to the turbidity of a McFarland Standard No. 1 (5 to 8 days), and two dilutions, 10^{-3} and 10^{-5}, are then used as inocula. For 7H12 broth cultures as a source of the inoculum, dilutions of 10^{-2} and 10^{-4} can be used when the daily radiometric growth index reaches 800 or higher.

The advantage of the direct over the indirect tests is that the results are available sooner (within 3 weeks on agar plates), and better represent the patient's original bacterial population. If the results of the direct test are not valid because there is insufficient or excessive growth in drug-free controls or heavy contamination, the test must be repeated with a pure culture, i.e., as an indirect test.

Antimicrobial agents to be incorporated into culture medium should be obtained in pure forms from the manufacturer (not from pharmacy). Appropriate stock solutions of the drugs should be made in accordance with the batch potency provided by the manufacturer. For example, if 25 ml of a stock solution of 10,000 µg/ml is needed and the drug has a potency of 940 mg/g, the following amount of drug powder is to be weighed and dissolved in 25 ml of the solvent: (10,000 x 25)/940 = 265.96 mg. Class A volumetric flasks should be used to make the stock solutions, and the drug powder should be weighed on a certified analytical balance. The diluent appropriate for each drug is indicated by the drug manufacturer or can be found listed in the Merck Index. For example, distilled water is recommended for isoniazid, streptomycin, PAS, kanamycin, amikacin, capreomycin, ethambutol, ofloxacin, and pyrazinamide. Rifampin should be dissolved in methanol, DMSO, or in 95% ethanol. Ethionamide and thiacetazone can be dissolved in ethylene glycol (analytical grade) or in dimethylsulfoxide. The stock solutions of the water-soluble drugs should be sterilized through a 0.45 µm pore size membrane filter. Aliquots of the stock solutions should be kept in special vials at either –70°C for no more than 12 months or at –20°C for not more than 2 months. When needed, one of these vials can be used to prepare the working solutions in sterile distilled water. After thawing, the stock solution vial must not be refrozen.

3. DRUG SUSCEPTIBILITY TESTS USING EGG-BASED MEDIUM

Three methods were originally suggested by the World Health Organization (WHO) panel for starch-free Lowenstein-Jensen (L-J) medium: a) the proportion method, b) the resistance ratio (RR) method, and c) the absolute concentration method [6,7].

3.1 The original proportion method (simplified variant)

The appropriate drug solutions are added to the medium before coagulation. Both drug-containing and drug-free (control) media are distributed into tubes that are placed in a slope position for coagulation at

85°C for 50 minutes. Afterwards, the tubes are left at room temperature overnight, and then stored in the refrigerator for no more than two months. The final concentrations of drugs incorporated into this medium for a simplified variant of the test are shown in Table 1. The original standard variant, not presented in this chapter, requires additional concentrations [4,7]. The inocula are prepared from a well-dispersed bacterial suspension adjusted to the optical density of a standard containing 1 mg/ml wet weight of bacterial harvest, after which 10^{-3} and 10^{-5} dilutions are inoculated in two sets of drug-containing and drug-free tubes, 0.1 ml per each slope. The tubes, with caps slightly ajar, are left for 24-48 hrs in a sloped position that allows the inoculum to be absorbed by the medium, after which the caps are tightened, and the tubes are incubated at 37°C in an upright position. After 28 days of incubation the colonies on the drug-containing and drug-free slopes are counted to calculate the proportion of resistant bacteria. Any proportion that exceeds 1% for isoniazid, rifampin and para-aminosalicylic acid (PAS), or 10% for the remaining drugs, indicates "resistant" and the results are final. If the proportion is less than this, a second reading is required at the 42nd day of cultivation in order to determine whether the isolate is, in fact, "susceptible."

Table 1. Critical concentrations (μg/ml) for *M. tuberculosis* in different media

Drug	LJ (proportion method)	7H10 agar	7H11 Agar	BACTEC® 7H12[a]
Isoniazid	0.2	0.2, 1.0	0.2, 1.0	0.1
Rifampin	40.0	1.0	1.0	0.5
Rifapentine		0.5	0.5	0.5
Streptomycin	4.0	2.0	2.0, 10.0	4.0
Pyrazinamide	100.0[b]			300.0[c]
Ethambutol	2.0	5.0	7.5	4.0
Ethionamide	20.0	5.0	10.0	2.5
Kanamycin	20.0	5.0	6.0	5.0
Amikacin			4.0	5.0
Capreomycin	20.0	10.0	10.0	5.0
Thiacetazone				3.0
PAS[d]	0.5	2.0	8.0	
Cycloserine		20.0	60.0	
Ofloxacin			4.0	2.0
Ciprofloxacin			4.0	2.0

[a] concentrations in use at the National Jewish Medical and Research Center; [b] at pH 5.5; [c] at pH 6.0; [d] PAS, para-aminosalicylic acid.

3.2   The resistance-ratio (RR) method

The RR is defined as a ratio of the MIC for the patient's strain to the MIC for the drug-susceptible reference strain, H37Rv, both tested in the same experiment [6,7]. Inclusion of the reference strain in each experiment is not just for quality control, but also to standardize the results by taking into account the test variations within certain permissible limits. This feature made the RR method the most accurate, but, because of the use of large numbers of media units, also the most expensive among the three conventional methods performed on solid media. For example, for a test with isoniazid, five concentrations ranging from 0.025 to 1.0 µg/ml should be used for the $H_{37}Rv$ strain, while concentrations of 0.2, 1.0, 5.0, 50.0 µg/ml are needed for the tested isolates. The original description of the RR method includes details of preparation of the inoculum that ensures that the suspension contains mostly viable bacteria [6,7]. Reading after 4 weeks of incubation defines "growth" on any slope as the presence of 20 or more colonies, and MIC is defined as the lowest drug concentration in the presence of which the number of colonies is less than 20. "The range required for the test strain is determined by the variation in the minimal inhibitory concentration (MIC) of H37Rv, and by the need to determine a resistance ratio of 2 or less for sensitive strains and a resistance ratio of 8 or more for resistant strains" [7].

3.3 The absolute concentration method

The critical concentrations to be incorporated into the medium are similar to those used in the proportion method, but the actual drug concentration considered "critical" should be established for each laboratory. Growth of 20 or more colonies in the presence of these concentrations is an indication of resistance. For testing of the QC strain ($H_{37}Rv$), three additional concentrations are needed: isoniazid-1.0, 0.05, 0.01; streptomycin-10.0, 2.0, 1.0; PAS-2.0, 0.2, 0.1; thiacetazone-5.0, 0.5, 0.1; ethionamide-50.0, 10.0, 5.0.

Bacterial suspensions are adjusted by the optical standard to have the turbidity equivalent to 1.0 mg/ml of wet weight, and diluted 1:50, which gives about $2x10^5$ to 10^6 bacteria per ml. The actual inoculum per tube made with a loop should contain $5x10^3$ to 10^4 bacteria. The drug-containing cultures and two drug-free controls are incubated at 37^oC for 4 weeks, and for 5-6 weeks if the growth is insufficient at the four-week reading. The readings are reported as: ++++ for confluent growth, +++ and ++ for discrete colonies in large number, + for 50 to 100 colonies, and (+) for 20 to 49 colonies. The inhibition of growth is reported if the number of colonies is less than 20, with ++++ or +++ growth in the drug-free controls.

4.   DIRECT AND INDIRECT TESTS USING 7H10/7H11 AGAR

In addition to the basic equipment necessary for a test in L-J medium, cultivation on 7H10/7H11 agar requires an incubator that can provide 5-10% CO_2, and the plates should be sealed in CO_2-permeable plastic bags after inoculation. The advantage of performing tests in agar plates is that the final results can be reported within 3 weeks instead of 4 to 6 weeks or more, as required using Lowenstein-Jensen medium.

4.1   Original CDC version

The Centers for Disease Control (CDC) recommend that the test be performed on 7H10 agar [9], with the drug concentrations shown in Table 1. The critical proportion of bacteria in the population designating the strain "resistant" is 1% (rather than 10%) for all drugs tested by the agar proportion method.   The 7H10 or 7H11 agar medium is usually made from commercially available Middlebrook 7H10 agar base.   The powder is suspended in distilled water in sterile flasks, autoclaved at 121^oC for 10 minutes and cooled to $52-54^oC$ in a water bath. Oleic acid-albumin-dextrose-catalase (OADC) enrichment is added aseptically in the amount of 10% of the volume to the cooled agar solution. Each flask of the medium is used to prepare either a drug-free control or one of the drug-containing media.   The appropriate working solutions of the drugs, made from an aliquot of the stock solution, are added to ensure the final concentrations indicated in the Table. The contents of each flask are distributed to one of the quadrants in a set of sterile quadrant plates, about 5.0 ml per quadrant, one quadrant for a drug-free medium and three others for media containing drugs. Two quadrant plates (each with a drug-free quadrant) are necessary for a test with four first-line drugs, and four plates for 10 drugs. After overnight incubation in the dark at 37^oC, drug plates are stored protected from light, in the refrigerator and must be used within 4 weeks of preparation.

For each strain, two identical sets of plates are used, one inoculated with 10^{-3} and the other with 10^{-5} dilutions of the bacterial suspension (if it is an indirect test), adjusted to the optical density of the McFarland Standard No. 1, 0.1 ml per quadrant. The plates are incubated for three weeks at 35^oC to 37^oC in an atmosphere of 10% CO_2. The results can be reported earlier if they show that the strain is "resistant." The percentage of resistant bacteria in the population is reported on the basis of comparison of the number of colony-forming units (CFU) on drug-containing and drug-free quadrants. More details on this technique can be found in the CDC manual [9].

4.2   Disc version of the proportion method

The CDC version of the proportion method is feasible when a substantial number of strains are tested in the laboratory systematically. Another technique can be used when a small number of cultures have to be tested [10,11]. Drug-impregnated discs are placed aseptically into the centers of the quadrants of the plates, and <u>exactly</u> 5.0 ml of OADC-supplemented 7H10 agar is pipetted over the disc. The discs must remain submerged. The plates are left overnight at room temperature (5°C for ethambutol-containing plates) to allow the drugs to diffuse into the agar. The following commercially available discs can be used for this technique (μg per disc): isoniazid-1.0, streptomycin-10.0, ethambutol-25.0, rifampin-5.0, PAS-10.0, ethionamide-25.0, and kanamycin-30.0.

4.3   National Jewish modification of the proportion method

7H11 instead of 7H10 agar is used in our laboratory because it provides better growth for multidrug-resistant strains that may not grow at all on the 7H10 agar. Critical concentrations developed for 7H11 agar [12] are different for five drugs as shown in Table 1.

5.   INDIRECT TEST IN LIQUID MEDIUM (BACTEC® METHOD)

New liquid medium systems (MB/BacT, MGIT, ESP) have been introduced recently, but so far, only the radiometric BACTEC-460® system (Becton Dickinson, Sparks, MD) has been approved by the Food and Drug Administration (FDA) for drug susceptibility testing in the United States. The liquid medium for this system, 7H12 broth, currently manufactured in the so-called 12B vials (4.0 ml in each), contains 7H9 broth base, casein hydrolysate, bovine serum albumin, catalase, and ^{14}C-fatty acid. Consumption of the ^{14}C-substrate by the growing bacteria results in release of the $^{14}CO_2$, the amount of which is expressed by the instrument as a growth index (GI) on a scale of 0 to 999. In the presence of an antimicrobial agent, susceptibility is detected by the inhibition of daily GI increases [4,13,14]. The major advantage of this technique is the ability to detect growth and its inhibition earlier than by any other means. In our laboratory, an indirect DST in this system required an average of 9.3 days [15]. The overall mean time for primary isolation plus indirect test was 18 days in a cooperative study by five institutions [13]. The major disadvantage of the BACTEC®

system is the problem of disposal of a large volume of radioactive materials (12B vials), though of very low radioactivity. Another disadvantage is the cost, which is much higher than for any of the solid media, though it is less expensive than the newer non-radioactive liquid medium systems [2].

The BACTEC® method, using 12B vials containing standard 7H12 broth (pH 6.8), has been approved by the FDA as a qualitative test with four first-line drugs: isoniazid, rifampin, ethambutol, and streptomycin. An additional test with pyrazinamide requires special BACTEC® medium (PZA vials) of pH 6.0. The manufacturer has been changing over time the critical concentrations of some drugs to improve the outcome of the test: streptomycin from 4.0 to 2.0 µg/ml, and ethambutol from 7.5 to 2.5 µg/ml. According to a number of reports, the new concentrations, especially of ethambutol 2.5 µg/ml, appear to be too low, and it may take an extended period of time until the company will be able to make another change in their official documents. In the meantime, based on our many years of experience with this system, we have been successfully using different drug-concentrations [4], which are shown in Table 1. Another difference from the manufacturer's manual is the concentration of pyrazinamide – we use 300.0 instead of 100.0 µg/ml [16]. In addition, as shown in Table 1, we have established critical concentrations for other drugs to be used in this system: ethionamide, kanamycin/amikacin, capreomycin, thiacetazone, ofloxacin/ciprofloxacin and rifapentine [4,17]. Besides the qualitative test with one critical concentration, there is also an option for a quantitative test for MIC determination, which requires at least two additional concentrations of each drug [4].

To perform a test, the appropriate working drug solutions (40-fold concentrates of the required final target concentrations) are added to the vials, 0.1 ml of each, using allergist syringes with fixed 27 1/2 G needle (BD catalog No. 5540). Lyophilized drugs can be purchased from the BACTEC® manufacturer. The original 12B culture can be used undiluted as the inoculum, 0.1 ml per vial, if the GI is between 300 and 800. If GI is 800 or higher, the culture in the "seed vial" (4.0 ml) should be diluted by adding 2.0 ml of diluting fluid. Two drug-free controls are required: the first is inoculated with the same suspension as for the drug-containing vials, and the second control is inoculated with 1:100 diluted bacterial suspension (1:10 for the pyrazinamide test). The curves of daily-recorded GIs in drug-containing vials are compared with those in two drug-free controls. It is assumed that the culture contains more than 1% resistant bacteria (10% in a test with pyrazinamide) if growth in the drug-containing vial progresses to a higher level than that in the 1:100 control (1:10 for pyrazinamide). On the other hand, the culture is considered "susceptible" if there are no significant daily GI increases in the presence of the critical drug concentration and the GI in the diluted control reaches a higher level than that in the drug-containing vial. Even assuming that this technique has the ability to distinguish between fully susceptible isolates and those containing 1% (10% for pyrazinamide) or more resistant bacteria, this method cannot determine the actual proportion of resistant bacteria in a culture. Therefore, it is a misnomer to call this technique the "BACTEC proportion method" as it has been labelled in one of the NCCLS documents [18]. In addition, there is evidence that the BACTEC® method may not be a reliable tool for detecting resistance in cultures containing less than 10% of drug-resistant bacteria [17]. Drug susceptibility testing in the BACTEC® system is reasonable if the same system is also used for the primary culture isolation. The total TAT of an indirect test with four drugs (including primary isolation) for most isolates is usually less than three weeks.

The manufacturer of the BACTEC® system has proposed using this system for a direct DST as well. This approach did not find practical application in clinical laboratories for the following reasons:
1. an extended TAT, not different in most cases from a combination of isolation plus an indirect test (21 days),
2. a proposed new standard of 10% instead 1% of the "critical proportion" of resistant bacteria to call the isolate "resistant",
3. the unknown effect of five antibiotics (PANTA), which were added to prevent the growth of contaminants, and
4. the excessive cost of unnecessary testing of unidentified nontuberculous mycobacteria (NTM) in areas with high rates of NTM.

Taking into account these well known problems with the direct test in the BACTEC® system, one should be even more cautious with any temptation to use other liquid medium systems (for example, MGIT) for direct susceptibility testing. In these media, which are richer than 7H12 broth, the rates of contamination may be much higher. In addition, if such an attempt is made in conjunction with a decontamination procedure, which is less vigorous than the NALC-NaOH method (for example, with 10% trisodium phosphate), the rate of contamination may become even higher.

6. CONCLUSIONS

Conventional methods provide an opportunity to select from a variety of protocols, depending on the number of DSTs to be performed, the availability of funds and the estimated cost-effectiveness, the equipment available, the particular drug resistances to be detected, etc. Here are some options ranked by increasing cost.

1. A "one plate strategy" to detect resistance to just two drugs may be the least expensive option using one 7H10/7H11 agar quadrant plate for either a direct test with smear-positive specimens, or an indirect test with cultures isolated from smear-negative specimens or when the direct test fails. The drug-free quadrant is for primary isolation but also serves as a 'no antibiotic' control, while the agar in the three other quadrants contains rifampin (1.0 µg/ml), and isoniazid (0.2 and 1.0 µg/ml). An agar bi-plate (with plain and selective 7H11 agar) can be used to attempt culture isolation from smear-negative specimens. The cost of supplies per test is about $1.00, if the medium is made in the laboratory. Turnaround time for the direct test is 3-4 weeks.

2. A similar approach, combining direct and indirect test by a proportion method with an attempt of culture isolation, can be done using L-J medium. Disadvantages: longer turnaround time, use of multiple tubes for each specimen, difficulties in reading the direct test results. Advantage: no need for a CO_2 incubator. The cost of supplies is about the same as in option 1. Turnaround time for the direct test is 4-6 weeks.

3. Testing on either of the solid media with the four first-line drugs.

4. Testing on either of the solid media with all drugs.

5. Inclusion of the BACTEC® system (in addition to solid media) for: a) rapid culture isolation, b) indirect test in case of failure of the direct test on a solid medium, c) indirect test with cultures isolated from smear-negative specimens, d) the pyrazinamide susceptibility test.

REFERENCES

1. Farmer PE, Shin SS, Bayona J, et al. DOTS-plus, Chapter 19, 285-306. In: Bastian I, Portaels F (eds.), Multidrug-resistant tuberculosis. Kluwer Academic Publ., The Netherlands, 2000.

2. Heifets L, Cangelosi GA. Drug susceptibility testing of *Mycobacterium tuberculosis* -- a neglected problem at the turn of the century. Int J Tuber Lung Dis 1999; 3: 564-581.

3. Foulds J, O'Brien R. New tools of the diagnosis of tuberculosis: the perspective of developing countries. Int J Tuberc Lung Dis 1998; 2: 778-83.

4. Heifets LB. Drug susceptibility tests in the management of chemotherapy of tuberculosis, Chapter 3, 89-121. In: Heifets LB (ed.), Drug susceptibility in the chemotherapy of mycobacterial infections. CRC Press, Boca Raton 1991.

5. Heifets L. Drug susceptibility testing in mycobacteriology. Clin Lab Med 1996; 16: 641-56.

6. Canetti G, Froman S, Grosset J, et al. Mycobacteria: laboratory methods for testing drug sensitivity and resistance. Bull World Hlth Org 1963; 29: 565-78.

7. Canetti G, Fox W, Khomenko A, et al. Advances in techniques of testing mycobacterial drug sensitivity and the use of sensitivity tests in tuberculosis control programs. Bull World Hlth Org 1969; 41: 21-43.

8. Telenti A. Genetics of drug resistance in tuberculosis. Clin Chest Med 1997: 18: 55-64.

9.   Kent PT, Kubica GP. Public Health Mycobacteriology. A guide for the Level III Laboratory. Centers for Disease Control, Atlanta, GA, 1985.

10. Wayne LG, Krasnow I. Preparation of tuberculosis susceptibility testing medium by means of impregnated discs. Am J Clin Pathol 1966; 45: 769-71.

11. Griffith DE, Barrett HL, Bodily HL, Wood RM. Drug susceptibility tests for tuberculosis using drug impregnated discs. Am J Clin Pathol 1967; 47: 812-17.

12. McClatchy JK. Susceptibility testing of mycobacteria. Lab Med 1978; 9: 47-52.

13. Roberts G, Goodman NL, Heifets L, et al. Evaluation of the BACTEC radiometric method for recovery of mycobacteria and drug susceptibility testing of *M. tuberculosis* from acid-fast smear-positive specimens. J Clin Microbiol 1983; 18: 689-96.

14. Siddiqi SH, Libonati JP, Middlebrook G. Evaluation of rapid radiometric method for drug susceptibility testing of *M. tuberculosis*. J Clin Microbiol 1981; 13: 908-12.

15. Heifets L. Rapid automated methods (BACTEC system) in clinical mycobacteriology. Sem Respir Inf 1986, 1; 242-249.

16. Heifets LB. Pyrazinamide, 668-76. In: Yu V, Merigan TC, Barriere SL. (eds.), Antimicrobial Therapy and Vaccines. Williams and Wilkins (Waverly Company), Baltimore 1999.

17. Heifets L, Sanchez T, Vanderkolk J, Pham V. Development of rifapentine susceptibility tests for *Mycobacterium tuberculosis*. Antimicrob Agents Chemother 1999; 43: 25-8.

18. National Committee for Clinical Laboratory Standards. Antimycobacterial susceptibility testing for *M. tuberculosis*. Tentative standard M2-T, Villanova, PA , 1995.

Chapter 9

Novel rapid antimicrobial susceptibility tests for *Mycobacterium tuberculosis*

Juan Carlos Palomino
Mycobacteriology Unit, Institute of Tropical Medicine, Antwerp, Belgium

1.   INTRODUCTION

Recent advances in the field of molecular biology and progress in the understanding of the molecular basis of *Mycobacterium tuberculosis* drug resistance have provided new tools for the rapid detection of drug resistance. However, partly due to the costs involved in their implementation, these novel techniques have not been applied in most clinical mycobacteriology laboratories, especially in low-income countries where tuberculosis (TB) constitutes a more serious health problem. Conventional methods such as the proportion method [1], the absolute concentration method, and the resistance-ratio method [2], are based on the measurement of growth in culture media containing antibiotics, and usually take several weeks to obtain results. The introduction of the BACTEC® radiometric system, and its adaptation for performing drug susceptibility testing (DST) of *M. tuberculosis* (BACTEC® TB-460), was therefore a major breakthrough for the rapid detection of mycobacterial growth and for the detection of drug resistance in tuberculosis [3,4]. BACTEC® is now used in numerous laboratories around the world but unfortunately mainly in developed countries or in reference laboratories with the necessary resources to implement this expensive mechanised technology as a routine procedure. With the current increase in drug resistance of *M. tuberculosis* [5], rapid and

145

I. Bastian and F. Portaels (eds.), Multidrug-Resistant Tuberculosis, 145-162.
© 2000 *Kluwer Academic Publishers. Printed in the Netherlands.*

reliable DST methods are urgently required in the clinical mycobacteriology laboratory. Such techniques would not only aid patient management but also facilitate drug resistance surveillance, which is important in planning and evaluating TB control programmes.

TB diagnostics can be classified in two broad classes: genotypic methods and phenotypic methods. This chapter will review some techniques from both classes that have been developed recently for *M. tuberculosis* DST. Their applicability in different settings will also be discussed. The current conventional methods for DST are addressed in another chapter [6].

2.   NOVEL GENOTYPIC TECHNIQUES

Insights into the molecular basis of drug resistance [7], combined with the availability of new molecular biology tools, have led to the development of several novel genotypic techniques for the rapid detection of *M. tuberculosis* drug resistance. Some of them make use of expensive equipment and laborious techniques, while others employ less sophistication, but all of them involve DNA extraction, gene amplification, and detection of a mutation. These techniques have several advantages: rapid turn-around time (TAT) of days instead of weeks, no need for growth of the organism, the possibility for direct application to clinical specimens, reduction in biohazard risks, and feasibility for automation. Unfortunately, the molecular tests also have disadvantages, including problems with inhibitors when attempting to apply these techniques directly to clinical samples. Following are some of the novel genotypic techniques described for detection of *M. tuberculosis* drug resistance.

2.1   Automated DNA sequencing

Among the molecular techniques available to detect *M. tuberculosis* drug resistance, DNA sequencing of PCR amplified products has been the most widely used, becoming a gold standard for this purpose. It has been performed by both manual and automated procedures although the latter has been the most commonly used [8-10]. Kapur et al. [11,12] described the application of automated DNA sequencing for characterizing mutations in the *rpo*B gene in rifampicin-resistant strains of *M. tuberculosis* and for the rapid identification of *M. tuberculosis* and *Mycobacterium* species. More recently Pai et al. [13] have confirmed the utility of the technique for *Mycobacterium* species assignment and for surrogate rifampicin susceptibility testing in a hospital-based clinical laboratory, where the rifampicin susceptibility phenotype was correctly predicted for all strains evaluated. Automated DNA sequencing has also been used to detect mutations responsible for resistance to INH, ciprofloxacin and streptomycin [8,14,15].

2.2   PCR-single strand conformation polymorphism (PCR-SSCP)

PCR-SSCP is based on the property of single-stranded DNA to fold into a tertiary structure whose shape depends on its sequence. Single strands of DNA differing by only one or a few bases will fold into different conformations with different mobilities on a gel, producing what is called single strand conformation polymorphisms (SSCP). After PCR amplification of the gene region of interest, the amplified DNA strands are separated by heat denaturation followed by cooling to allow single DNA strands to fold into a characteristic conformation, whose different electrophoresis mobility is detected on a gel.

In combination with PCR, SSCP has been applied for the detection of resistance to rifampicin, isoniazid, streptomycin and ciprofloxacin [8, 14-16]. More recently, Pretorius et al. [17] applied PCR-SSCP for rapid detection of rifampicin resistance in clinical isolates of *M. tuberculosis* and were able to detect 95% of the resistant isolates. Scarpellini et al. [18] also used PCR-SSCP to detect rifampicin resistance in cerebrospinal fluid samples, correctly identifying the rifampicin susceptibility phenotype of isolates from all patients for whom susceptibility tests were available.

As with automated sequencing, SSCP by automated methods seems more suitable for large reference laboratories in developed countries. An alternative approach using silver staining has also been proposed [9], which could probably be implemented in laboratories with limited resources.

2.3   PCR-heteroduplex formation (PCR-HDF)

This assay described by Williams et al. [19] is performed by mixing amplified DNA from test organisms and susceptible control strains to obtain hybrid complementary DNA. If a resistant strain is present, the mutation will produce a heteroduplex which has a different electrophoretic mobility compared with the homoduplex hybrid (no mutation present). PCR-HDF was employed to detect all rifampicin resistant isolates having mutations within a 305-bp region of the *rpo*B gene. The test does not require radioactive compounds and may be appropriate for clinical laboratories. More recently, Williams et al. [20] have applied a procedure utilizing a single tube hemi-nested PCR amplification generating a *M. tuberculosis*-specific *rpo*B fragment that is annealed to a synthetic universal heteroduplex generator (UHG) derived from *rpo*B gene region where mutations encoding rifampicin resistance occur. From 44 *M. tuberculosis* culture-positive strains, 5 out of 6 rifampicin resistant strains were detected by the PCR-UHR assay. The specimen giving a susceptible result by the PCR-UHG assay but resistant by culture, did not contain a mutation in the *rpo*B region. As stated by the authors, the most cost-effective application of this assay would be at reference laboratories receiving large numbers of specimens since this would decrease the cost of the test per specimen.

2.4   Solid phase hybridization assay

The Line Probe Assay (LiPA) (Innogenetics N.V., Zwijndrecht, Belgium) is a commercial test for the rapid detection of the *M. tuberculosis* complex and rifampicin resistance. LiPA is based on the hybridization of amplified DNA from cultured strains or clinical samples to ten probes encompassing the core region of the *rpo*B gene of *M. tuberculosis*, which are immobilized on a nitrocellulose strip [21]. Absence of hybridization of the amplified DNA to any of the sensitive sequence-specific probes indicates mutations that may encode resistance; likewise, if hybridization to the mutation-specific probes occur, the mutation is present. In the original study by De Beenhouwer et al. [21], LiPA results matched classical testing in 65 out of 67 specimens. Further evaluation of this assay by Cooksey et al. [22] with a collection of 51 rifampicin-resistant strains gave an overall concordance of 90.2% with phenotypic susceptibility testing. Rossau et al. [23] evaluated 107 *M. tuberculosis* isolates with known *rpo*B sequences, 52 non-*M. tuberculosis* complex strains, and 61 sensitive and 203 resistant clinical isolates, and their results indicated that the probe was 100% specific for the *M. tuberculosis* complex; no discrepancies were observed with the results of nucleotide sequencing. Furthermore, all strains sensitive by in vitro susceptibility testing were identified correctly, and among the resistant strains only 2 % yielded conflicting results. More recently, Gamboa et al. [24] evaluated the LiPA with 59 *M. tuberculosis* culture-positive specimens (most of respiratory origin) and found a concordance of 98.3% with the DST of the isolated strains. As with all commercial methods however, the cost of the kit may limit its use in many developing countries.

2.5 Emerging new technologies for rapid detection of MDRTB

2.5.1 DNA Microarrays

One recent approach for genotypic detection of resistance is based on hybridization of amplified DNA to high density oligonucleotide arrays on a glass miniaturized support giving the possibility to examine large amounts of sequence in a single hybridization step. Gingeras et al. [25] designed an array to determine the specific nucleotide sequence of a 705-bp fragment of the *rpo*B gene, detecting rifampicin resistance in 44 clinical isolates evaluated. Additionally, they were able to simultaneously genotype and speciate non-tuberculous isolates. More recently Troesch et al [26] have used this same technology for *Mycobacterium* species identification and rifampicin resistance detection using two sequence databases. By hybridizing fluorescent-labelled amplified genetic material from mycobacterial colonies, 27 different species were detected, as was rifampicin resistance in 15 evaluated strains. To circumvent some of the limitations of the original technique such as high cost, complexity and difficulty for interpretation, Head et al. [27] have reported the use of a moderate density array, allowing efficient and easy to interpret sequence information. They detected and characterized mutations in nine resistant isolates evaluated, while no mutation was found in the one susceptible strain tested. The potential to include additional probes for other drugs in the same solid support would be an added advantage to the technique; however, there is still the concern about the costs, complexity and requirement of skilled personnel, that hampers the application of these technologies in standard mycobacteriology laboratory settings.

2.5.2 Reporter systems

Two main approaches for the use of reporter systems have been proposed. Firstly, Cooksey et al. [28] described the construction of plasmids containing the firefly luciferase gene that were used to transform an avirulent strain of *M. tuberculosis*. The production of light was then detected 48 hours after these transformants had been incubated in the presence or absence of drugs. Later on, Arain et al. [29] employed reporter strains of *M. tuberculosis* and *M. bovis* BCG endogenously expressing luciferase to test the activity of rifampicin and isoniazid. They also developed a standardized system (Bio-Siv) for bioluminescence assay of several antimicrobials, including isoniazid, ethambutol, rifampicin, amikacin, streptomycin and ciprofloxacin, where MICs values correlated with conventional methods in the BACTEC® system [30]. Similarly, Hickey et al. [31] have used an enhanced luciferase-expressing mycobacterium for evaluating antimycobacterial activity directly in mice. More recently, Shawar et al. employed recombinant strains of *M. bovis* BCG and *M. intracellulare* in a 96-well mini-tube format for detecting antimycobacterial activity in the extracts of natural products [32].

The other approach with reporter systems has been the use of phages as vectors to introduce the luciferase gene. For example, Jacobs and collaborators [33] cloned the luciferase gene into the genome of mycobacteriophages and expressed the gene in *M. tuberculosis*; DST was performed by assessing the production of light by viable phage-infected mycobacteria. The light was detectable minutes after infection. Cultivation of susceptible *M. tuberculosis* strains in the presence of rifampicin or isoniazid caused extinction of the light signal. This same group has modified the system using another phage (phAE88), which produces increased intensity and enhanced duration of the light signal, allowing detection of drug activity within one day [34]. A further modification allows detection of the emitted light with a custom-made Polaroid® film box, termed the Bronx box [35].

Reporter systems other than luciferase have also been described [36,37]. For example, the green fluorescence protein (GFP) of the jellyfish *Aequorea victoria* has been used as a reporter molecule. This reporter system does not require cofactors or substrates due to the intrinsically fluorescent nature of GFP. However, these alternative reporter systems have generally only been used for the screening of new compounds with activity against *M. tuberculosis* and not for clinical AST [38-40].

Although the reporter systems described above have shown in general good sensitivity and reproducibility, there is still the issue of the cost of implementation in endemic countries and at the level of the clinical mycobacteriology laboratory.

2.5.3   Miscellaneous genotypic techniques

Several other new genotypic techniques have been proposed for the rapid detection of drug resistance in *M. tuberculosis*: cleavase fragment length polymorphism (CFLP) [41], dideoxy fingerprinting (ddF) [42,43], hybridization protection assays [44-46], a method based on reverse transcriptase-strand displacement amplification of mRNA [47], RNA/RNA duplex base-pair mismatch assay [48], and DNA sequence analysis using fluorogenic reporter molecules (ie. molecular beacons) [49]. However, these techniques have not been extensively studied and have not been further validated with clinical isolates. Although they share the high specificity common to all sequencing techniques, most of them rely on technically demanding procedures and in some cases need specialized and costly equipment precluding their use at the clinical laboratory level, not to mention mycobacteriology laboratories in developing countries where TB is more prevalent.

3. NOVEL PHENOTYPIC TECHNIQUES

Phenotypic techniques have generally relied on culture methods that require the visual detection of *M. tuberculosis* colonies for interpretation of results. Due to the slow growth rate of *M. tuberculosis*, these phenotypic methods require several weeks before completion. A novel group of phenotypic methods are being introduced that provide 'rapid' results by detecting earlier signs of mycobacterial growth using various technologies: measurement of metabolism with the aid of color indicators, detection of oxygen consumption, or early visualization of microcolonies.

3.1 Mycobacteria growth indicator tube (MGIT)

Among the commercial systems recently developed for the rapid detection of mycobacterial growth, the MGIT system (Becton Dickinson, USA) has been evaluated in several comparative studies for the early detection of *M. tuberculosis* and other mycobacteria [50-52]. The system was subsequently adapted for *M. tuberculosis* DST. The MGIT system consists of glass tubes containing a modified Middlebrook 7H9 liquid medium together with a fluorescence quenching-based oxygen sensor embedded at the bottom of each tube. When inoculated with *M. tuberculosis*, consumption of the dissolved oxygen will produce fluorescence when illuminated by a UV lamp. For DST, a set containing a growth control and drug-containing tubes is inoculated with the isolate under study, and after a period of incubation at 37°C, growth is compared in the drug-containing and control tubes allowing determination of susceptibility or resistance. Several evaluations have been reported of MGIT for the rapid detection of drug resistant *M. tuberculosis*. Reisner et al. [53] compared the reliability of MGIT for isoniazid and rifampicin DST with the BACTEC® system for 29 isolates. They reported a TAT of 3-8 days (median 6 days) for MGIT and 4-10 days (median 6 days) for BACTEC®, and obtained full agreement for isoniazid and for 28/29 isolates with rifampicin. In other studies, the MGIT system has compared fairly well with the proportion method on Löwenstein-Jensen (LJ) medium, agar-based medium, and BACTEC® [54-59], especially for rifampicin and isoniazid; however, further standardization is still needed for ethambutol and streptomycin. No MGIT DST studies have been done with second-line antibiotics for *M. tuberculosis*. Very recently, an automated system using the MGIT tubes has been introduced by the manufacturer [60], which claims to reduce the time to detection and to facilitate the manipulation and reading of large numbers of samples. However, unnecessary introduction of this equipment would increase the cost of the procedure, preventing its use in laboratories with limited resources.

3.2   The PhaB assay

A new phenotypic culture-based DST, the phage amplified biologically (PhaB) assay, has been recently introduced [61]. This test is based on the ability of viable *M. tuberculosis* to support the replication of an infecting mycobacteriophage; non-infecting exogenous phages are inactivated by chemical treatment. The number of endogenous phages, which is an indication of the original number of viable *M. tuberculosis*, is then determined after cycles of infection, replication and release in a rapidly-growing mycobacteria. When evaluated with 46 *M. tuberculosis* clinical isolates, the assay correctly identified susceptibility or resistance to rifampicin in 44 isolates (95.7%), and to isoniazid in 40 of 46 isolates (87%). Results were available within 3-4 days. The test could theoretically be performed directly on patient samples, reducing even further the time for drug susceptibility results. One limitation of the assay, however, is the specificity of the mycobacteriophage (D29) used in the procedure. This phage can infect other mycobacteria. This problem could be overcome by choosing an alternative bacteriophage or by altering the specificity of D29. Additional studies are needed to evaluate the performance of the test in different laboratory settings [62].

3.3   E-test

The E-test, another commercial system (AB BIODISK, Sweden), is based on determination of drug susceptibility using strips containing gradients of impregnated antibiotics. Strips containing the drug of choice are applied on the surface of an agar medium inoculated with the test strain; after a period of incubation, the minimum inhibitory concentration (MIC) is read from the point at which the ellipse (formed by the inhibition of growth) intersects the strip [63]. The test has been applied to a variety of difficult-to-grow microorganisms including rapidly growing mycobacteria [64-67]. Wanger & Mills have compared the E-test with the BACTEC® and agar proportion methods for testing the susceptibility of *M. tuberculosis* to four first-line anti-tuberculosis drugs and reported equivalent interpretive results for all the strains evaluated [68,69]. Although the values were within $\pm 2 \log_2$ dilutions, agreement was found to be 93, 100, 90, and 94% for isoniazid, rifampicin, ethambutol, and streptomycin, respectively. Results were obtained within 5 to 10 days using a rather high inoculum, equivalent to a McFarland 3.0 standard. More recently, Hausdorfer et al. [70] have evaluated the E-test with the proportion method on LJ and BACTEC® for the same four drugs; of 81 isolates evaluated, 73 (90.1%) gave concordant results for the four drugs (69 susceptible and 4 resistant). The eight remaining isolates were susceptible by the proportion method, but resistant by the E-test, five resistant to ethambutol, two resistant for isoniazid and one resistant to both ethambutol and streptomycin. The authors concluded that due to the high rate of false resistance, the method could not be recommended for use in clinical laboratories. No further studies have been performed to clarify the usefulness of the E-test for the routine mycobacteriology laboratory. The cost of the strips is also a disadvantage.

3.4   Rapid metabolic tests

Tetrazolium salts have been used to study metabolism and viability in a number of microorganisms [71-73], and to measure toxicity for eucaryotic and procaryotic cells [74,75]. Yajko et al. [76] were the first to describe a colorimetric method based on an oxidation-reduction dye, Alamar blue, for the quantitative measurement of drug susceptibility in *M. tuberculosis*. The dye in the oxidized state is blue but is pink when reduced. The change is easily discernible visually, or can be measured spectrophotometrically or fluorometrically. For DST, a group of tubes containing dilutions of each antituberculous drug and a control tube without any drug are inoculated with the isolate under study. After a period of incubation (ie. 7, 10 and 14 days), the Alamar blue is added and the   tubes again incubated for color development; those tubes supporting growth of the bacteria (ie. resistant to the drug) reduce the indicator, changing the color from blue to pink. Yajko et al studied 50 isolates of *M. tuberculosis* determining the MICs of isoniazid, rifampicin, ethambutol and streptomycin, and comparing the results with those obtained by the agar proportion method; interpretive agreement between the two methods was 98% for isoniazid, rifampicin and ethambutol and 94% for streptomycin. Collins & Franzblau [77] adapted the test to a microtiter format, and compared this format with the BACTEC® system for high throughput screening of compounds against *M. tuberculosis* and *M. avium*. They subsequently used the microtiter system in a laboratory in a low-income country to determine the MICs of isoniazid, rifampicin, ethambutol and streptomycin for 34 clinical isolates of *M. tuberculosis* [78]. The microtiter results were available within 8 days and had an overall agreement of 93.6% (after re-testing 12 of 17 samples with discrepant results) with results obtained using the BACTEC® system. More recently, Palomino & Portaels [79] have evaluated a similar test using one critical concentration of each of the four drugs. Compared with the proportion method on LJ, they found an overall agreement of 97% for all four drugs (100% for isoniazid and rifampicin); results were available after 8 days of incubation.

Mshana et al. [80] and Abate et al. [81] have proposed a similar colorimetric system, which uses 3-(4,5-dimethylthiazol-2-yl)-2,5-diphenyl tetrazolium bromide (MTT) as the viability indicator, for the rapid detection of rifampicin resistance. In this case, the dye changes from yellow to blue, and this color change can also be visually differentiated. In a tube macro-method with Dubos broth, they studied 92 clinical isolates and obtained full concordance for their assay compared with the BACTEC® system. Additional evaluations show that this system can be successfully adapted for the study of first and second-line antituberculous drugs (Julieta Luna, personal communication).

3.5   Microcolony detection method

Some studies have evaluated a method of microcolony detection on solid media. When inoculated on a thin layer of agar, such as Middlebrook 7H11 in a Petri plate, mycobacteria form typical microcolonies easily detectable with a microscope. In evaluations for the rapid detection and diagnosis of *M. tuberculosis*, this method has compared favorably with conventional culture on LJ [82-84]. When applied as a rapid method for *M. tuberculosis* DST, Schaberg et al. [85] found that microcolony detection produced shorter median TAT than conventional methods for 64 smear-positive (ie. 11 vs 62 days) and 133 smear-negative specimens (35 vs 72 days). All cases of single-drug and multi-drug resistance were correctly identified. Current evaluations of the microcolony detection method for rapid susceptibility testing of rifampicin, isoniazid and second-line drugs show a very good correlation with the proportion method. Microcolony detection therefore provides an alternative method for rapid DST in laboratories with limited resources (Jaime Robledo, personal communication); further evaluations of this low-cost methodology are necessary to assess its usefulness for clinical mycobacteriology laboratories in low-income countries.

3.6   Miscellaneous phenotypic procedures

Several other procedures have been proposed for the rapid detection of drug resistance in *M. tuberculosis*. For example, a bioluminescence assay has been used to detect ATP produced by viable *M. tuberculosis* in the presence and absence of antibiotics. The bioluminescence assay was evaluated with the first-line drugs and gave results in 5-7 days with good correlation with the resistance ratio method and BACTEC® [86, 87]. Another rapid DST method for isoniazid and streptomycin involves measurement of mycolic acid levels using high performance liquid chromatography [88]; standardization of the assay was done with *M. tuberculosis* H37Ra and results were obtained in 3 to 4 days. However, no evaluation of this test has been done with clinical isolates of *M. tuberculosis*. Drug susceptibility testing has also been attempted by flow cytometry using *M. tuberculosis* labelled with fluorescein diacetate; the procedure was evaluated on 17 clinical isolates with ethambutol, isoniazid and rifampicin and the results were available after 3 days [89,90]. The new ESP culture system II (Accumed International, USA), which detects pressure changes resulting from the consumption or production of gas by growing mycobacteria, has also been evaluated for DST of the four first-line drugs [91]. The agreement of the ESP results with BACTEC® ranged from 93 to 100 % in an evaluation of 20 clinical strains and 30 challenge strains of *M. tuberculosis*; additional studies will be necessary to assess the performance of this new ESP system. As with other automated methods, this system has the disadvantage of requiring sophisticated equipment, which is only available from one commercial source, thereby limiting its wider application in developing countries.

4.   CONCLUSIONS

Many new possibilities have arisen for detecting drug resistance in *M. tuberculosis* and for performing DST. These novel methods rely on new information concerning molecular mechanisms of drug resistance, or on new approaches in detecting mycobacterial growth. The first group of technologies, categorized as genotypic methods, has the advantage of being rapid and specific. However, not all of the molecular mechanisms of drug resistance are known; hence, the current molecular tools cannot detect all resistant strains. Furthermore, the sophistication of some of these methods and their requirement for expensive equipment restrict their implementation to laboratories in developed countries or to reference laboratories with the necessary resources of equipment and personnel (Figure 1). The second group of technologies, categorized as phenotypic methods, is more diverse. Some of them, although being simple in their procedure, still require expensive equipment not always available in laboratories in TB-endemic countries. Others involve uncomplicated procedures that could be easily implemented in routine mycobacteriology laboratories. However, these phenotypic methods require further careful evaluation and validation to obtain acceptable levels of sensitivity, specificity and reproducibility before they replace the current DST procedures.

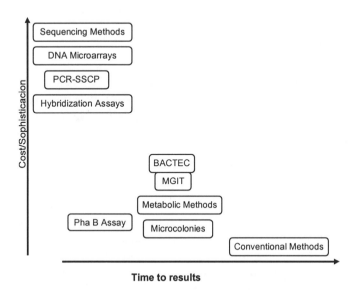

Figure 1. Comparisons of turnaround-time (TAT) versus cost and sophistication for various drug susceptibility testing methodologies. Each laboratory must consider their circumstances, their financial resources, and their expertise, before choosing the most appropriate technique for improving their detection of drug resistant *M. tuberculosis*.

REFERENCES

1. Canetti G, Fox W, Khomenko A, Mahler HT, Menon NK, Mitchison DA, Rist N, Smelev NA. Advances in techniques of testing mycobacterial drug sensitivity, and the use of sensitivity tests in tuberculosis control programmes. Bull World Health Organ 1969; 41: 21-43.
2. Kent PT, Kubica GP. (eds). Public Health Mycobacteriology: a guide for the level III laboratory. U.S. Department of Health and Human Services, Atlanta 1985.
3. Siddiqi SH, Libonati JP, Middlebrook G. Evaluation of rapid radiometric method for drug susceptibility testing of *Mycobacterium tuberculosis*. J Clin Microbiol 1981; 13: 908-12.
4. Roberts GD, Goodman NL, Heifets L, Larsh HW, Lindner TH, McClatchy JK, McGinnis MR, Siddiqi SH, Wright P. Evaluation of the BACTEC radiometric method for recovery of mycobacteria and drug susceptibility testing of *Mycobacterium tuberculosis* from acid-fast smear-positive specimens. J Clin Microbiol 1983; 18: 689-96.

5. Pablos-Mendez A, Raviglione MC, Laszlo A, Binkin N, Rieder HL, Bustreo F, Cohn DL, Lambregts-van Weezenbeek CS, Kim SJ, Chaulet P, Nunn P. Global surveillance for antituberculosis-drug resistance, 1994-1997. World Health Organization-International Union against Tuberculosis and Lung Disease Working Group on Anti-Tuberculosis Drug Resistance Surveillance. N Engl J Med 1998; 338: 1641-9.

6. Heifets L. Conventional methods for antimicrobial susceptibility testing of *Mycobacterium tuberculosis*, Chapter 8, 133-143. In: Bastian I, Portaels F (eds.), Multidrug-resistant tuberculosis. Kluwer Academic Publ., The Netherlands 2000.

7. Takiff H. Molecular mechanisms of drug resistance, Chapter 6, 77-114. In: Bastian I, Portaels F (eds.), Multidrug resistant tuberculosis. Kluwer Academic Publ., The Netherlands 2000.

8. Cooksey RC, Morlock GP, McQueen A, Glickman SE, Crawford JT. Characterization of streptomycin resistance mechanisms among *Mycobacterium tuberculosis* isolates from patients in New York City. Antimicrob Agents Chemother 1996; 40: 1186-8.

9. Delgado MB, Telenti A. Detection of mutations associated with quinolone resistance in *Mycobacterium tuberculosis*. In Persing DH. (ed), Selected PCR Protocols for Emerging Infectious Diseases, American Society for Microbiology, Washington D.C. 1996.

10. Telenti A, Imboden P, Marchesi F, Lowrie D, Cole S, Colston MJ, Matter L, Schopfer K, Bodmer T. Detection of rifampicin-resistance mutations in *Mycobacterium tuberculosis*. Lancet 1993; 341: 647-50.

11. Kapur V, Li LL, Iordanescu S, Hamrick MR, Wanger A, Kreiswirth BN, Musser JM. Characterization by automated DNA sequencing of mutations in the gene (*rpo*B) encoding the RNA polymerase beta subunit in rifampin-resistant *Mycobacterium tuberculosis* strains from New York City and Texas. J Clin Microbiol 1994; 32:1095-8.

12. Kapur V, Li LL, Hamrick MR, Plikaytis BB, Shinnick TM, Telenti A, Jacobs WR Jr, Banerjee A, Cole S, Yuen KY, Clarridge III JE, Kreiswirth BN, Musser JM. Rapid *Mycobacterium* species assignment and unambiguous identification of mutations associated with antimicrobial resistance in *Mycobacterium tuberculosis* by automated DNA sequencing. Arch Pathol Lab Med 1995; 119: 131-8.

13. Pai S, Esen N, Pan X, Musser JM. Routine rapid *Mycobacterium* species assignment based on species-specific allelic variation in the 65-kilodalton heat shock protein gene (*hsp*65). Arch Pathol Lab Med 1997; 121: 859-64.

14. Heym B, Honore N, Truffot-Pernot C, Banerjee A, Schurra C, Jacobs WR Jr, van Embden JD, Grosset JH, Cole ST. Implications of multidrug resistance for the future of short-course chemotherapy of tuberculosis: a molecular study. Lancet 1994; 344: 293-8.

15. Takiff HE, Salazar L, Guerrero C, Philipp W, Huang WM, Kreiswirth B, Cole ST, Jacobs WR Jr, Telenti A. Cloning and nucleotide sequence of *Mycobacterium tuberculosis* gyrA and gyrB genes and detection of quinolone resistance mutations. Antimicrob Agents Chemother 1994; 38: 773-80.

16. 14. Telenti A, Imboden P, Marchesi F, Schmidheini T, Bodmer T. Direct, automated detection of rifampin-resistant *Mycobacterium tuberculosis* by polymerase chain reaction and single-strand conformation polymorphism analysis. Antimicrob Agents Chemother 1993; 37: 2054-58.

17. Pretorius GS, Sirgel FA, Schaaf HS, van Helden PD, Victor TC. Rifampicin resistance in *Mycobacterium tuberculosis*--rapid detection and implications in chemotherapy. S Afr Med J 1996; 86: 50-5.

18. Scarpellini P, Braglia S, Brambilla AM, Dalessandro M, Cichero P, Gori A, Lazzarin A. Detection of rifampin resistance by single-strand conformation polymorphism analysis of cerebrospinal fluid of patients with tuberculosis of the central nervous system. J Clin Microbiol 1997; 35: 2802-6.

19. Williams DL, Waguespack C, Eisenach K, Crawford JT, Portaels F, Salfinger M, Nolan CM, Abe C, Sticht-Groh V, Gillis TP. Characterization of rifampin-resistance in pathogenic mycobacteria. Antimicrob Agents Chemother 1994; 38: 2380-6.

20. Williams DL, Spring L, Gillis TP, Salfinger M, Persing DH. Evaluation of a polymerase chain reaction-based universal heteroduplex generator assay for direct detection of rifampin susceptibility of *Mycobacterium tuberculosis* from sputum specimens. Clin Infect Dis 1998; 26: 446-50.

21. De Beenhouwer H, Lhiang Z, Jannes G, Mijs W, Machtelinckx L, Rossau R, Traore H, Portaels F. Rapid detection of rifampicin resistance in sputum and biopsy specimens from tuberculosis patients by PCR and line probe assay. Tuber Lung Dis 1995; 76: 425-30.

22. Cooksey RC, Morlock GP, Glickman S, Crawford JT. Evaluation of a line probe assay kit for characterization of *rpo*B mutations in rifampin-resistant *Mycobacterium tuberculosis* isolates from New York City. J Clin Microbiol 1997; 35: 1281-3.

23. Rossau R, Traore H, De Beenhouwer H, Mijs W, Jannes G, De Rijk P, Portaels F. Evaluation of the INNO-LiPA Rif. TB assay, a reverse hybridization assay for the simultaneous detection of *Mycobacterium tuberculosis* complex and its resistance to rifampin. Antimicrob Agents Chemother 1997; 41: 2093-8.

24. Gamboa F, Cardona PJ, Manterola JM, Lonca J, Matas L, Padilla E, Manzano JR, Ausina V. Evaluation of a commercial probe assay for detection of rifampin resistance in *Mycobacterium tuberculosis* directly from respiratory and nonrespiratory clinical samples. Eur J Clin Microbiol Infect Dis 1998; 17: 189-92.

25. Gingeras TR, Ghandour G, Wang E, Berno A, Small PM, Drobniewski F, Alland D, Desmond E, Holodniy M, Drenkow J. Simultaneous genotyping and species identification using hybridization pattern recognition analysis of generic *Mycobacterium* DNA arrays. Genome Res 1998; 8: 435-48.

26. Troesch A, Nguyen H, Miyada CG, Desvarenne S, Gingeras TR, Kaplan PM, Cros P, Mabilat C. *Mycobacterium* species identification and rifampin resistance testing with high-density DNA probe arrays. J Clin Microbiol 1999; 37: 49-55.

27. Head SR, Parikh K, Rogers Y, Bishai W, Goelet P, Boyce-Jacino MT. Solid-phase sequence scanning for drug resistance detection in tuberculosis. Mol Cell Probes 1999; 13: 81-7.

28. Cooksey RC, Crawford JT, Jacobs WR Jr, Shinnick TM. A rapid method for screening antimicrobial agents for activities against a strain of *Mycobacterium tuberculosis* expressing firefly luciferase. Antimicrob Agents Chemother 1993; 37: 1348-52.

29. Arain TM, Resconi AE, Singh DC, Stover CK. Reporter gene technology to assess activity of antimycobacterial agents in macrophages. Antimicrob Agents Chemother 1996; 40: 1542-44.

30. Arain TM, Resconi AE, Hickey MJ, Stover CK. Bioluminescence screening in vitro (Bio-Siv) assays for high-volume antimycobacterial drug discovery. Antimicrob Agents Chemother 1996; 40: 1536-41.

31. Hickey MJ, Arain TM, Shawar RM, Humble DJ, Langhorne MH, Morgenroth JN, Stover CK. Luciferase in vivo expression technology: use of recombinant mycobacterial reporter strains to evaluate antimycobacterial activity in mice. Antimicrob Agents Chemother 1996; 40: 400-7.

32. Shawar RM, Humble DJ, Van Dalfsen JM, Stover CK, Hickey MJ, Steele S, Mitscher LA, Baker W. Rapid screening of natural products for antimycobacterial activity by using luciferase-expressing strains of *Mycobacterium bovis* BCG and *Mycobacterium intracellulare*. Antimicrob Agents Chemother 1997; 41: 570-4.

33. Jacobs WR Jr, Barletta RG, Udani R, Chan J, Kalkut G, Sosne G, Kieser T, Sarkis GJ, Hatfull GF, Bloom BR. Rapid assessment of drug susceptibilities of *Mycobacterium tuberculosis* by means of luciferase reporter phages. Science 1993; 260: 819-22.

34. Carriere C, Riska PF, Zimhony O, Kriakov J, Bardarov S, Burns J, Chan J, Jacobs WR Jr. Conditionally replicating luciferase reporter phages: improved sensitivity for rapid detection and assessment of drug susceptibility of *Mycobacterium tuberculosis.* J Clin Microbiol 1997; 35: 3232-39.

35. Riska PF, Su Y, Bardarov S, Freundlich L, Sarkis G, Hatfull G, Carriere C, Kumar V, Chan J, Jacobs WR Jr. Rapid film-based determination of antibiotic susceptibilities of *Mycobacterium tuberculosis* strains by using a luciferase reporter phage and the Bronx Box. J Clin Microbiol 1999; 37: 1144-9.

36. Chung GA, Aktar Z, Jackson S, Duncan K. High-throughput screen for detecting antimycobacterial agents. Antimicrob Agents Chemother 1995; 39: 2235-8.

37. Srivastava R, Kumar D, Srivastava BS. Recombinant *Mycobacterium aurum* expressing *Escherichia coli* beta-galactosidase in high throughput screening of antituberculosis drugs. Biochem Biophys Res Commun 1997; 240: 536-9.

38. Kremer L, Baulard A, Estaquier J, Poulain-Godefroy O, Locht C. Green fluorescent protein as a new expression marker in mycobacteria. Mol Microbiol 1995; 17: 913-22.

39. Collins LA, Torrero MN, Franzblau SG. Green fluorescent protein reporter microplate assay for high-throughput screening of compounds against *Mycobacterium tuberculosis.* Antimicrob Agents Chemother 1998; 42 : 344-7.

40. Srivastava R, Deb DK, Srivastava KK, Locht C, Srivastava BS. Green fluorescent protein as a reporter in rapid screening of antituberculosis compounds in vitro and in macrophages. Biochem Biophys Res Commun 1998; 253: 431-6.

41. Sreevatsan S, Bookout JB, Ringpis FM, Mogazeh SL, Kreiswirth BN, Pottathil RR, Barathur RR. Comparative Evaluation of Cleavase Fragment Length Polymorphism With PCR-SSCP and PCR-RFLP to Detect Antimicrobial Agent Resistance in *Mycobacterium tuberculosis.* Mol Diagn 1998; 3: 81-91.

42. Felmlee TA, Liu Q, Whelen AC, Williams D, Sommer SS, Persing DH. Genotypic detection of *Mycobacterium tuberculosis* rifampin resistance: comparison of single-strand conformation polymorphism and dideoxy fingerprinting. J Clin Microbiol 1995; 33: 1617-23.

43. Liu YC, Huang TS, Huang WK, Chen CS, Tu HZ. Dideoxy fingerprinting for rapid screening of *rpo*B gene mutations in clinical isolates of *Mycobacterium tuberculosis.* J Formos Med Assoc 1998; 97: 400-4.

44. Miyamoto J, Koga H, Kohno S, Tashiro T, Hara K. New drug susceptibility test for *Mycobacterium tuberculosis* using the hybridization protection assay. J Clin Microbiol 1996; 34: 1323-6.

45. Koga H, Miyamoto J, Ohno H, Ogawa K, Tomono K, Tashiro T, Kohno S. A rapid drug susceptibility test for *Mycobacterium tuberculosis* using the hybridization protection assay. J Antimicrob Chemother 1997; 40: 189-94.

46. Martin-Casabona N, Xairo Mimo D, Gonzalez T, Rossello J, Arcalis L. Rapid method for testing susceptibility of *Mycobacterium tuberculosis* by using DNA probes. J Clin Microbiol 1997; 35 2521-5.

47. Hellyer TJ, DesJardin LE, Teixeira L, Perkins MD, Cave MD, Eisenach KD. Detection of viable *Mycobacterium tuberculosis* by reverse transcriptase-strand displacement amplification of mRNA. J Clin Microbiol 1999; 37: 518-23.

48. Nash KA, Gaytan A, Inderlied CB. Detection of rifampin resistance in *Mycobacterium tuberculosis* by use of a rapid, simple, and specific RNA/RNA mismatch assay. J Infect Dis 1997; 176: 533-6.

49. Piatek AS, Tyagi S, Pol AC, Telenti A, Miller LP, Kramer FR, Alland D. Molecular beacon sequence analysis for detecting drug resistance in *Mycobacterium tuberculosis*. Nat Biotechnol 1998; 16: 359-63.

50. Hanna BA, Walters SB, Bonk SJ, Tick LJ. Recovery of mycobacteria from blood in mycobacteria growth indicator tube and Lowenstein-Jensen slant after lysis-centrifugation. J Clin Microbiol 1995; 33: 3315-6.

51. Badak FZ, Kiska DL, Setterquist S, Hartley C, O'Connell MA, Hopfer RL. Comparison of mycobacteria growth indicator tube with BACTEC 460 for detection and recovery of mycobacteria from clinical specimens. J Clin Microbiol 1996; 34: 2236-9.

52. Pfyffer GE, Welscher HM, Kissling P, Cieslak C, Casal MJ, Gutierrez J, Rusch-Gerdes S. Comparison of the Mycobacteria Growth Indicator Tube (MGIT) with radiometric and solid culture for recovery of acid-fast bacilli. J Clin Microbiol 1997; 35: 364-8.

53. Reisner BS, Gatson AM, Woods GL. Evaluation of mycobacteria growth indicator tubes for susceptibility testing of *Mycobacterium tuberculosis* to isoniazid and rifampin. Diagn Microbiol Infect Dis 1995; 22: 325-9.

54. Palaci M, Ueki SY, Sato DN, Da Silva Telles MA, Curcio M, Silva EA. Evaluation of mycobacteria growth indicator tube for recovery and drug susceptibility testing of *Mycobacterium tuberculosis* isolates from respiratory specimens. J Clin Microbiol 1996; 34: 762-4.

55. Walters SB, Hanna BA. Testing of susceptibility of *Mycobacterium tuberculosis* to isoniazid and rifampin by mycobacterium growth indicator tube method. J Clin Microbiol 1996; 34: 1565-7.

56. Bergmann JS, Woods GL. Mycobacterial growth indicator tube for susceptibility testing of *Mycobacterium tuberculosis* to isoniazid and rifampin. Diagn Microbiol Infect Dis 1997; 28: 153-6.

57. Bergmann JS, Woods GL. Reliability of mycobacteria growth indicator tube for testing susceptibility of *Mycobacterium tuberculosis* to ethambutol and streptomycin. J Clin Microbiol 1997; 35: 3325-7.

58. Morcillo N, Scipioni S, Vignoles M, Trovero A. Rapid diagnosis and susceptibility of *Mycobacterium tuberculosis* to antibiotics using MGIT system. Rev Argent Microbiol 1998; 30: 155-62.

59. Palomino JC, Traore H, Fissette K, Portaels F. Evaluation of Mycobacteria Growth Indicator Tube (MGIT) for drug susceptibility testing of *Mycobacterium tuberculosis*. Int J Tuberc Lung Dis 1999; 3: 344-8.

60. Hanna BA, Ebrahimzadeh A, Elliott LB, Morgan MA, Novak SM, Rusch-Gerdes S, Acio M, Dunbar DF, Holmes TM, Rexer CH, Savthyakumar C, Vannier AM. Multicenter evaluation of the BACTEC MGIT 960 system for recovery of mycobacteria. J Clin Microbiol 1999; 37: 748-52.

61. Wilson SM, al-Suwaidi Z, McNerney R, Porter J, Drobniewski F. Evaluation of a new rapid bacteriophage-based method for the drug susceptibility testing of *Mycobacterium tuberculosis*. Nat Med 1997; 3: 465-8.

62. McNerney R. TB: the return of the phage. A review of fifty years of mycobacteriophage research. Int J Tuberc Lung Dis 1999; 3: 179-84.

63. AB BIODISK. Susceptibility testing of mycobacteria. Etest technical guide no. 5 AB BIODISK, N.A., Inc. Piscataway, N.J. 1996.

64. Lebrun L, Onody C, Vincent V, Nordmann P. Evaluation of the Etest for rapid susceptibility testing of *Mycobacterium avium* to clarithromycin. J Antimicrob Chemother 1996; 37: 999-1003.

65. Biehle JR, Cavalieri SJ, Saubolle MA, Getsinger LJ. Evaluation of Etest for susceptibility testing of rapidly growing mycobacteria. J Clin Microbiol 1995; 33: 1760-4

66. Hoffner SE, Klintz L, Olsson-Liljequist B, Bolmstrom A. Evaluation of Etest for rapid susceptibility testing of *Mycobacterium chelonae* and *M. fortuitum*. J Clin Microbiol 1994; 32:1846-9.

67. Koontz FP, Erwin ME, Barrett MS, Jones RN. Etest for routine clinical antimicrobial susceptibility testing of rapid-growing mycobacteria isolates. Diagn Microbiol Infect Dis 1994; 19: 183-6.

68. Wanger A, Mills K. Etest for susceptibility testing of *Mycobacterium tuberculosis* and *Mycobacterium avium-intracellulare*. Diagn Microbiol Infect Dis 1994; 19: 179-81.

69. Wanger A, Mills K. Testing of *Mycobacterium tuberculosis* susceptibility to ethambutol, isoniazid, rifampin, and streptomycin by using Etest. J Clin Microbiol 1996; 34: 1672-6.

70. Hausdorfer J, Sompek E, Allerberger F, Dierich MP, Rusch-Gerdes S. E-test for susceptibility testing of *Mycobacterium tuberculosis*. Int J Tuberc Lung Dis 1998; 2: 751-5.

71. Novak SM, Hindler J, Bruckner DA. Reliability of two novel methods, alamar and E test, for detection of methicillin-resistant *Staphylococcus aureus*. J Clin Microbiol 1993; 31: 3056-7.

72. Zabransky RJ, Dinuzzo AR, Woods GL. Detection of vancomycin resistance in enterococci by the Alamar MIC system. J Clin Microbiol 1995; 33: 791-3.

73. Pfaller MA, Barry AL. Evaluation of a novel colorimetric broth microdilution method for antifungal susceptibility testing of yeast isolates. J Clin Microbiol 1994; 32: 1992-6.

74. Ahmed SA, Gogal Jr. RM, Walsh JE. A new rapid and simple non-radioactive assay to monitor and determine the proliferation of lymphocyte: an alternative to H^3-thymidine incorporation assay. J Immunol Methods 1994; 170: 211-24.

75. Page B, Mage M, Noel C. A new fluorometric assay for cytoxicity measurements in vitro. Int J Oncol 1993; 3: 473-6.

76. Yajko DM, Madej JJ, Lancaster MV, Sanders CA, Cawthon VL, Gee B, Babst A, Hadley WK. Colorimetric method for determining MICs of antimicrobial agents for *Mycobacterium tuberculosis*. J Clin Microbiol 1995; 33: 2324-7.

77. Collins L, Franzblau SG. Microplate alamar blue assay versus BACTEC 460 system for high-throughput screening of compounds against *Mycobacterium tuberculosis* and *Mycobacterium avium*. Antimicrob Agents Chemother 1997; 41: 1004-9.

78. Franzblau SG, Witzig RS, McLaughlin JC, Torres P, Madico G, Hernandez A, Degnan MT, Cook MB, Quenzer VK, Ferguson RM, Gilman RH. Rapid, low-technology MIC determination with clinical *Mycobacterium tuberculosis* isolates by using the microplate Alamar Blue assay. J Clin Microbiol 1998; 36: 362-6.

79. Palomino JC, Portaels F. Simple Procedure for Drug Susceptibility Testing of *Mycobacterium tuberculosis* Using a Commercial Colorimetric Assay. Eur J Clin Microbiol Infect Dis 1999; 18: 380-383.

80. Mshana RN, Tadesse G, Abate G, Miorner H. Use of 3-(4,5-dimethylthiazol-2-yl)-2,5-diphenyl tetrazolium bromide for rapid detection of rifampin-resistant *Mycobacterium tuberculosis*. J Clin Microbiol 1998; 36: 1214-9.

81. Abate G, Mshana RN, Miorner H. Evaluation of a colorimetric assay based on 3-(4,5-dimethylthiazol-2-yl)-2,5-diphenyl tetrazolium bromide (MTT) for rapid detection of rifampicin resistance in *Mycobacterium tuberculosis*. Int J Tuberc Lung Dis 1998; 2: 1011-6.

82. Mejia GI, Castrillon L, Trujillo H, Robledo JA. Microcolony detection in 7H11 thin layer culture is an alternative for rapid diagnosis of *Mycobacterium tuberculosis* infection. Int J Tuberc Lung Dis 1999; 3: 138-42.

83. Idigoras P, Perez-Trallero E, Alcorta M, Gutierrez C, Munoz-Baroja I. Rapid detection of tuberculous and non-tuberculous mycobacteria by microscopic observation of growth on Middlebrook 7H11 agar. Eur J Clin Microbiol Infect Dis 1995; 14: 6-10.

84. Welch DF, Guruswamy AP, Sides SJ, Shaw CH, Gilchrist MJ. Timely culture for mycobacteria which utilizes a microcolony method. J Clin Microbiol 1993; 31: 2178-84.

85. Schaberg T, Reichert B, Schulin T, Lode H, Mauch H. Rapid drug susceptibility testing of *Mycobacterium tuberculosis* using conventional solid media. Eur Respir J 1995; 8: 1688-93.

86. Nilsson LE, Hoffner SE, Ansehn S. Rapid susceptibility testing of *Mycobacterium tuberculosis* by bioluminescence assay of mycobacterial ATP. Antimicrob Agents Chemother 1988; 32: 1208-12.

87. Beckers B, Lang HR, Schimke D, Lammers A. Evaluation of a bioluminescence assay for rapid antimicrobial susceptibility testing of mycobacteria. Eur J Clin Microbiol 1985; 4: 556-61.

88. Garza-Gonzalez E, Guerrero-Olazaran M, Tijerina-Menchaca R, Viader-Salvado JM. Determination of drug susceptibility of *Mycobacterium tuberculosis* through mycolic acid analysis. J Clin Microbiol 1997; 35: 1287-9.

89. Moore AV, Kirk SM, Callister SM, Mazurek GH, Schell RF. Safe determination of susceptibility of *Mycobacterium tuberculosis* to antimycobacterial agents by flow cytometry. J Clin Microbiol 1999; 37: 479-83.

90. Kirk SM, Schell RF, Moore AV, Callister SM, Mazurek GH. Flow cytometric testing of susceptibilities of *Mycobacterium tuberculosis* isolates to ethambutol, isoniazid, and rifampin in 24 hours. J Clin Microbiol 1998; 36: 1568-73.

91. Bergmann JS, Woods GL. Evaluation of the ESP culture system II for testing susceptibilities of *Mycobacterium tuberculosis* isolates to four primary antituberculous drugs. J Clin Microbiol 1998; 36: 2940-3.

Chapter 10

Pharmacology of the second-line antituberculosis drugs

Charles A. Peloquin and Barbara Auclair
Infectious Disease Pharmacokinetics Laboratory, National Jewish Medical and Research Center Denver, Colorado

1. INTRODUCTION

The so-called second-line antituberculosis drugs are a diverse group of agents that share one or two features: modest activity against *Mycobacterium tuberculosis,* or a fairly high potential for producing adverse effects. Because of these features, they are reserved for cases of tuberculosis (TB) that cannot be treated with the first-line agents. The principles of treatment for multidrug-resistant TB (MDRTB) using these drugs are similar to those for the treatment of TB with the first-line drugs. Combination chemotherapy is used to prevent the emergence of drug-resistant mutants already present among the population of organisms infecting the patient. Because most mutations are drug-specific, spontaneously occurring mutants are generally resistant only to one drug.

2. AMINOGLYCOSIDES AND POLYPEPTIDES

The aminoglycosides used for TB are amikacin (AK), kanamycin (KM), and streptomycin (SM). In SM, the aminocyclitol ring is streptidine; in AK

I. Bastian and F. Portaels (eds.), Multidrug-Resistant Tuberculosis, 163-174.
© 2000 *Kluwer Academic Publishers. Printed in the Netherlands.*

and KM, it is 2-deoxystreptamine [1,2]. Aminoglycosides irreversibly bind to the 30S ribosomal subunit in susceptible aerobic organisms, leading to the termination of protein synthesis. Additional mechanisms are being studied. Typical minimal inhibitory concentrations (MICs) for *M. tuberculosis* are 1-2 µg/ml in liquid media and 10-20 µg/ml in solid media [3,4]. In gram-negative bacteria, resistance results from the incorporation of plasmids, leading to enzymatic inactivation. However, spontaneous, single-step mutations leading to altered drug binding are relevant in mycobacteria. In general, resistance to KM and to AK occur simultaneously, but are independent of SM resistance, and independent of capreomycin (CM) and viomycin (VM) resistance [5].

CM and VM are chemically distinct polypeptides [1]. CM and VM appear to inhibit the translocation of peptidyl-tRNA and the initiation of protein synthesis [3-5]. Unlike the aminoglycosides, CM and VM apparently do not cause misreading of the genetic code. Typical agar MICs for CM are in the range of 15-20 µg/ml [6]. Resistance mechanisms are not well described.

In general, CM and VM behave pharmacokinetically like the aminoglycosides [7]. All are poorly absorbed orally, but intramuscular injections are generally absorbed over 30-90 minutes. Intravenous infusions in 100 ml of 5% dextrose in water or normal saline can be given over 30 minutes. Aminoglycosides distribute primarily into the extracellular water (volume of distribution Vd of 0.25 L/Kg), and plasma protein binding is limited (0-34%) [2,6]. Aminoglycosides and polypeptides are eliminated by glomerular filtration, and no metabolites have been identified. The typical elimination half-lives are 2-4 hours, and renal clearances parallel the creatinine clearance. Doses (adult and pediatric) are typically 12-15 mg/Kg 5 to 7 times weekly, or 20-27 mg/Kg 2 to 3 times weekly. Daily doses produce maximum serum concentrations (C_{max}) of 35-45 µg/ml, and the higher doses produce C_{max} of 65-80 µg/ml. These C_{max} values are back-calculated to the end of the infusion using linear regression upon two post-infusion concentrations.

These drugs can adversely affect vestibular, auditory, and renal function. Reported differences in the incidence of these toxicities among the agents reflect, in part, differences in the sizes and frequencies of doses studied. Elevated serum creatinine levels due to non-oliguric acute tubular necrosis are usually reversible; renal wasting of cations also may occur [2,6]. Periodic monitoring (every 2-4 weeks) of the serum blood urea nitrogen, creatinine, calcium, potassium, and magnesium should be considered. Vestibular changes may be noted on physical exam, and may occur independently of, or in conjunction with, tinnitus and auditory changes. The latter is best detected by monthly audiograms for those patients requiring prolonged treatment.

Less common toxicities include eosinophilia, skin rashes, and drug fever [6]. CM is not expected to cross-sensitize with the aminoglycosides. Aminoglycosides and polypeptides can potentiate other nephrotoxins, such as amphotericin B, or the neuromuscular blocking agents.

3.   CLOFAZIMINE

Clofazimine (CF) is a riminophenazine derivative originally synthesized in 1957. CF is commercially available as a capsule containing micronized drug suspended in an oil-wax base. CF may inhibit replication and growth by binding selectively to mycobacterial DNA at the guanine base [8]. CF appears bactericidal against *M. tuberculosis in vitro*, compared to its bacteriostatic activity against other mycobacteria. CF MICs ranged from 0.06 to 2.0 µg/ml when tested in 7H9 BACTEC [9]. CF's intracellular activity against *M. tuberculosis* is reported to be good due to its ability to accumulate in macrophages in high concentrations. The issue of resistance and cross-resistance with CF has not been fully investigated.

The absorption of CF varies depending on the formulation. Oral bioavailability of the microcrystalline formulation of CF is approximately 70%, and is increased by high-fat meals. The time to C_{max} (T_{max}) is 4 to 12 hours [10]. Oral administration of single 200 mg dose of CF results in a C_{max} of 0.47 µg/ml. Multiple daily doses produce concentrations of 0.5 to 2.0 µg/ml. CF is widely distributed into body fluids and tissues, principally in adipose tissues and in the reticuloendothelial system. Crystal deposition has been reported in virtually all organs. The Vd and protein binding of CF have not been determined. CF is excreted into breast milk, and is found in placental tissues. It does not seem to cross the intact blood-brain barrier [11]. The elimination of CF is best described by a bi-exponential decay in plasma concentrations with an elimination half-life ranging from 7 to 10 days in the initial phase, and an estimate of 70 days for the terminal phase. Very little is known on the metabolism of CF. We have recently found that CF is unaffected by hemodialysis; the effect of hepatic dysfunction on CF is unknown [12]. The usual dosage of CF for MDRTB is 50 to 200 mg once daily. Pediatric doses are not clearly established, but can be estimated at 2-3 mg/Kg.

Since CF is a lipophilic dye, it causes a dose-related red-brown or bronze discoloration of body tissues and fluid that usually appears within 1 to 4 weeks. Discoloration disappears within 6 to 12 months after CF is discontinued. A similar hyperpigmentation in the conjunctiva, cornea, and lacrimal fluid has been reported. Ichthyosis and dryness of the skin is also common with this drug, but can be prevented by the application of oil, petrolatum, or 25% urea emollient lotion. The most serious adverse reactions associated with CF are dose-related gastrointestinal (GI) toxicities. CF can produce a statistically significant increase in rifampin's T_{max}, but this interaction is unlikely to be clinically significant.

4.   CYCLOSERINE

Cycloserine (CS), a structural analog of D-alanine, was discovered in 1955 [1,13]. The chemically derived terizidone is similar to CS in antibacterial activity and toxicity profile. CS disrupts D-alanine incorporation into peptidoglycan during bacterial cell wall synthesis, and produces a loss of acid-fastness in mycobacteria. Cycloserine's MICs against *M. tuberculosis* are 6.2 to 25 µg/ml in liquid media and Lowenstein-Jensen medium [14]. It is generally bacteriostatic at achievable concentrations, and appears to act slowly. Cross-resistance with the other antimycobacterial drugs has not been demonstrated.

CS has a C_{max} of 18.5 ± 6.6 µg/ml after single 500 mg doses, and a T_{max} of 1.0 ± 0.7 hours following 250-500 mg doses [13]. With chronic dosing, concentrations of 20-35 µg/ml are normal. Food reduces and delays cycloserine absorption. CS's Vd and protein binding are not clearly established. CS diffuses into most body fluids and tissues, including human breast milk. Cerebrospinal fluid (CSF) concentrations are approximately 54-79% of plasma concentrations. CS is primarily eliminated by urinary excretion (47-84%), with a reported serum half-life of 8-25 hours. The usual dose of CS ranges from 250-750 mg per day, typically divided every 12 hours. Pediatric doses of 10-20 mg/Kg/day (maximum 1000 mg) in 2 equally divided doses have been used. CS is best tolerated if the dose is increased gradually over several days, and serum concentrations are helpful for guiding dosing. CS dosages need to be adjusted in renal impairment [7]. Doses may be given once daily for moderate impairment. Patients on hemodialysis probably should receive the drug 3 times per week. CS should be given after hemodialysis sessions because of significant removal, and serum concentrations should be monitored closely [12]. Hepatic failure should not require a dose change. CS has been used safely in pregnant women, although it should be avoided during the first trimester if possible [13,15,16].

CS can cause neurotoxicity, including anxiety, confusion, memory loss, dizziness, lethargy, and depression, including suicidal tendencies. Both focal and grand mal seizures may occur, but are rare with careful dosing [11]. Although CNS effects are more frequent with elevated serum CS concentrations (>35 µg/ml), some CNS disturbances are seen at "normal' concentrations. Pyridoxine (vitamin B-6, 50-60 mg per day) is often given in an attempt to prevent some of the CNS effects. CS may have additive CNS effect with other agents, including isoniazid and the fluoroquinolones.

5. ETHIONAMIDE

Ethionamide (ETA) was first synthesized in 1956 [1,17]. ETA's free carbothionamide group, also found on thiacetazone, and its pyridine ring, also found on INH, appear to be essential for activity [3,4]. Prothionamide, the n-propyl derivative of ETA, might have fewer gastrointestinal (GI) toxicities [6]. ETA is only active against mycobacteria, especially *M. tuberculosis*, *M. avium-intracellulare* and *M. leprae*. The MICs for *M. tuberculosis* in 7H12 broth MIC's range from 0.3-1.2 µg/ml, and in 7H11 agar, 2.5-10 µg/ml. Under clinical conditions, ETA is probably bacteriostatic. In animals and in man, 10 mg/Kg appears to be the minimally effective dose. *In vitro*, sustained concentrations above the MIC appear to be the most effective. ETA is in some ways like isoniazid and thiacetazone, affecting mycolic acid production and showing some cross-resistance with the latter. It is active versus both extra- and intracellular mycobacteria in monocytes [17].

ETA's absorption appears to be nearly complete [7,18]. The C_{max} after single 500-mg oral doses is 2.24 ± 0.82 µg/ml, and the T_{max} is 1.75 ± 0.75 hours. We recently have found that ETA can be given with orange juice, a high-fat breakfast, or antacids, with only small reductions in C_{max} AUC (area under the serum concentration-versus-time curve)(authors' unpublished data). Rectal doses of 500 mg ETA produced an AUC 57.3% and a C_{max} of 33% of those from oral doses. ETA has an estimated Vd of 1.5-4.0 L/Kg, CSF concentrations are close to those in the plasma, and only 10-30% of the drug is protein-bound. ETA crosses the placenta, and probably into human breast milk [17]. ETA is extensively metabolized. The sulfoxide metabolite appears be active, and may interconvert with the parent compound. Only 5% or less of the dose is excreted in the urine. The elimination half-life of ETA ranges from 1.5 to 3.0 hours. The usual dose of ETA ranges from 250-1000 mg per day. Most patients tolerate doses of 250-500 mg every 12 hours if introduced gradually over several days. ETA may also be dosed in children at 15-20 mg/Kg/day, typically up to 1000 mg, divided into two doses. No dosage adjustment is necessary in renal impairment, and little ETA is removed by hemodialysis [12]. Serum concentrations of ETA should be monitored in patients with severe hepatic impairment. ETA use during pregnancy has been associated with premature delivery, congenital delivery, congenital deformities and Down's Syndrome, and generally should be avoided in women who are pregnant [7,11].

ETA is famous for its GI intolerance, primarily nausea or vomiting. ETA suppositories, alone or combined with smaller oral doses, may reduce this problem. ETA may be given with food or prior to bedtime to reduce GI intolerance. ETA may cause CNS effects, including headache, drowsiness, giddiness, depression, psychosis, and visual changes, although a causative role has not been established. ETA also may cause peripheral neuritis, hepatotoxicity, and goiter, with or without hypothyroidism; the latter is compounded by the concurrent use of para-aminosalicylic acid (PAS) [17]. Thyroid-stimulating hormone (TSH) concentrations should be monitored periodically. ETA is associated with gynecomastia, alopecia, impotence, menorrhagia, photodermatitis, acne, arthritis, and elevated serum glucose concentrations. ETA and PAS may have additive thyroid toxicities, and ETA will exacerbate the GI toxicities of other drugs.

6. FLUOROQUINOLONES

Ciprofloxacin (CIP), ofloxacin (OFL), levofloxacin (LEVO), and sparfloxacin (SPAR) are the most active quinolones against *M. tuberculosis*. LEVO is the optical S-(-) isomer of the racemic mixture OFL. The fluoroquinolones exert their antimycobacterial effects through the inhibition of DNA gyrase (bacterial topoisomerase II) [19]. The carboxylate group at position 3 and the carbonyl group at position 4 are necessary for antibacterial activity, while addition of a fluorine atom in position 6 greatly broadens the antibacterial spectrum of activity [20]. Fluoroquinolones show bactericidal activity against *M. tuberculosis*, with MBC/MIC ratios generally between 2 and 4 [21,22]. CIP and OFL inhibit *M. tuberculosis* at concentrations of 0.25 to 2.0 µg/ml and 0.5 to 2.0 µg/ml, respectively. LEVO is twice as active as its racemic mixture. SPAR is the most potent with MICs ranging from 0.2 to 0.5 µg/ml. The most common mechanisms of resistance to quinolones involve point mutations in DNA gyrase, particularly in the gyrA gene, and alterations in cell membrane permeability are also possible. Cross-resistance has been reported between quinolones.

CIP, OFL, LEVO, and SPAR display linear pharmacokinetics. Absorption of the latter 3 exceeds 90% [19,23]. The absorption of CIP is lower, ranging from 56 to 77%. The T_{max}'s are 1 to 2 hours for CIP, OFL and LEVO; 2 to 6 hours for SPAR. Fluoroquinolones are widely distributed in body fluids and tissues. The Vd ranges from 1 to 2 L/Kg for CIP, OFL, and LEVO, to 3.6 L/Kg for SPAR, and their intracellular concentrations usually greatly exceed those in the serum. The use of SPAR for the treatment of tuberculous meningitis is limited, since it penetrates poorly into the CSF. Concentrations of CIP and OFL in inflamed meninges are 40 to 90% of concomitant serum concentrations; LEVO's penetration may be somewhat lower than the racemic mixture based on available data. CIP, OFL, SPAR, and probably LEVO cross the placenta and penetrate into breast milk. These four quinolones are only moderately bound to plasma proteins, 20 to 52%.

OFL and LEVO are primarily excreted unchanged in the urine via glomerular filtration and tubular secretion. CIP is eliminated by renal (66%) and non-renal (33%) pathways [11,19]. Four CIP metabolites have been isolated with only minimal antibacterial activity compared to the parent compound. SPAR is mainly eliminated by non-renal mechanisms. The elimination half-life of CIP is short (3-4 hours) in comparison with OFL and LEVO (6-8 hours). SPAR has a long terminal half-life of 15 to 20 hours. Based on current information, LEVO has the best combination of good *in vitro* activity and low toxicity. We use large doses oncedaily to maximize the C_{max} to MIC ratio. Our usual once-daily doses for adults are CIP 750-1000 mg, OFL 800-1000 mg, or LEVO 750-1000 mg. SPAR generally cannot be dosed over 200 mg because of toxicity. Comparable pediatric doses would be roughly 10 mg/Kg for CIP, OFL, and LEVO. We have not used SPAR in children to date. Food modestly reduces C_{max} but not AUC; however, concomitant ingestion of dairy products or drugs containing di- or trivalent cations should be avoided. Dose adjustment in renal insufficiency is recommended for all of these drugs. Dose adjustments for CIP, OFL, and LEVO are probably unnecessary in patients with hepatic impairment. The pharmacokinetic disposition of SPAR is not altered in presence of liver dysfunction. Fluoroquinolones are not recommended in pregnant or lactating women or in children unless absolutely necessary.

The most common reported side effects involved the central nervous system and the GI tract [11,19,24]. These agents should be used with caution in patient with prior history of seizure, since quinolones appear to have some pro-convulsant activity. Phototoxicity and cardiotoxicity (QT interval prolongation) are concerns with the administration of SPAR. Oral absorption of all the quinolones is significantly impaired due to chelation when co-administered with aluminum, magnesium, iron, zinc, and calcium. Concomitant administration with antacids, sulcralfate, and multivitamins containing minerals should be avoided or at least spaced by 4 to 6 hours. CIP significantly increased theophylline and caffeine serum concentrations by inhibiting the cytochrome P-450 isoenzyme IA2. OFL, LEVO, and SPAR have only minimal effects on methylxanthine metabolism. Drugs known to prolong QT interval should be avoided with SPAR.

7.   PARA-AMINOSALICYLIC ACID

PAS, discovered in the mid-1940's by Lehmann, is a synthetic structural analog of aminobenzoic acid [1,25]. PAS has bacteriostatic activity, primarily against *M. tuberculosis* and *M. bovis*. Depending on the media and inoculum size, MICs (in this case >90% inhibition) are 0.5-2.0 µg/ml (liquid media) or 1-10 µg/ml (agar). PAS may not work within macrophages, and para-aminobenzoic acid (PABA) competitively antagonizes the action of PAS *in vitro* [25]. PAS is fairly slow to act, taking more than 24 hours to show inhibition, even at high concentrations. The threshold dose is 210 mg/Kg/day in guinea pigs, with higher doses producing no greater effect. Dosing guinea pigs with PAS 3 times per week was less effective than daily doses. PAS was initially thought to inhibit the synthesis of folic acid, but later the biosynthesis of coenzyme F in the folic acid pathway was proposed as the target. Other theories about the action of PAS include interference with the uptake and utilization of salicylic acid, and thus iron transfer, or interference with mycobactin synthesis. PAS has shown cross-resistance with thiacetazone, although the mechanism of this cross-resistance is not known.

PAS and its sodium salt are extensively absorbed from the GI tract, producing C_{max} of 70-80 µg/ml within 1-2 hours [7]. Urinary recovery is 80-88% of the dose (PAS and metabolite). In the US, PAS is now available as enteric-coated, sustained-release granules (Paser®, Jacobus Pharmaceuticals). This granular preparation avoids high PAS concentrations in the stomach, has a C_{max} of 20-60 µg/ml, and has a T_{max} of about 6 hours post dose, provided that it is administered with an acidic food or beverage. The granules should not be chewed [25]. PAS is widely distributed in the body, especially the kidney, lung and liver, but to a lesser degree in the CNS. Its Vd has been broadly estimated at 1-4 L/Kg. PAS is 50-73% bound to plasma protein. The serum half-life of PAS is 45-60 minutes following oral tablets. PAS is rapidly acetylated to two main metabolites, N-acetyl-PAS, and p-aminosalicyluric acid, neither of which is active versus *M. tuberculosis*. The acetylation of PAS is a saturable process.

The U.S. Food and Drug Administration (FDA) approved adult dose of PAS granules is 12 grams/day in 3 divided doses, although twice daily dosing may be sufficient [26]. Some clinicians have tried 6-8 grams once daily as part of directly observed therapy, or DOT. The recommend pediatric dose is 50 mg/Kg 3 times daily. PAS's half-life is not altered in renal disease, but those of the metabolites are prolonged 6-fold. Hemodialysis removes small amounts of the parent compound, but also removes acetyl-PAS [12]. An extended dosing interval for PAS (every 12-24 hours) may be reasonable in severe renal dysfunction. There is no significant alteration of the PAS clearance in patients with liver disease, but given occasional hepatotoxicity, PAS should be used with caution [25]. Although PAS has been used safely in pregnant women, its safety profile has not been established completely [25].

GI disturbances from PAS are the most common adverse effects [6,11,25]. With standard tablets, nausea, vomiting, abdominal pain and diarrhea were very common. The new Paser® granules have offered significant relief from pain; however, diarrhea remains a significant problem. This diarrhea is usually self-limited over the first 2 weeks of therapy. Patients should be notified that the empty granules will appear in the stool. Various types of malabsorption with PAS are common, including steatorrhea, vitamin B_{12}, folate, xylose and iron. Hypersensitivity reactions with fever, conjunctivitis and rash occur in 5-10% of patients on PAS, and may include eosinophilia, leukopenia, thrombocytopenia, and hepatitis. Desensitization to PAS-hypersensitivity is not recommended [25]. PAS-induced hepatitis most commonly begins with a rash, followed by fever, anorexia and diarrhea. Early recognition is critical, as the mortality can be as high as 21% [25]. Patients with glucose-6-phosphate dehydrogenase deficiency may experience hemolytic anemia. PAS is known to produce goiter, with or without myxedema, and is more frequent with concomitant ethionamide therapy. This can be prevented or treated with thyroxine. Previous forms of PAS that contained bentonite reduced serum rifampin concentrations; this is not a problem with the new granules. Reduced serum digoxin concentrations have been reported. Ammonium chloride should not be used with PAS.

8. OTHER DRUGS

Amoxicillin-clavulanic acid has been used for MDRTB, although its role remains uncertain. This combination, as well as other ß-lactamase-stable compounds such as cefoxitin, might be more effective if they could be delivered into the macrophages. Perhaps liposomal formulations could achieve this aim. New rifamycins, including rifapentine and rifalazil (KRM-1648), are options primarily for the treatment of rifampin-susceptible TB. PA-824, under development at Pathogenesis Corporation in Seattle, WA, is a nitroimidazopyran, chemically related to metronidazole. It is hoped that this compound will prove to be safe and effective for TB in humans. The new macrolides clarithromycin and azithromycin have very limited activity against *M. tuberculosis*, and are better options for *M. avium* infections. Finally, thiacetazone is an inexpensive but weak drug against TB. It remains an option for desperate cases of MDRTB. Its use is limited by severe rashes that are more prevalent in HIV-positive patients.

9.   THERAPEUTIC DRUG MONITORING

Therapeutic drug monitoring (TDM) of the second-line drugs is our standard of practice at National Jewish [27]. With these weak agents, obtaining adequate serum concentrations is critical. Some agents, like cycloserine, are associated with concentration-related toxicities. Also, patients with altered clearance may be overdosed with agents like the aminoglycosides, cycloserine and ethambutol. We typically measure 2- and 6-hours post-dose concentrations to detect delayed absorption or malabsorption. Two- and 10-hour concentrations can be used to estimate the half-life for cycloserine. Thereafter, patients are monitored periodically, particularly if they experience a change in renal function. Given the long treatment durations of MDRTB (> 24 months), we believe that it is important to determine the proper dose early.

10.   SUMMARY

The second-line drugs are not routinely used, because more potent and less toxic alternatives exist for drug-susceptible TB. However, these drugs are critical for the management of the growing global problem of MDRTB.

REFERENCES

1. Offe HA. Historical introduction and chemical characteristics of antituberculosis drugs, p 1-30. In: Bartmann K (ed.), Antituberculosis Drugs. Springer-Verlag, Berlin, 1988.
2. Nicolau DP, Quintiliani R. Aminoglycosides, p 621-637. In: Yu VL, Merigan TC, Barriere S, White NJ (eds.), Antimicrobial Chemotherapy. Williams and Wilkins, Baltimore, MD, 1998.
3. Verbist L. Mode of action of antituberculous drugs (Part I). Medicon Intl 1974; 3: 11-23.
4. Verbist L. Mode of action of antituberculous drugs (Parts II). Medicon Intl 1974; 3: 3-17.
5. Winder FG. Mode of action of the antimycobacterial agents and associated aspects of the molecular biology of the mycobacteria, p 353-438. In: Ratledge C, Stanford J, (eds.), The Biology of Mycobacteria: Vol 1 — Physiology, Identification, and Classification. Academic Press, London, 1982.
6. Kucers A, Bennett N McK. The Use of Antibiotics. 4th ed. JB Lippencott Co, Philadelphia, PA, 1988.

7. Peloquin CA. Antituberculosis drugs: pharmacokinetics, p 89-122. In: Heifets LB (ed.), Drug Susceptibility in the Chemotherapy of Mycobacterial Infections. CRC Press, Boca Raton, FL, 1991.

8. Arbiser JL, Moschella SL. Clofazimine: A review of its medical uses and mechanisms of action. J Am Acad Dermatol 1995; 32: 241-7.

9. Reddy VM, Nadaahur G, Daneluzzi D, O'Sullivan JF, Gangadharam PRJ. Antituberculosis activities of clofazimine and its new analogs B4154 and B4157. Antimicrob Agents Chemother 1996; 40: 633-636.

10. Schaad-Lanyi Z, Dieterle W, Dubois JP, Theobald W, Vischer W. Pharmacokinetics of clofazimine in healthy volunteers. Int J Lepr 1987; 55: 9-15.

11. McEvoy GK, Ed. AHFS Drug Information 1999. American Society of Health-Systems Pharmacists, Bethesda, MD, 1999.

12. Malone RS, Fish DN, Spiegel DM, Childs JM, Peloquin CA. The effect of hemodialysis on cycloserine, ethionamide, para-aminosalicylate, and clofazimine. Chest 1999; 116: 984-990.

13. Berning SE, Peloquin CA. Antimycobacterial Agents: Cycloserine, p 638-642. In: Yu VL, Merigan TC, Barriere S, White NJ (eds.), Antimicrobial Chemotherapy. Williams and Wilkins, Baltimore, MD, 1998.

14. Heifets LB: Antituberculosis Drugs: Antimicrobial activity *in vitro*, p 27-41. In: Heifets LB (ed.), Drug Susceptibility in the Chemotherapy of Mycobacterial Infections. CRC Press, Boca Raton, FL, 1991.

15. Hamadeh MA, Glassroth J. Tuberculosis and pregnancy. Chest 1992; 101: 1114-1120.

16. Vallejo JG, Starke JR. Tuberculosis and pregnancy. Clin Chest Med 1992; 13: 693-707.

17. Berning SE, Peloquin CA. Antimycobacterial Agents: Ethionamide, p 650-654. In: Yu VL, Merigan TC, Barriere S, White NJ (eds.), Antimicrobial Chemotherapy. Williams and Wilkins, Baltimore, MD, 1998.

18. Iwainsky H. Mode of action, biotransformation and pharmacokinetics of antituberculosis drugs in animals and man, p 399-553. In: Bartmann K (ed.), Antituberculosis Drugs. Springer-Verlag, Berlin, 1988.

19. Schentag JJ, Scully BE. Quinolones, p 621-637. In: Yu VL, Merigan TC, Barriere S, White NJ (eds.), Antimicrobial Chemotherapy. Williams and Wilkins, Baltimore, MD, 1998.

20. Bryskier A, Chantot JF. Classification and structure-activity relationships of fluoroquinolones. Drugs 1995; 49 (suppl 2): 16-28.

21. Garcia-Rodriguez JA, Gomez Garcia AC. In-vitro activities of quinolones against mycobacteria. J Antimicrob Chemother 1993; 32: 797-808.

22. Rastogi N, Goh KS. In vitro activity of the new difluorinated quinolones sparfloxacin (AT-4140) against Mycobacterium tuberculosis compared with activities of ofloxacin and ciprofloxacin. Antimicrob Agents Chemother 1991; 35: 1933-36.

23. Martin SJ, Meyer JM, Chuck SK, Jung R, Messick CR, Pendland SL. Levofloxacin and sparfloxacin: new quinolone antibiotic. Ann Pharmacother 1998; 32: 320-36.

24. Berning SE, Madsen L, Iseman MD, Peloquin CA. Long-term safety of ofloxacin and ciprofloxacin in the treatment of mycobacterial infections. Am J Respir Crit Care Med 1995; 151: 2006-9.

25. Berning SE, Peloquin CA. Antimycobacterial Agents: Para-aminosalicylic acid, p 663-668. In: Yu VL, Merigan TC, Barriere S, White NJ (eds.), Antimicrobial Chemotherapy. Williams and Wilkins, Baltimore, MD, 1998.

26. Peloquin CA, Berning SE, Huitt GA, Childs JM, Singleton MD, James GT. Once-daily and twice-daily dosing of p-aminosalicylic acid (PAS) granules. Am J Respir Crit Care Med 1999; 159: 932-4.

27. Peloquin CA. Using therapeutic drug monitoring to dose the antimycobacterial drugs. Clin Chest Med 1997; 18: 79-87.

Chapter 11

Treatment of multidrug-resistant tuberculosis

Michael D. Iseman and Gwen A. Huitt
National Jewish Medical and Research Center, Denver, Colorado

1.   INTRODUCTION

The modern era of effective tuberculosis chemotherapy began in 1952. Since then, strains of *Mycobacterium tuberculosis* have acquired resistance to various drugs. The rising prevalence of multidrug-resistant strains (resistant to isoniazid and rifampicin, with or without resistance to other drugs) is most ominous and has resulted in many cases of marginally treatable, often fatal, disease. The World Health Organization (WHO) noted in 1997 that not only is tuberculosis a global emergency, but that several "hot spots" exist where multidrug-resistant tuberculosis (MDRTB) prevalence is so high that control programs are threatened [1]. These "hot spots", in conjunction with rising HIV prevalence, pose a serious threat to tuberculosis control programs. Many still consider MDRTB a focal problem that need not be addressed on a global scale. The contrary view, eloquently stated by Farmer et al, is that "… in choosing to ignore MDRTB as a global priority, we are setting our sights too low. Unambitious goals will insure millions of deaths and the persistence, in the human population, of resistant *M. tuberculosis*" [2]. In this chapter we will focus on the care of patients with MDRTB as well as examine the origins, biologic mechanisms, and epidemiology of drug resistance, its impact on the outcome of therapy, and the implications of MDR-TB for standard initial therapeutic regimens.

I. Bastian and F. Portaels (eds.), Multidrug-Resistant Tuberculosis, 175-190
© 2000 *Kluwer Academic Publishers. Printed in the Netherlands.*

2.   INADEQUATE TREATMENT PROGRAMS AND ACQUIRED DRUG RESISTANCE

Streptomycin was introduced for the management of tuberculosis 45 years ago. Soon it became evident that monotherapy frequently resulted in treatment failure that was associated with *in vitro* resistance to the drug [3,4]. Aminosalicylic acid and isoniazid were subsequently combined with streptomycin in a regimen that was nearly universally curative. Treatment was highly successful because it was done in hospitals, assuring compliance and preventing acquired drug resistance. In the 1960's, however, therapy was shifted to the outpatient setting. Unfortunately, this shift reduced adherence, leading to rising rates of failure, relapse, and acquired drug resistance [5-9]. These factors, coupled with rising HIV rates, were associated with increases in both morbidity and drug resistance in the United States in the period 1984-1992. In response, federal and other governmental agencies funnelled over $1 billion into restructuring tuberculosis control programs and broadly expanding directly observed therapy (DOT) capacity [10]. The results have been dramatic: total cases have dropped from 26,673 in 1992 to 18,361 in 1998 (-31%); and, MDR cases have fallen from 3.5% in 1992 to less than 1% in 1998 [11]. Attention must now be focused on the global community to pursue similar results [12].

3.   BIOLOGIC MECHANISMS OF RESISTANCE

Mycobacteria utilize three basic strategies to achieve drug resistance:
(a) a lipid rich cell wall which greatly reduces permeability for many compounds;
(b) production of degrading and drug-modifying enzymes which render certain compounds useless; and,
(c) most significantly, modification by spontaneous chromosomal mutations of key target genes.

These mutations are unlinked; hence, resistance to a drug is not associated with resistance to an unrelated drug. At least eight such resistance genes have been characterized [13]. The emergence of drug resistance represents the survival of random pre-existing mutations, not a change caused by exposure to the medication. That the mutations are unlinked is the cardinal principle underlying modern chemotherapy. For example, resistance mutations to isoniazid or rifampicin occur in roughly 1 in 10^8 to 10^9 replications of bacteria [14]. The likelihood of spontaneous mutations causing resistance to both isoniazid and rifampicin is the product of these probabilities or 1 in 10^{16}. Patients with tuberculosis, even those with extensive cavitary disease, harbour far fewer mycobacteria than this, so the development of spontaneous, dual resistance is highly improbable.

This model breaks down when chemotherapy is inadequate, however. In the circumstances of monotherapy [15], erratic drug ingestion, omission of one or more of the prescribed agents, sub-optimal dosage, poor drug absorption, or an insufficient number of active agents in a regimen [16], a susceptible strain of *M. tuberculosis* may become resistant to multiple drugs within a matter of months.

4.   CURRENT EPIDEMIOLOGY OF RESISTANCE

MDRTB is a global problem with focal emergencies. The WHO estimates that 50 million people may be infected with strains of *M. tuberculosis* resistant to at least one of the standard agents [1]. In a 1994-7 study by the International Union Against Tuberculosis and Lung Disease (IUATLD) and the WHO, 34 of 35 countries surveyed were experiencing increased prevalence of MDRTB. "Hot spots" included Russia, Latvia, Estonia, the Dominican Republic, the Ivory Coast, and Argentina. In Russia, MDRTB is a major health emergency in prison populations, with death rates from 11-24%, the disease causing 50-80% of prison deaths [17-19].

The most powerful predictor of MDRTB in these studies was a history of prior treatment. Inadequate therapy is the most common means by which resistance is acquired, and patients who have previously undergone therapy should be presumed to harbour drug-resistant organisms until proved otherwise. Additionally, patients with cavitary lesions are at greater risk of resistance [4, 20], presumably because they harbour greater numbers of rapidly multiplying mycobacteria.

In the past, most cases of MDRTB evolved through multiple, ineffectual courses of treatment. This is commonly referred to as acquired drug resistance. Recently, however, a new pattern has emerged: transmission of MDRTB to contacts, which results in primary drug resistance. Epidemics of MDRTB have been described mainly among populations with pre-existing acquired immunodeficiency syndrome (AIDS) or human immunodeficiency virus (HIV) infection. But, transmission of infection following exposure to MDRTB cases has been reported in substantial numbers of HIV-negative health care workers and institutional personnel [21-24]. And, outbreaks of MDR-TB have been described among HIV-negative groups exposed in institutions such as hospitals, prisons, and schools [25-27].

5. **EFFECTS OF DRUG RESISTANCE ON TREATMENT OUTCOME**

5.1 HIV-negative immunocompetent patients

The best data on the influence of drug-resistance on treatment outcome comes from trials conducted in East Africa, Hong Kong, and Singapore [28]. For patients treated for six months or longer, the presence of drug-resistant organisms at the start of therapy was associated with an 83-fold greater risk (11.6 percent vs. 0.15 percent) of treatment failure, defined as the failure of treatment to produce negative cultures. There was also a twofold (11 percent vs. 5 percent) greater risk of relapse, defined as recurrence of disease after treatment was stopped. Infections with organisms resistant to single drugs such as isoniazid or streptomycin could be treated successfully with four-drug regimens featuring the extended use of rifampicin. The success rate was much lower among patients with organisms resistant to rifampin and isoniazid: eight of 11 patients (73 percent) with isoniazid-and rifampicin-resistant bacilli did not respond to treatment or relapsed.

Results from a recent study in Korea indicate that sustained bacterial and clinical response was achieved in 82% (52/63) of HIV-negative MDRTB patients who received individually tailored regimens [29]. Treatment failure was associated with initial resistance to a greater number of drugs. Results from 171 HIV-negative patients studied at NJC from 1976-1983 were not as favourable. All patients had extensive pulmonary tuberculosis resistant to isoniazid and rifampicin as well as various other drugs; the average strain was resistant to 5.8 drugs [16]. The usual duration of the hospital stay was seven months, and the patients received an average of 5.7 drugs. Adjunctive surgical resection was used in nine patients. After discharge, nearly all patients returned to their home communities to complete therapy under close supervision. Oral medications were given for an average of 24 months after the organisms could no longer be detected in the sputum. This approach yielded a disappointing 65% initial rate of sputum conversion and, because of subsequent relapses, a long-term cure rate of only 56%. We believe that a major adverse factor in outcome in these patients was the chronicity of disease. The great majority of cases had been treated for many years before referral to our facility. We reason that extensive fibrotic changes limited drug penetration and prevented closure of cavities.

5.2 Patients with HIV Infection / AIDS / Immunosuppression

Numerous reports have portrayed the dismal outcome of HIV-infected individuals with MDRTB. Many of the reports document nosocomial outbreaks in hospitals and correctional institutions [21,23,30,31]. In all studies, survival was significantly improved if therapy with at least 4 drugs with *in vitro* activity was instituted within one month of diagnosis. Other important factors associated with treatment success were higher CD-4 lymphocyte counts, no prior AIDS diagnosis, and adequate serum drug concentrations [32-34].

Critical observations have been made through careful analyses of these outbreaks. First is the need for appropriate environmental controls to prevent nosocomial transmission. Second, a high index of suspicion for MDRTB must be maintained for HIV-infected individuals. Third, prompt initiation of appropriate drug therapy clearly reduces mortality. And, fourth, patients with advanced AIDS at the time of presentation have a much shorter median survival than HIV seropositive individuals with no prior opportunistic infections (3.3 months vs. 10.6 months) [32].

Patients with other immunosuppressed states (eg. insulin-dependent diabetes mellitus, connective tissue disorders, vasculitis, long-term glucocorticoid therapy, and cancer) are also potentially at great risk for poor outcomes if they become infected with MDRTB. Drug toxicity, drug malabsorption, and drug-drug interactions all pose significant treatment difficulties for both the patient and the clinician.

6. IMPLICATIONS OF MULTIDRUG RESISTANCE FOR INITIAL THERAPY

Currently, United States guidelines advocate an initial four-drug regimen: isoniazid, rifampicin, pyrazinamide and ethambutol (pyrazinamide is given for two months, isoniazid and rifampicin for six months, and ethambutol may be discontinued when there is laboratory documentation of isoniazid and rifampicin susceptibility)[35,36]. This regimen is recommended on the premise that ethambutol will act as an "insurance policy" to protect rifampicin while awaiting susceptibility results. Similar concerns have led WHO to deem this initial 4-drug regimen as the standard of care.

In much of the world where TB is rampant, drug susceptibility testing is not available. Even in the industrialized nations, the results of susceptibility tests commonly are not available for two to four months, although the test can be done far more rapidly [37,38]. Obtaining susceptibility tests rapidly allows treatment to be modified in a timely manner to protect against further acquired drug resistance and to diminish the potential toxicity of empirical five or six-drug regimens. In addition, cumulative data on the prevalence of drug resistance within communities is crucial for guiding empirical choices for initial therapy.

7. TREATMENT OF PATIENTS WITH MULTIDRUG-RESISTANT TUBERCULOSIS

As well as reliable drug-susceptibility testing, a careful history of previous treatment must be taken to provide optimal treatment for MDRTB. The importance of a prior history of drug usage was highlighted in a review of patients with MDRTB treated at National Jewish Hospital from 1976 through 1983; this analysis demonstrated that previous therapy with a drug for more than a month was associated with diminished efficacy of that drug regardless of apparent *in vitro* susceptibility.

Table 1. Dosages and pharmacokinetics of antituberculosis medications

Drug	Usual adult daily dosage[a]	Peak serum concentration µg/ml	Usual MIC range[b] µg/ml
First-line oral drugs			
Pyrazinamide	30 mg/kg	20-60	6.2-50
Ethambutol	15-25 mg/kg	3-5	0.5-2.0
Injectable drugs			
Streptomycin	15 mg/kg	35-45	0.25-2.0
Amikacin	15 mg/kg	35-45	0.5-1.0
Kanamycin	15 mg/kg	35-45	1.5-3.0
Capreomycin	15 mg/kg	35-45	1.25-2.5
Second-line drugs			
Ciprofloxacin	750 mg q.d.	3-5	0.25-2.0
Ofloxacin	600 mg q.d.	8-10	0.25-2.0
Levofloxacin	750 mg q.d.	8-12	< 1.0
Ethionamide	250 mg b.i.d. or 500 mg q.d.	1-5	0.3-1.2
Aminosalicylic acid	4 gm b.i.d.	40-70	Not known
Cycloserine	250 mg b.i.d. or 500 mg q.d.	20-35	Not known

[a]q.d., once daily dose; b.i.d., twice a day. [b]data from reference 39; MIC, minimum inhibitory concentration.

7.1 Initiation of Retreatment for MDRTB

An MDRTB retreatment regimen should include at least four but, possibly, as many as six or seven drugs. The number of drugs used varies depending on the extent of disease and the potency of the available agents. Ideally, therapy should be initiated in the hospital to permit observation of toxicity and intolerance and to allow a change of regimen before strongly aversive conditioning makes the patient psychologically as well as physically intolerant of the medications. At our institution, we usually initiate treatment with small doses of each drug and increase to the planned dose over three to 10 days. Drug dosages as well as optimal timing of administration achieve maximal serum concentrations in the target range with minimal side effects (Tables 1 & 2). We have employed pharmacokinetic studies to optimize therapy since the bioavailability and clearance of the retreatment antituberculosis drugs are not predictable. Persons at relatively greater risk for malabsorption include persons with AIDS, insulin-dependent diabetes mellitus, haemodialysis, or a history of gastro-intestinal resection [40]. These measures may seem tedious and time-consuming, but we believe they offer the most effective way to institute retreatment. This approach seems justified because of the implications of retreatment failure, not only for the patient with a life-threatening disease, but also for the public, in terms of the financial and social costs of extended, repeated hospitalizations and the transmission of potentially incurable tuberculosis to others [27]. Some strategies for treating patients with proven MDRTB are shown in Table 3.

The treatment of patients with documented drug resistance is straightforward in contrast to that of patients for whom susceptibility results are not available. When treatment fails or a relapse occurs, the original regimen should be continued or resumed until new susceptibility data are obtained. However, these important variables must be considered.

a) <u>was drug susceptibility determined initially?</u> If so, and the appropriate drugs were used, the unsuccessful outcome was probably caused by non-compliance. If not, primary resistance to one or more of the initially employed drugs may have contributed to the unfavourable result.

b) <u>was therapy self-administered or directly observed?</u> If the latter, primary resistance was probably the dominant factor; less likely, malabsorption may be involved.

c) <u>is the patient particularly vulnerable to tuberculosis?</u> For example, a patient with advanced AIDS and TB who experiences treatment failure or relapse might die if an inadequate regimen is used. Hence, the re-treatment regimen should include new drugs.

d) how long will it take to obtain new susceptibility results? If the results will be available in two weeks, one might continue the prior medications. If the results will not be available for two to four months, however, it might be prudent to add several new drugs to prevent the development of further drug resistance.

Table 2. Side effects of antituberculosis medications

Drug	Side effects[a]
Pyrazinamide	Hepatitis, rash, arthritis/arthralgia, hyperuricaemia, abdominal distress
Ethambutol	Optic neuritis, abdominal distress
Injectable drugs Streptomycin, Amikacin, Kanamycin, Capreomycin	Hearing loss, ataxia, nystagmus, proteinuria, azotaemia, serum electrolyte abnormalities, eosinophila
Quinolones Ofloxacin , Levofloxacin, Ciprofloxacin	Arthralgia, tendonitis, headache, anxiety, tremulousness, abdominal distress, thrush
Ethionamide	Abdominal distress, dysgeusia, hypothyroidism, diarrhoea, glucose intolerance, sexual dysfunction, rash
Aminosalicylic acid	Abdominal distress, nausea, diarrhoea, bloating, rash, hypothyroidism, oedema
Cycloserine	Mood and cognitive deterioration, psychosis, seizures

[a]a partial listing; for more information, see the Physicians' Desk Reference or the package insert provided with each medication.

7.2   Drugs Used in Retreatment Regimens

Retreatment agents are generally less potent, often require multiple daily doses, and typically are less well tolerated than the first-line medications. These agents are summarized in tables 1 and 2. The mainstays of most retreatment regimens would be a fluoroquinolone, an aminoglycoside, and 2 or 3 other agents [41-45].

Other drugs not included in the table, but used in some desperate situations include clofazimine, amoxicillin-clavulanate, clarithromycin, and azithromycin [46]. These agents have been used successfully in cases involving mycobacteria other than tuberculosis, although their clinical efficacy in tuberculosis has not been established. Amithiozone, or thioacetazone, used in the developing nations because of its low price, has modest tuberculostatic activity. The side effects of amithiozone are similar to those of ethionamide; particularly problematic is erythema multiforme or toxic epidermal necrolysis in patients with AIDS. For this reason, amithiozone has been deemed inappropriate for use in HIV-infected individuals [47].

Immunomodulation is now being targeted as an important adjunct for treatment of MDRTB. Interferon gamma activates macrophages and helps potentiate killing of tubercle bacilli. Condos et al [48] have reported clinical and radiographic improvement in patients who received interferon gamma via aerosol. IL-2 is also being actively studied as an immunomodulatory agent [49].

Table 3. Potential regimens for patients with tuberculosis with various patterns of drug resistance

Resistance	Suggested regimen	Duration of therapy	Comments
Isoniazid, streptomycin	Rifampicin Pyrazinamide Ethambutol Amikacin[a]	6 to 9 months	Anticipate 100% response rate and less than 5% relapse rate
Isoniazid and ethambutol (± streptomycin)	Rifampicin Pyrazinamide Amikacin[a] Quinolone[b]	6 to 12 months	Efficacy should be comparable to above regimen
Isoniazid and rifampicin (± streptomycin)	Pyrazinamide Ethambutol Amikacin[a] Quinolone[b]	18 to 24 months	Consider surgery
Isoniazid, rifampicin, and ethambutol (± streptomycin)	Pyrazinamide Amikacin[a] Quinolone[b] plus 2 other drugs[c]	24 months after conversion	Consider surgery
Isoniazid, rifampicin, and pyrazinamide (± streptomycin)	Ethambutol Amikacin[a] Quinolone[b] plus 2 other drugs[c]	24 months after conversion	Consider surgery
Isoniazid, rifampicin, pyrazinamide, and ethambutol (± streptomycin)	Amikacin[a] Quinolone[b] plus 3 other drugs[c]	24 months after conversion	Surgery, if possible

[a]Capreomycin is a reasonable alternative if there is resistance to amikacin, kanamycin and streptomycin. If toxicity does not intervene, injectable agents are continued for four to six months. All of the injectable agents may be given intravenously or intramuscularly, and are given daily (or 2-3 times per week). [b]Quinolones include ciprofloxacin, ofloxacin, and levofloxacin. [c]Second-line drugs include ethionamide, cycloserine, or aminosalicylic acid. Clofazimine and amoxicillin-clavulanate may also be considered but their efficacy remains unconfirmed. Clarithromycin, azithromycin, and rifabutin are unlikely to be of benefit.

7.3 Monitoring re-treatment

Sputum specimens should be obtained for semi-quantitative smear and culture weekly during the initial phase of therapy in order to determine the baseline mycobacterial burden. Improvement in the results of bacteriologic testing of sputum is the main marker of response, but decreased fever, cough, sputum, as well as weight gain are important indirect markers of success.   Improvement on the chest radiograph may lag behind other changes.

The optimal duration of retreatment has not been clearly identified. At NJC we usually administer injectable drugs for six months after sputum conversion or surgical resection if toxicity does not intervene. Patients infected with organisms that are resistant to all or most of the first-line drugs are treated with oral medications for 24 months after the sputum culture becomes negative. This duration of treatment is based on the impression, not rigorously documented, that discontinuation of treatment before this time increases the risk of reactivation. Among the patients we cared for from 1973-1983, approximately 20% who initially responded to therapy with sustained negative sputum cultures experienced reactivation after discontinuation of therapy [16] (this observation led us to more aggressive use of surgery).

Generally, if chemotherapy is to achieve sputum conversion, it will do so within four months in most patients. If sputum conversion does not occur or the patient relapses, further acquired resistance to the agents being used will appear. Hence, if chemotherapy is not successful, the potential benefits of resectional surgery should be considered.

7.4   The Role of Resectional Surgery

In view of disastrous adverse consequences of treatment failure, we have become more aggressive with resectional surgery as an adjunct to medical treatment [50]. Patients are considered for resectional surgery if their pattern of drug resistance and extent of disease indicate a significant risk of medical treatment failure. Criteria for surgery include localized pulmonary disease, adequate cardiopulmonary reserve and optimal medical therapy for at least six weeks [51]. We attempt to render the patient sputum smear negative prior to surgery but this is not an absolute criterion. Adequate nutritional support must be maintained prior to surgery, and a serum albumin of at least 3.0 gm/dl will help promote wound healing. The surgery must be performed by a thoracic surgeon with adequate experience to cope with the severely distorted anatomy.

From 1983-1998, we have performed 153 resectional surgeries on patients with tuberculosis [52]. Among these patients, there have been 22 deaths, 5 of which were related to surgery. Overall, however, the clinical and bacteriologic responses have been gratifying: 125 of 136 (92%) long-term survivors have had consistently negative sputum smears and cultures. Because the great majority of these patients had active disease despite extended retreatment, substantially fewer were deemed likely to be cured with only chemotherapy.

7.5 What to Do in Cases of Ultimate Treatment Failure?

In spite of aggressive management, there inevitably will be some patients who remain sputum culture positive with MDRTB. If improved chemotherapy cannot be provided and if surgery is not feasible or available, we must address the elements of care that can provide optimal quality and duration of life for these unfortunate patients. Yet, we must be mindful of the mandate to minimize the public risk of transmission of an untreatable, potentially lethal infection.

Our limited experience suggests that, despite clear-cut failure and high levels of drug resistance, total discontinuation of treatment is not prudent. We believe that in some proportion of cases, ongoing use of medications may act to suppress the infection. At the point when it becomes clear that "cure" is not achievable, one might reconsider the drug regimen, perhaps abandoning some of the more poorly tolerated or expensive agents, but leaving the patient on a maintenance program—perhaps including isoniazid, rifampicin, and ethambutol. If therapy reduction is undertaken, the patient should be observed lest unanticipated, abrupt worsening occurs. Suffering from constitutional or respiratory distress must also be alleviated by the use of antipyretics, analgesics, cough suppressants, and supplemental oxygen.

To lessen the likelihood of transmission of infection, patients and families should be counselled to minimize indoor exposure of uninfected or particularly vulnerable contacts. Patients must be instructed to cover their mouths and noses during coughing spells, and home ventilation should be maximized.

8. PREVENTION OF TUBERCULOSIS IN THE CONTACTS OF MDRTB PATIENTS

Patients with advanced MDRTB are typically treated initially in the hospital, where the risk of transmission of tuberculous infection to health care workers and other patients is substantial [53,54]. Because infection with drug-resistant tubercle bacilli is especially hazardous, special precautions should be taken to minimize the risk [55]. Theoretically, this could be accomplished by proper ventilation, but studies of a recent tuberculosis outbreak in an office building indicated that there are practical limits to this method [56]. We believe that the use of ultraviolet germicidal irradiation devices is both theoretically and practically the best means to curtail tuberculosis transmission [57,58]; the value of masks, respirators, and filtration devices is unproved and highly problematic. One nosocomial epidemic appeared to be curtailed by an aggressive program of rigorous isolation policies, negative-pressure ventilation of patients' rooms, filtration of major air conduits, use of submicron moulded masks, and the use of ultraviolet fixtures in areas where negative-pressure ventilation could not be achieved [59].

Isoniazid is the only medication proven efficacious for the prevention of tuberculosis [34,60,61]. But, on the basis of various *in vitro* data and animal studies, rifampicin is believed to have equal or greater efficacy [62]. But for contacts thought to be infected with tubercle bacilli resistant to both these agents, there is no obvious choice for preventive chemotherapy. The CDC has developed a complex but thoughtful set of recommendations for the care of persons exposed to MDRTB [63]. The document helps clinicians assess the likelihood that there is new infection, that the infecting strain is drug-resistant, and the probability that the newly infected person will develop active tuberculosis--vital elements in decision making about preventive therapy. For contacts deemed likely to be newly infected with MDRTB and at high risk for active disease, treatment with ethambutol and pyrazinamide or, alternatively, levofloxacin, ofloxacin or ciprofloxacin and pyrazinamide was proposed. However, the fluoroquinolone/PZA regimen has been associated with an unexpectedly high risk of adverse effects including hepatitis, nausea, and skin rash; therefore, this approach must be regarded with caution [64].

Given the lack of attractive drugs for preventive treatment, there has been renewed interest in the use of BCG (the bacillus of Calmette and Guérin) vaccine for health professionals or others at high risk of exposure to tuberculosis, including multidrug-resistant strains [65]. BCG vaccine has not been clearly shown to be effective in adults, however. Its strongest protective effects are in infants and children [65]; two recent studies that included adults failed to show protection [66,67]. Hence, we have been reluctant to use a vaccine of uncertain efficacy, which would confound the results of tuberculin skin-test surveillance and create a potentially false sense of security among those who work in facilities where patients with tuberculosis are treated. In addition, vaccination with BCG--an attenuated but living strain of *M. bovis*--poses a potential risk of disseminated disease or progressive local infection among immunocompromised recipients.

9.   SUMMARY

The frequency of tuberculosis resistant to standard antituberculous medications is rising in many areas of the world. This increase is a major threat to treatment and control programs. To prevent this situation from worsening, initial treatment programs that entail directly observed therapy supported by effective inducements or enforcement must be used [68-71]. Re-treatment of patients with documented MDRTB ideally should be carried out in programs with comprehensive microbiological, psychosocial, and nutritional support systems. Regimens of multiple drugs, which generally are poorly tolerated and more toxic than traditional regimens, must be administered for 18 to 24 months. Resectional surgery may be required for substantial numbers of patients. For patients with AIDS who acquire tuberculosis caused by MDR strains, the disease may prove lethal before effective therapy can be implemented.

REFERENCES

1. World Health Organization. Anti-tuberculosis drug resistance in the world: the WHO/IUATLD global project on anti-tuberculosis drug resistance surveillance 1994-1997. WHO, Geneva, 1997.
2. Farmer P, Kim J. Community based approaches to the control of multidrug resistant tuberculosis: introducing "DOTS-plus". Brit Med J 1998; 317: 671-674.
3. Mitchison DA. Development of streptomycin resistant strains of tubercle bacilli in pulmonary tuberculosis: results of simultaneous sensitivity tests in liquid and on solid media. Thorax 1950; 5: 144-161.
4. Canetti G. Present aspects of bacterial resistance in tuberculosis. Am Rev Respir Dis 1965; 92: 687-703.
5. Hobby GL. Primary drug resistance in tuberculosis: a review. Am Rev Respir Dis 1962; 86: 839-846.
6. *Idem.* Primary drug resistance in tuberculosis: a review. Am Rev Respir Dis 1963; 87: 29-36.
7. Doster B, Caras GJ, Snider DE. A continuing survey of primary drug resistance in tuberculosis, 1961 to 1968: a U.S. Public Health Service cooperative study. Am Rev Respir Dis 1976; 113: 419-425.
8. Kopanoff DE, Kilburn JO, Glassroth JL, Snider DE Jr, Farer LS, Good RC. A continuing survey of tuberculosis primary drug resistance in the United States: March 1975 to November 1977: a United States Public Health Service cooperative study. Am Rev Respir Dis 1978; 118: 835-842.
9. Snider DE, Cauthen GM, Farer LS, et al. Drug-resistant tuberculosis. Am Rev Respir Dis 1991; 144: 732.
10. Park MM, Davis AL, Schluger NW, Cohen H, Rom WN. Outcome of MDR-TB patients, 1983-1993: prolonged survival with appropriate therapy. Am J Resp Crit Care Med 1996; 153: 317-324.
11. Moore M, Onorato IM, McCray E, Castro KG. Trends in drug-resistant tuberculosis in the United States, 1993-1996. JAMA 1997; 278: 833-837.
12. Iseman MD, Sbarbaro JA. The increasing prevalence of resistance to antituberculosis chemotherapeutic agents: implications for global tuberculosis control. Curr Clin Top Infect Dis 1992; 12: 188-207.
13. Telenti A. Genetics of drug resistance in tuberculosis. Clin Chest Med 1997; 18: 55-64.
14. David HL. Drug-resistance in *M. tuberculosis* and other mycobacteria. Clin Chest Med 1980; 1: 227-230.

15. Costello HD, Caras GJ, Snider DE Jr. Drug resistance among previously treated tuberculosis patients, a brief report. Am Rev Respir Dis 1980; 121: 313-316

16. Goble M, Iseman MD, Madsen LA, Waite D, Ackerson L, Horsburgh CR Jr. Treatment of 171 patients with pulmonary tuberculosis resistant to isoniazid and rifampin. N Engl J Med 1993; 328: 527-532.

17. Coninx R, Pfyffer GE, Mathieu C, Savina D, Debacker M, Jafarov F, Jabrailow, Ismailov A, Mirzoev F, de Haller R, Portaiels F. Drug resistant tuberculosis in prisons in Azerbaijan: case study. BMJ 1998; 316: 1423-1425.

18. Coninx R, Mathieu C, Debacker M, Mirzoev F, Ismaelov A, de Haller R, Meddings DR. First-line tuberculosis therapy and drug-resistant *Mycobacterium tuberculosis* in prisons. Lancet 1999; 353: 969-973.

19. Khomenko A, and Medécins sans Frontières, cited in Reyes H, Conninx R. Pitfalls of tuberculosis programmes in prisons. Br Med J 1997; 315:1447-1450.

20. Ben-Dov I, Mason GR. Drug-resistant tuberculosis in a southern California hospital: trends from 1969 to 1984. Am Rev Respir Dis 1987; 135: 1307-1310.

21. Kenyon TA, Ridzon R, Luskin-Hawk R, Schultz C, Paul WS, Valway SE, Onorato IM, Castro K. A nosocomial outbreak of multidrug-resistant tuberculosis. Ann Int Med 1997; 127: 32-36.

22. Pitchenik AE, Burr J, Laufer M, et al. Outbreaks of drug-resistant tuberculosis at an AIDS center. Lancet 1990; 335: 440-1.

23. Fischl MA, Uttamchandani RB, Daikos GL, et al. An outbreak of tuberculosis caused by multiple-drug resistant tubercle bacilli among patients with HIV infection. Ann Intern Med 1992; 117: 177-183.

24. Snider DE Jr, Kelly GD, Cauthen GM, Thompson NJ, Kilburn JO. Infection and disease among contacts of tuberculosis cases with drug-resistant and drug-susceptible bacilli. Am Rev Respir Dis 1985; 132: 125-132.

25. Reves R, Blakey D, Snider DE Jr, Farer LS. Transmission of multiple drug-resistant tuberculosis: report of a school and community outbreak. Am J Epidemiol 1981; 113: 423-430.

26. Nardell E, McInnis B, Thomas B, Weidhaas S. Exogenous reinfection with tuberculosis in a shelter for the homeless. N Engl J Med 1986; 315: 1570-1575.

27. Outbreak of multidrug-resistant tuberculosis --- Texas, California, and Pennsylvania. MMWR Morb Mortal Wkly Rep 1990; 39: 369-372.

28. Mitchison DA, Nunn AJ. Influence of initial drug resistance on the response to short-course chemotherapy of pulmonary tuberculosis. Am Rev Respir Dis 1986; 133: 423-430.

29. Park SK, Kim CT, Song SD. Outcome of chemotherapy in 107 patients with pulmonary tuberculosis resistant to isoniazid and rifampin. Int J Tuberc Lung Dis 1998; 2; 877-884.

30. Dooley SW, Villarino ME, Lawrence M, Salinas L, Amil S, Rullan JV, et al. Nosocomial transmission of tuberculosis in a hospital unit for HIV-infected patients. JAMA. 1992; 267: 2632-2634.

31. Edlin BR, Tokars JI, Grieco MH, Crawford JT, Williams J, Sordillo EM, et al. An outbreak of multidrug-resistant tuberculosis among hospitalized patients with the acquired immunodeficiency syndrome. N Engl J Med. 1992; 326: 1514-1521.

32. Park MM, Davis AL, Schluger NW, Cohen H, Rom WN. Outcome of MDR-TB patients, 1983-1993: prolonged survival with appropriate therapy. Am J Resp Crit Care Med 1996; 153: 317-324.

33. Peloquin CA, Nitta AT, Burman WJ, et al. Low anti-tuberculosis drug concentrations in patients with AIDS. Ann Pharmacother 1996; 30: 919-925.

34. Berning SE, Huitt GA, Iseman MD, Peloquin CA. Malabsorption of antituberculosis medications by a patient with AIDS. N Engl J Med 1992; 327: 1817-1818.
35. American Thoracic Society/Centers for Disease Control. Treatment of tuberculosis and tuberculosis infection in adults and children. Am J Respir Crit Care Med 1994; 149: 1359-1374.
36. Initial therapy for tuberculosis in the era of MDR-TB: recommendations of the Advisory Council for the Elimination of Tuberculosis. MMWR Morb Mortal Wkly Rep 1993; 42(RR-7): 1-8.
37. Heifets LB. Drug susceptibility in the chemotherapy of mycobacterial infections. CRC Press, Boca Raton, Fl, 1991.
38. Heifits L. Drug susceptibility testing. Clinc Lab Med 1996; 16: 641-656.
39. Heifits L. Qualitative and quantitative drug-susceptibility tests in mycobacteriology. Am Rev Respir Dis 1988; 137: 1217-1222.
40. Berning SE, Madsen L, Iseman MD, Peloquin CA. Long-term safety of ofloxacin and ciprofloxacin in the treatment of mycobacterial infections. Am J Resp Crit Care Med 1995; 151: 2006-2009.
41. Sirgel FA, Botha FJ, Parkin DP, Van de Wal BW, Schall R, Donald PR, Mitchison DA. The early bactericidal activity of ciprofloxacin in patients with pulmonary tuberculosis. Am J Respir Crit Care Med 1997; 156: 901-905.
42. Hong Kong Chest Service/British Medical Research Council. A controlled study of rifabutin and an uncontrolled study of ofloxacin in the retreatment of patients with pulmonary tuberculosis resistant to isoniazid, streptomycin, and rifampicin. Tuber Lung Dis 1992; 73: 59-67.
43. Tsukamura M. *In vitro* antituberculosis activity of a new antibacterial substance ofloxacin (DL8280). Am Rev Respir Dis 1985; 131: 348-351.
44. Heifets LB, Lindholm-Levy PJ. Bacteriostatic and bactericidal activity of ciprofloxacin and ofloxacin against *Mycobacterium tuberculosis* and Mycobacterium avium complex. Tubercle 1987; 68: 267-276.
45. Chen C-H, Shih J-F, Lindholm-Levy PJ, Heifets LB. Minimal inhibitory concentrations of rifabutin, ciprofloxacin, and ofloxacin against *Mycobacterium tuberculosis* isolated before treatment of patients in Taiwan. Am Rev Respir Dis 1989; 140: 987-989.
46. Nadler JR, Berger J, Nord JA, Cofsky R, Saxena M. Amoxicillin-clavulanic acid for treating drug-resistant Mycobacterium tuberculosis. Chest 1991; 99: 1025-1026.
47. Nunn P, Kibuga D, Gathua S, et al. Cutaneous hypersensitivity reactions due to thiacetazone in HIV-1 seropositive patients treated for tuberculosis. Lancet 1991; 337: 627-630.
48. Condos R, Rom WN, Schluger NW. Treatment of multidrug resistant pulmonary tuberculosis with interferon-gamma via aerosol. Lancet 1997; 349: 1513-1515.
49. Johnson BJ, Bekker LG, Rickman R, Brown S, Lesser M, Ress S, Willcox P, Steyn L, Kaplan G. rhuIL-2 adjunctive therapy in multidrug resistant tuberculosis: a comparison of two treatment regimens and placebo. Tubercle and Lung Dis 1997; 78: 195-203.
50. Iseman MD, Madsen L, Goble M, Pomerantz M. Surgical intervention in the treatment of pulmonary disease caused by drug-resistant Mycobacterium tuberculosis. Am Rev Respir Dis 1990; 141: 623-625.
51. Mahmoudi A, Iseman MD. Surgical intervention in the treatment of drug-resistant tuberculosis: update and extended follow-up (Abstract). Am Rev Respir Dis 1992; 145 Suppl: 1816.
52. Pomerantz M, personal communication, 1998.

53. Pearson ML, Jereb JA, Frieden TR, et al. Nosocomial transmission of multidrug-resistant *Mycobacterium tuberculosis*: a risk to patients and health care workers. Ann Intern Med 1992;117:191-6.

54. Di Perri G, Cadeo GP, Castelli F, et al. Transmission of HIV-associated tuberculosis to health-care workers. Lancet 1992; 340: 682.

55. Dooley SW Jr, Castro KG, Hutton MD, Mullan RJ, Polder JA, Snider DE Jr. Guidelines for preventing the transmission of tuberculosis in health-care settings, with special focus on HIV-related issues. MMWR Morb Mortal Wkly Rep 1990; 39: 1-29.

56. Nardell EA, Keegan J, Cheney SA, Etkind SC. Airborne infection: theoretical limits of protection achievable by building ventilation. Am Rev Respir Dis 1991; 144: 302-306.

57. Riley RL, O'Grady F. Airborne infection: transmission and control. Macmillan, New York, 1961.

58. Iseman MD. A leap of faith: what can we do to curtail intrainstitutional transmission of tuberculosis? Ann Intern Med 1992; 117: 251-253.

59. Otten J, Chan J, Cleary T. Successful control of an outbreak of multidrug-resistant tuberculosis in an urban teaching hospital (Abstract). In: Proceedings and abstracts of the World Congress on Tuberculosis, Bethesda, Md., November 16-19, 1992.

60. Ferebee SH. Controlled chemoprophylaxis trials in tuberculosis: a general review. Bibl Tuberc Med Thorac 1970; 26: 28-106.

61. International Union against Tuberculosis Committee on Prophylaxis. Efficacy of various durations of isoniazid preventive therapy for tuberculosis: five years of follow-up in the IUALT trial. Bull World Health Organ 1982; 60: 555-564.

62. Iseman MD, Sbarbaro JA (eds). National ACCP Consensus Conference on Tuberculosis. Chest 1985; 87 Suppl.

63. Management of persons exposed to multidrug-resistant tuberculosis. MMWR Morb Mortal Wkly Rep 1992; 41: 61-71.

64. Ridzon R, Meador J, Maxwell R, Higgins K, Weismuller P, Onorato IM. Asymptomatic hepatitis in persons who received alternative preventive therapy with pyrazinamide and ofloxacin. Clin Infect Dis, 1997; 24: 1264-1265.

65. Greenberg PD, Lax KG, Schechter CB. Tuberculosis in house staff: a decision analysis comparing the tuberculin screening strategy with the BCG vaccination. Am Rev Respir Dis 1991; 143: 490-495.

66. Clemens JD, Chuong JJ, Feinstein AR. The BCG controversy: a methodological and statistical reappraisal. JAMA 1983; 249: 2362-2369.

67. Trial of BCG vaccines in south India for tuberculosis prevention: first report. Bull Int Union Against Tuberc 1980; 55: 14-22.

68. Ponnighaus Jm, Fine PE, Sterne JA, et al. Efficacy of BCG vaccine against leprosy and tuberculosis in northern Malawi. Lancet 1992; 339: 636-639.

69. Sbarbaro JA. Compliance: inducements and enforcements. Chest 1979; 76 Suppl: 750-756.

70. Cohn DL, Catlin BJ, Peterson KL, Judson FN, Sbarbaro JA. A 62-dose, 6-month therapy for pulmonary and extrapulmonary tuberculosis: a twice-weekly, directly observed, and cost-effective regimen. Ann Intern Med 1990; 112: 407-415.

71. Iseman MD, Cohn DL, Sbarbaro JA. Directly observed treatment of tuberculosis --- we can't afford not to try it. N Engl J Med 1993; 328: 576-578.

Chapter 12

Treatment of multidrug-resistant tuberculosis in developing countries

Sir John Crofton[1] and Armand Van Deun[2]

[1]*Professor Emeritus of Respiratory Diseases and Tuberculosis, University of Edinburgh, Scotland*

[2]*Mycobacteriology Unit, Institute of Tropical Medicine, Antwerp, Belgium*

1. INTRODUCTION

Health professionals are only beginning to address the problems of treating multidrug-resistant tuberculosis (MDRTB) in developing countries. Experience both in developed and developing countries has confirmed that MDRTB can be prevented by a good National Tuberculosis Programme (NTP) with mass treatment by reliable regimens [1-4]. However, there is almost no experience in developing countries of mass treatment of MDRTB. Indeed there is very limited experience even in developed countries [2,5-7]. The problem has only recently begun to be widely discussed internationally. This chapter is based on some personal participation in these discussions by one of us (JC), and the other (AVD) has provided personal experience and preliminary results from MDRTB treatment programmes in Rwanda and Bangladesh. Any recommendations must therefore be provisional until more experience is gained in this field.

2. CAUSES OF MDRTB IN DEVELOPING COUNTRIES

If genuinely new TB patients are treated with internationally-approved standardised drug combinations [8], new drug resistance should only rarely

191

I. Bastian and F. Portaels (eds.), Multidrug-Resistant Tuberculosis, 191-203.

emerge unless the patient has been infected with an already resistant strain [1-4]. The prevalence of MDRTB in a country is an important indication of the effectiveness of the local NTP. A high prevalence of drug resistance suggests the consistent failure to ensure that all new patients are cured by good drug combinations [9].

Clinical mismanagement and other factors producing MDRTB are discussed extensively by Pablos-Mendez and Lessnau in another chapter in this book [10]. In developing countries the following factors are of particular significance [11,12]:

1. Careless or ignorant prescribing owing to poor undergraduate or postgraduate education (in some countries, even non-Western-trained doctors can prescribe and therefore misuse Western drugs)[13,14];
2. Easy access to treatment is limited by financial constraints (treatment may not be free, either in the private sector, or, often because of corruption, in the public sector);
3. Drug shortages owing to poor management or budgetary limitations;
4. Inappropriate or unsafe regimens and/or indications for their use in the NTP [9,15,16];
5. The use of drugs or drug combinations of unproven bioavailability;
6. Poor case management, particularly in the initial intensive phase when bacillary load is high. With intermittent regimens, omission of doses by patients may result in resistance even when using standard drug regimens [17].

3.   THE EXTENT OF MDRTB IN DEVELOPING COUNTRIES

The World Health Organization (WHO) and the International Union against Tuberculosis and Lung Disease (IUATLD) have carried out a first attempt at a global survey of drug resistance covering 35 countries on 5 continents [9,18]. This global survey may have under-estimated the MDRTB problem in developing countries. For example, the participating countries probably had better control programmes than had non-participants. On the other hand, the MDRTB problem may be relatively limited still, since it is usually not severe in really poor, rural populations [19]. Our experience in Bangladesh is that levels of resistance, including MDRTB, were not that high [15]. Patients were simply were too poor to afford the amount of drugs necessary to create resistance.

4.   MISDIAGNOSIS OF MDRTB

It is often assumed that all apparent failure of treatment is due to the emergence of drug resistance. With good regimens, it is far more often due to failure to take full treatment. Even in a well-implemented NTP, the supervision of every dose is practically impossible. Although most failures, particularly after category II treatment (ie. 2SEHRZ/1EHRZ/5(EHR)$_3$), carry resistant strains, a study in Bangladesh has found that 18% of patients failing category 1 treatment and 7% of category II failures had *M. tuberculosis* strains that were fully sensitive (Table 1).

Table 1. Resistance observed after Category I and II treatment regimens, Damien Foundation Bangladesh 1995-1998

	After Category I treatment 2EHRZ/6HT		After Category II treatment 2SEHRZ/1EHRZ/5(HER)$_3$	
	Relapses (n=136)	Failures (n=163)	Relapses (n=43)	Failures (n=86)
Any resistance	74 (54%)	131 (82%)	35 (83%)	80 (93%)
Resistance to H	69 (51%)	123 (76%)	33 (77%)	80 (93%)
Resistance to H + R	8 (6%)	36 (22%)	25 (58%)	75 (87%)

H, isoniazid; R, rifampicin

Misdiagnosis may also be due to laboratory error. Any laboratory delivering results of TB drug susceptibility testing (DST) should participate in national or international quality control evaluations. A network of supranational reference laboratories has been created to make this possible [9]. Even when laboratory methods are reliable there can be an error in labelling specimens, transient resistance or other vagaries in DST. Any laboratory report of resistance must be considered in its clinical context. If clinical and bacteriological progress has been satisfactory under the current regimen, treatment should not be immediately changed. The DST should be repeated.

5.   PARTICULAR PROBLEMS IN DEVELOPING COUNTRIES

In most developing countries health services are short of finance and of technical and organisational skills. The top priority must be to establish a good, reliable NTP based on the WHO-recommended strategy known as DOTS (directly observed therapy, short-course) [8] and so prevent MDRTB. It is morally and operationally indefensible to try to cope with MDRTB resulting from a poor or non-existing DOTS programme without stemming the MDRTB inflow by addressing this basic priority.

Where an MDR treatment programme is contemplated, the following very difficult problems have to be effectively addressed:
1. Cost and logistics of reliably providing all the necessary reserve drugs [12];
2. Ensuring that these second-line drugs are only made available to special units with staff highly trained in requisite clinical, social and organisational skills [12]. If these very expensive drugs with unpleasant side-effects are made available to the unskilled, the results could be disastrous. Additional resistance could develop to these reserve drugs leading to an untreatable epidemic.
3. Ensuring that the drugs are only used on patients with genuine MDRTB, not on patients whose "failed" treatment is due to cryptic default or a false laboratory result.

Accurate records of previous treatments should be available for MDRTB patients treated in a well-established NTP. For patients coming from outside the NTP (eg. those treated in private), a diagnosis of MDRTB should await laboratory confirmation or clinical diagnosis based on the failure of supervised treatment. MDRTB treatment programmes will therefore require laboratory support. The minimal facilities required would be a local laboratory providing reliable AFB-microscopy for identification of suspect MDRTB cases and close follow-up of patients on MDRTB treatment regimens. DST could be done by a laboratory at a distance, or even overseas, if no such facility is available locally.

Directly observed therapy (DOT) is an absolute prerequisite to treat these very difficult cases, to deal with side effects, and to avoid waste of very limited resources. DOT requires meticulous organisation, and careful and continuous supervision of the patient observers, whether in hospital or in the community.

6.   POTENTIAL APPROACHES TO THE PROBLEM

We reiterate that so far there is little experience of mass treatment of MDRTB in developing countries. At present there is much discussion as to the appropriate policies. Two major approaches are under consideration:

6.1   The individualised approach

This is the classical method long used by experienced experts for treating MDRTB patients in developed countries [5-7,20-22]. The patient's probable pattern of resistance is estimated by careful clinical consideration of the errors in his/her previous treatment and the successive episodes of failure that indicate probable acquisition of resistance. This estimate of resistance is confirmed in due course by laboratory testing. The regimen is then designed to consist of drugs to which that patient's bacilli are first estimated and later confirmed to be sensitive. This policy has been successfully implemented by Farmer and his colleagues in Peru [22,23]. Farmer et al had considerable independent financial support for drugs and for DST by an experienced laboratory in the USA. Currently the policy is being extended to other areas in Peru and, hopefully, trialed in some centres in the former Soviet Union. In the Peru project, MDRTB patients were treated in their own homes with highly organised DOT supervision by paid members of the local community. It should be mentioned that Peru already had a successful DOTS programme for new patients, but this had not previously included the treatment of MDR patients.

6.2 The standardised approach

Some experts with extensive experience in a range of developing countries have argued that such a meticulous programme, with strong financial, technical and expatriate support, could not be generalised to many Third World countries. A simpler and more standardised approach would be required.

Such an approach has, of course, been highly successful in dealing with newly diagnosed cases under the WHO/IUATLD DOTS programmes. Standardised re-treatment of failures, relapses and defaulters from primary treatment has been almost as successful in some countries, suggesting that few failures were due to MDRTB (unpublished personal analysis of 1995 WHO figures for DOTS programmes in 9 developing countries and WHO 1996 results). For example, systematic testing in a rural Bangladeshi population showed that only 22% of culture-positive Category I treatment failures (2EHRZ/6HT) had MDRTB (Table 1). However, virtually all failures of the re-treatment regimen (2SEHRZ/1EHRZ/5(EHR)$_3$) had resistance to at least one drug. Of the re-treatment failures, 87% had MDRTB compared with "only" 58% of the re-treatment relapses.

The proportion of true MDRTB cases among patients failing re-treatment regimens will depend on the number of such patients who have received unreliable unsupervised treatment outside the DOTS programme (where failure is due to non-adherence not resistance). To put the Bangladesh experience into context, the programme treated 9,000 smear-positive patients in 1998 and the cohort of 1997 achieved 85% cure by the first-line regimen and 80% by the re-treatment regimen.

The Bangladesh experience suggests that, in a well-run programme with reliable smear microscopy and treatment records, it might be possible to make an educated guess of the probability of MDRTB in individual patients. This is an important observation because there are risks to withholding MDRTB treatment pending DST results. For example, an MDRTB trial in Rwanda found that about half of the patients disappeared or died while waiting for these results to arrive from an international reference laboratory (data not shown). In contrast, of 41 Bangladeshi patients commenced on MDRTB treatment based on clinical and sputum smear evidence of failure of standard re-treatment, subsequent DST found only two (4.9%) not to have MDRTB. Unfortunately, clinical history and smear status did not have the same predictive value for detecting MDRTB among relapse cases following Category II treatment. Of six such patients enrolled into the MDRTB treatment programme prior to initial DST results, three (50.0%) were subsequently shown not to have MDRTB. Hence, in a well-run programme, we suggest that rapid results on rifampicin susceptibility are required from a reference laboratory only for cases relapsing after standard re-treatment, not for Category II failures.

Another argument in favour of standardised re-treatment is the limited choice of drugs available and required in a low-income country. The more-effective reserve drugs (eg. quinolones, kanamycin) will have been misused only rarely because of their unavailability. Furthermore, the less effective and/or less safe drugs, such as cycloserine or PAS, cannot be used for various reasons. For example, regular laboratory monitoring of patients for side effects (eg. cycloserine levels, renal and thyroid function tests) will usually be impossible.

MDRTB treatment requires the use of at least three drugs that the patient has never used before. Fortunately, pyrazinamide and ethambutol will often still be active because these drugs seem to be much less popular than isoniazid, streptomycin and rifampicin in poor populations. In developing countries, it may also be justifiable to use safe, cheap and readily available products of controversial activity, such as high-dose isoniazid and clofazimine. Given in addition to three unused and possibly some previously used drugs, such regimens may provide affordable treatment for a larger number of MDRTB patients in developing countries.

Logistically it will be much easier to train staff in the use of one MDRTB regimen employed within a standardised management framework. Drug procurement and supply will also be simplified because reliable supplies of only a limited number of second-line drugs will be required. A well-chosen standard regimen may therefore prove as successful as individualised treatment. Selection of the standard regimen will require information from a local DST survey that includes re-treatment failures and relapses, and investigates resistance to at least the main drugs. In most countries it might be wise also to test ofloxacin but not other reserve drugs unless there is evidence that they have been used regularly by failure cases.

The outline for MDRTB programmes using standardised regimens is contained in a WHO publication [12]. Such a programme is being introduced within the general Tuberculosis Control Programme in Peru where its effectiveness may in due course be compared with that of the individualised programme of Farmer and Kim [22,23].

Table 2. Sputum conversion results in standardised MRDTB treatment programme, Damien Foundation Bangladesh

	Sputum results in patients continuing/completing treatment	
	Smear conversion	Culture conversion
After 3 months	49/56 (87.5%)	49/51 (96.1%)
After 15 months	21/22 (95.5%)	14/15 (93.3%)
After 21 months	20/21 (95.2%)	3/4 (75.0%)

Sixty-four patients with MDRTB confirmed by drug susceptibility testing were enrolled to receive a standard regimen of 3KOPCHZE/12OPHZE/6PE (K, kanamycin; O, ofloxacin; P, prothionamide; C, clofazimine; H, isoniazid; Z, pyrazinamide; E, ethambutol). The tabulated results are incomplete because the study is on-going. Of the original cohort, 8 patients have died, 9 have defaulted, 36 remain on treatment, 10 have completed therapy, and one has failed.

Preliminary results are already available from the Damien Foundation Bangladesh TB programme which used a single standard regimen to treat 64 patients with MDRTB confirmed by DST (see Table 2). There is no evidence of the human immunodeficiency virus (HIV) in this Bangladeshi population so the HIV status of these patients was not ascertained. From the original cohort, there have been eight deaths; two of these deaths were attributed to severe drug side effects. One or more drugs had to be stopped for six patients. Prothionamide was the most common drug discontinued or reduced in dosage. Four patients defaulted during the first three months of treatment and another five patients refused to continue treatment after sputum conversion and clinical improvement, due to minor but troublesome side effects. Future MDRTB treatment programmes must recognise this high default rate and provide adequate education and supervision to ensure that a high proportion of enrolled patients complete their prolonged MDRTB treatment regimens.

Of 51 patients who continued treatment and had culture results available, sputum culture conversions were achieved in 49 (96.1%); the latest conversion occurred after six months treatment. Ten patients have successfully completed their 21-month treatment regimen while 36 patients remain on treatment. So far, only one patient has shown clinical or bacteriological evidence of failure.

7.   APPROPRIATE CONTEXTS FOR MDRTB
TREATMENT PROGRAMMES

The priority for an MDRTB treatment programme will vary from country to country. Two major factors will be the degree of success of the NTP and the extent of the national MDRTB problem, as established by sample surveys. Various mathematical models have been proposed to estimate the probable spread of MDRTB in a country. However, these models are based on some assumptions and on ill-defined values allotted to certain variables. Their results have therefore proved controversial. On the one hand, some experts believe that MDRTB presents a significant risk in many countries and that the utmost effort must be made to tackle the problem urgently [25], even diverting resources from the DOTS programme (while incidentally acknowledging the essential priority of the latter). An alternative view [26] is that the highest priority must be given to establishing an effective countrywide DOTS programme for new cases. DOTS will cure far more infectious patients, decrease attack rates, and prevent the development of MDRTB. Only when the programme is well established would it be justified to deviate resources to meet the vastly higher cost and greater skills needed to cure a patient with MDRTB. Few developing countries will be able to tackle the problem without substantial international help both in finance and expertise. Nevertheless, a judicial choice of drugs and suppliers may go far in cutting drug-costs, while other costs (eg. hospitalisation expenses), are often negligible. There are perhaps four contexts in which MDRTB treatment programmes may be justified.

7.1   Countries with successful DOTS programmes and
low MDRTB rates

"Clean-up" MDRTB treatment programmes could be established in countries with long-running successful DOTS programmes and low rates of MDRTB, such as the East African countries with good NTPs initiated in the 1980s with IUATLD assistance. The prerequisites for establishing an MDRTB treatment programme could be combined rates of cured patients, treatment completions and deaths of at least 85% for new cases and 80% in re-treatment cases.

The small number of MDRTB patients could be managed in a special centre with international support. In most cases, a standardised approach would probably be justified. Irrespective of the NTP's good record, the diagnosis of MDRTB must be confirmed by carefully checking the treatment records and verifying re-treatment failures. Selection of patients based on motivation (ie. by insisting on long-term hospitalisation) will further guard against starting non-MDRTB cases on unnecessary treatment.

Some of the first line drugs might still be active in a high proportion of cases (because of the negligible influence of private treatments outside of the NTP). Most MDRTB patients in these circumstances will demonstrate resistance to rifampicin, isoniazid, streptomycin and occasionally ethambutol. Pyrazinamide resistance is less likely [12]. The following standard regimen is therefore suggested: kanamycin (or amikacin or capreomycin according to cost and availability), plus ethionamide, plus ofloxacin, plus pyrazinamide. Ethambutol, being at less risk, should also be given unless resistance is proven. Also addition of high dose INH and clofazimine might prove beneficial with little risk of side effects. Cycloserine and PAS should be used on evidence of more extensive resistance only, since cost as well as side effects will usually be excessive.

The regimen should be given for 3 months, or until sputum has been negative on direct smear for 2 months (as shown by monthly smears), whichever is the longer. This intensive phase should be followed by 18 months of ethionamide, ofloxacin plus ethambutol, though other variations aiming to reduce costs and/or side effects might be as effective.

7.2 Countries with recently-introduced, effective DOTS programmes

Countries that have only recently established effective DOTS programmes will produce little new MDRTB but the poor practices of earlier programmes may have left a substantial residual MDRTB problem. Potential examples of such countries include Peru, Vietnam, and the rural areas of China.

An initial DST survey should be performed to determine the common resistance profiles of MDRTB patients. These surveys may also need to test reserve drugs if they have been available and used. Capreomycin, though more expensive, must be used if kanamycin or amikacin resistance proves common. Otherwise, the "clean-up" regimen recommended above could be used, with addition of cycloserine since resistance to ethambutol must be expected. Unacceptable side effects make PAS a poor alternative drug in regimens containing ethionamide. In some countries, it may be feasible to tailor the regimen using rapid susceptibility tests with the assistance of a reference centre.

7.3   The former Soviet Union

Due to gross shortages in the former Soviet Union, patients have been
treated with whatever drugs were available or could be bought privately.
Preliminary results of resistance surveys and the poor outcome of standard
WHO regimens suggest that MDRTB rates are high in many areas. The
situation is particularly disturbing in prisons [27,28].

External funding of an ambitious MDRTB treatment programme has
been promised. There is an extensive and trained infrastructure, but the
USSR Tuberculosis Control Programme used a complex and expensive
methodology. The WHO methods are now being trialed in pilot areas with
international help in drug provision and training. Once an effective DOTS
programme has been assured, it should be possible to graft on a programme
for the treatment of MDRTB. With trained medical manpower available,
individualised treatment may prove possible in some areas/countries though
standardised regimens may have to be used in others. This will also depend
on the extent of resistance to reserve drugs that may already exist. With the
political and economic situation in flux, it will be essential to ensure that the
reserve drugs are only made available to units highly trained in their use.
Otherwise, increasing private practice may lead to ignorant misuse and
widespread resistance to the reserve drugs. As HIV increases in these
countries, an untreatable epidemic could result.

7.4   Countries with high MDRTB rates and no DOTS
             programme.

The main problem often lies with ignorant or unscrupulous treatment by
private doctors who may not even be Western trained [13,14]. Drug firm
representatives may try to persuade doctors to use reserve drugs that may or
may not be reliable.

In such countries the highest priority must be to expand a national DOTS
programme as quickly as possible. But even when an effective DOTS
programme has taken off, it may take time before the often ill-reputed
Government services attract the majority of the patients. There should be
intensive undergraduate and postgraduate training so that all doctors give
reliable treatment to new patients. Once an effective NTP has been
established, international aid could be sought to institute pilot expert
MDRTB units. The initial intensive phase of treatment could be
administered in hospital by the MDRTB unit. Local health professionals
specially trained in the use of these reserve drugs could then supervise the
continuation phase.

8.   SURGERY FOR MDRTB CASES

Thoracic surgery may or may not be available in some of the above mentioned countries. In practice, demand on these scarce facilities is high; hence it will only rarely be available for TB patients, who are often very poor. If available it has a limited place but requires careful timing [5-7,12,21,22].

9.   CONCLUSIONS

As indicated at the beginning of this chapter, there is little experience of managing MDRTB in developing countries. We have only been able to outline some of the problems and potential solutions. MDRTB treatment in developing countries will not be possible without major international funding and technical support. This chapter can be no more than a basis for discussion.

Finally, it must be realised that a high MDRTB rate in developing countries is a threat not only to local populations but also to the rest of the world. Tuberculosis knows no frontiers. Nor does MDRTB. Politicians and administrators, national and international, must be persuaded that urgent action is required to prevent a global disaster.

REFERENCES

1.   Chaisson RE, Coberly JS, De Cock K. DOTS and drug resistance: a silver lining to a darkening cloud. Int J Tuberc Lung Dis 1999; 3: 1-3.
2.   Frieden TR, Fujiwara PI, Washko RM, Hamburg MA. Tuberculosis in New York City - turning the tide. N Engl J Med 1995; 333: 229-33.
3.   Weiss SE, Slocum PC, Blais FX, King B, Nunn M, Matney GB, Gomez E, Foresman BH. The effect of directly observed therapy on rates of drug resistance and relapse in tuberculosis. N Engl J Med 1994; 330: 1179-84.
4.   Kenyon TA, Mwasekaga MJ, Huebner R, Rumisha D, Binkin N, Maganu E. Low levels of drug resistance amidst rapidly increasing tuberculosis and human immunodeficiency co-epidemics in Botswana. Int J Tuberc Lung Dis 1999; 3: 4-11.
5.   Goble M, Iseman MD, Madsen LA, Waite D, Ackerson L, Horsburgh CR. Treatment of 171 patients with pulmonary tuberculosis resistant to isoniazid and rifampicin. N Engl J Med 1993; 328: 527-532.
6.   Iseman M D. Treatment of multidrug resistant tuberculosis. N Engl J Med 1993; 329: 781-91.
7.   Iseman MD, Huitt G. Treatment of multidrug-resistant tuberculosis, Chapter 11, 175-190. In: Bastian I, Portaels F (eds.), Multidrug-resistant tuberculosis. Kluwer Academic Publ., The Netherlands 2000.

8.   Maher D, Chaulet P, Spinaci S, Harries A. Treatment of tuberculosis. Guidelines for national programmes. Geneva: WHO, 1997.
9.   Pablos-Mendez A, Laszlo A, Bustreo F et al. Anti-tuberculosis drug resistance in the world. The WHO/IUATLD global project on anti-tuberculosis drug resistance surveillance. WHO, Geneva 1997.
10. Pablos-Mendez A, Lessnau K. Clinical mismanagement and other factors producing anti-tuberculosis drug resistance, Chapter 5, 59-76. In: Bastian I, Portaels F (eds.), Multidrug-resistant tuberculosis. Kluwer Academic Publ., The Netherlands 2000.
11. Crofton J. Multidrug resistance: Danger for the Third World, Chapter 11, 231-3. In: Porter JDH, McAdam KPWJ (eds.), Tuberculosis: Back to the future. Wiley, Chichester UK 1994.
12. Crofton J, Chaulet P, Maher D. Guidelines for the management of drug-resistant tuberculosis. WHO, Geneva 1997.
13. Upelkar MW, Shepard DS. Treatment of tuberculosis by private practitioners in India. Tubercle 1991; 72: 284-90.
14. Mudur G. Private doctors in India prescribe wrong tuberculosis drugs. Br Med J 1998; 317: 904.
15. Van Deun A, Aung KJM, Chowdhury S, Saha S, Pankaj A, Ashraf A, Rigouts L, Fissette K, Portaels F. Drug-susceptibility of Mycobacterium tuberculosis in a rural area of Bangladesh and its relevance to the national treatment regimens. Int J Tuberc Lung Dis 1999; 3: 143-48.
16. Datta M., Radhamani MP, Selvaraj R, Paramasivan CN, Gopalan BN, Sudeendra CR, Prabhakar R. Critical assessment of smear-positive pulmonary tuberculosis patients after chemotherapy under the district tuberculosis programme. Tubercle Lung Dis 1993; 74: 180-6.
17. Mitchison DA. How drug resistance emerges as the result of poor compliance during short course chemotherapy for tuberculosis. Int J Tuberc Lung Dis 1998; 2: 10-15.
18. Espinal M. Epidemiology of multidrug-resistant tuberculosis in resource-poor countries, Chapter 3, 29-44. In: Bastian I, Portaels F (eds.), Multidrug-resistant tuberculosis. Kluwer Academic Publ., The Netherlands 2000.
19. Chaulet P, Zidouni N. Evaluation of applied strategies of tuberculosis control in the developing world, 601-27. In: Reichman LB, Hershfield ES (eds.), Tuberculosis, a comprehensive international approach. Marcel Dekker Inc, New York 1993.
20. Crofton J. The prevention and management of drug resistant tuberculosis. Bull Int Union Tuberc Lung Dis 1987; 62: 6-11.
21. Harkin TJ, Harris HW. Treatment of multidrug resistant tuberculosis, Chapter 70, 843-50. In: Rom W N, Stuart G (eds.), Tuberculosis. Little Brown, New York 1996.
22. Farmer P, Kim JY. Community-based approaches to the control of multidrug resistant tuberculosis: introducing "DOTS-plus". Br Med J 1998; 317: 671-4.
23. Farmer PE, Shin SS, Bayona J, et al. DOTS-plus, Chapter 19, 285-306. In: Bastian I, Portaels F (eds.), Multidrug-resistant tuberculosis. Kluwer Academic Publ., The Netherlands 2000.
24. WHO. Global tuberculosis control: WHO report 1999. WHO, Geneva 1999.
25. Blower S, Small P, Hopewell P. Control strategies for tuberculosis epidemics: new models for old problems. Science 1996; 273: 497-500.
26. Frieden TR. What should be the response to a reported rise in drug-resistant tuberculosis? (Abstract). Global Congress on Lung Health / 29th World Conference of the IUATLD, Bangkok 23-26 November 1998. Int J Tuberc Lung Dis 1998; 2: S180-1.

27. Coninx R, Pfyffer GE, Mathieu C, Savina D, Debacker M, Jafarov F, Jabrailov I, Ismailov A, Mirzoev F, de Haller R, Portaels F. Drug resistant tuberculosis in prisons in Azerbaijan: case study. Br Med J 1998; 316: 1423-5.

28. Maher D, Grzemska M, Coninx R, Reyes H. Guidelines for the control of tuberculosis in prisons. WHO and International Committee of the Red Cross, Geneva 1998.

Chapter 13

Treatment outcome of multidrug-resistant tuberculosis

Edward E. Telzak
Division of Infectious Diseases, Bronx-Lebanon Hospital Center, and the Albert Einstein College of Medicine, New York

1.   INTRODUCTION

Cases of multidrug-resistant tuberculosis (MDRTB), defined as resistance to at least isoniazid and rifampin, increased sharply in the early 1990s [1-3]. The rise in MDRTB was associated with previous treatment for tuberculosis, human immunodeficiency virus (HIV) infection, and in some inner city communities, recently transmitted disease [1,4,5]. Case fatality rates in early outbreak investigations often exceeded 80%, with a median survival of between 4 and 16 weeks [6-11]. Subsequent data documented a substantial decline in the number of new MDRTB cases and improvement in clinical outcomes, even among severely immunocompromised patients [12-15]. Drug resistant tuberculosis, however, is not a new phenomenon. In fact, almost immediately after the introduction of streptomycin in 1944, streptomycin-resistant *Mycobacterium tuberculosis* was described [16,17]. Patients who initially had responded to treatment later relapsed as a result of streptomycin-resistant strains. The development of effective therapy followed by drug resistance and clinical failure is a recurrent theme in the history of tuberculosis. This chapter will focus specifically on studies that have provided data on the expected outcome of patients with MDRTB. The treatment of MDRTB in both the industrial and developing world, the

I. Bastian and F. Portaels (eds.), Multidrug-Resistant Tuberculosis, 205-212.
© 2000 *Kluwer Academic Publishers. Printed in the Netherlands.*

pharmacology of second-line antituberculosis chemotherapy and new chemotherapeutic agents and strategies are discussed elsewhere in this volume [18-21].

2.   HIV-NEGATIVE PATIENTS

The most comprehensive data on the effects of drug resistance on treatment outcome derive from a series of 12 controlled trials conducted by the British Medical research Council in Africa, Hong Kong and Singapore [22]. However, given the rarity of initial rifampin resistance, and thus MDRTB, limited conclusions could be drawn about treatment outcome of MDRTB. Of 8,212 patients enrolled in these trials, 1,041 (12.7%) had tuberculosis with initial resistance to at least one drug, including 447 (5%) with initial isolates resistant to isoniazid alone and 256 (3%) resistant to isoniazid and streptomycin. Initial resistance to rifampin was present in only 11 patients, 8 of whom had MDRTB. For patients treated for a minimum of 6 months, treatment failure occurred in only 4 of 2691 patients (0.15%) with drug sensitive isolates compared with 52 of 449 patients (12%) among those with drug resistant isolates. Relapse, defined as recurrence of positive cultures, occurred twice as often among those with resistant isolates (11% vs. 5%). Failure during chemotherapy occurred in 5 of the 8 patients with MDRTB, and 2 of the remaining 3 relapsed after therapy was stopped.

The series summarizing the experience at National Jewish Hospital of 171 HIV-uninfected patients treated for MDRTB over an 11-year period from 1973 to 1983 is the most extensive to date [23]. Patients in this series were referred from throughout the United States and abroad after treatment by physicians in their own communities had failed. These patients had tuberculosis for a median of six years and had received a median of six drugs before being referred to Denver. Not unexpectedly, the disease was usually advanced with 144 patients (84%) having bilateral disease with at least one cavity. Patient hospital stays exceeded seven months. Outcomes in this group were poor: of 134 patients for whom adequate follow-up data were available, 87 (65%) initially responded to chemotherapy with sputum cultures becoming negative. Treatment failure, defined as persistently positive cultures despite chemotherapy, occurred in 47 patients (35%). The overall response rate, including relapses, was 56%, and the mortality attributable to tuberculosis was 22%. Many antituberculous regimens were used with the most frequent consisting of pyrazinamide, ethionamide, cycloserine, aminosalicylic acid and one of the injectable aminoglycosides or polypeptide antimicrobial agents. Though the large number of regimens used precluded an analysis of treatment efficacy according to particular regimens, prior use of a greater number of drugs predicted treatment failure.

The Denver series and their approach to the treatment of MDRTB provided the foundation for other groups involved in the treatment of MDRTB. Subsequent case series of MDRTB among HIV-uninfected patients have documented better response rates. In a series from Bellevue Medical Center, 173 patients treated from 1983 to 1994 had a median survival of 22 months [15]. However, for the 41 HIV-uninfected patients, median survival was greater than 120 months: the mortality rate was 29% for those in whom the vital status was known so the median survival had not yet been reached. For the 23 patients who completed therapy, 2 (9%) expired after completing treatment; in one, the cause of death was attributed to tuberculosis. There was a significant difference in duration of survival between patients who received appropriate therapy, defined as treatment with at least two drugs to which the infecting strain was susceptible, compared with those who received inadequate or no therapy (median survival > 120 months vs. 68 months, p <0.01).

Seven New York City hospitals also reported on their experience with MDRTB among HIV-uninfected patients [24]. Of the 25 patients, which represented complete case finding at each of the hospitals, 24 had clinical responses and all 17 patients for whom data on microbiologic response were available had such a response. The one patient who did not have a favorable clinical response died five days after standard doses of isoniazid, rifampin, ethambutol, and pyrazinamide were initiated. Results of susceptibility tests of her isolate became available post-mortem and indicated resistance to all five first-line antituberculosis agents. The patient died from overwhelming tuberculosis. Subsequent follow-up of this cohort has shown that 22 (88%) patients responded to at least 3 drugs with in-vitro activity against the isolate and remain free of disease a median of 45 months after the initiation of therapy [25]. One patient relapsed after 17 months of treatment and responded to re-treatment with 3 drugs with in-vitro activity against the original isolate. MDRTB resolved in another patient without treatment and remains in remission 6 years after diagnosis. Thus, these data indicate that HIV-negative patients with MDRTB can be expected to respond to medical therapy and that response is usually durable.

The difference in success rates between the Denver series and subsequent series from New York can readily be explained by the different patient characteristics at entry [26,27]. The Denver study included only referred patients with the most severe clinical manifestations in whom treatment had failed elsewhere, whereas only 8 of 25 patients from the New York City case series had received previous therapy. Compared with the New York group, the Denver patients had more extensive pulmonary disease, a greater degree of drug resistance (resistance to a median of 6 drugs vs. 3.5 drugs), lower rates of primary disease and both more intensive and longer duration of prior treatment. In addition, all patients who responded to treatment in the New York series received prolonged treatment with quinolones, a class of drug that was largely unavailable to the Denver patients.

3.   HIV-POSITIVE PATIENTS

MDRTB gained widespread recognition after several outbreaks in the United States in hospitals and the prison system were widely publicized [6-11]. These outbreaks were most notable for a prevalence of HIV co-infection that frequently exceeded 80% and an extremely high mortality rate (72% to 89%) associated with rapid disease progression from diagnosis to death (median interval, 4 to 16 weeks). Subsequent to these outbreaks, improved outcomes for HIV-infected patients have been documented.

Numerous retrospective case series have substantiated the initial reports that improvement in clinical outcome with decreased mortality can be achieved when immunocompromised, HIV-infected patients are started on at least two drugs with in-vitro activity against the MDRTB isolate. Of 34 HIV-infected patients with MDRTB reported from an inner city hospital in the South Bronx, New York City, 20 (59%) initially responded to treatment [13]. Four patients relapsed, and only one of these responded to re-treatment. Thus, the overall response rate was 50%. The median survival for these 34 patients was 315 days (range, 1 - 1,027 days). Multivariate analysis revealed that receipt of appropriate therapy (at least 2 drugs with in-vitro activity against the isolate) for at least 2 consecutive weeks was the only variable associated with both initial and overall response. For the 20 patients who received 2 or more active drugs for at least 2 weeks, the cumulative probability of survival at 12 months was 82%. Though there appeared to be some clustering of cases based on RFLP data, the authors concluded that these cases occurred in a non-outbreak setting.

In a smaller series of HIV-associated MDRTB reported from New York City, 14 (82%) of 17 patients survived at least 4 months, and 10 (59%) survived at least one year after initial diagnosis of MDRTB [14]. Thirteen of these patients were identified prospectively and 11 received at least two agents that were active in vitro. All 11 had a favorable clinical response to therapy and all 9 patients with initially positive sputum cultures became culture negative. Eight became culture negative with antimycobacterial therapy alone and one required surgical intervention. The investigators also confirmed that severe HIV-associated immunosuppression was a predictor of increased mortality for all patients with tuberculosis.

The largest series of HIV-infected patients with MDRTB is from Bellevue Hospital [15]. The overall median survival for the 90 patients was 6.8 months. However, 35 (39%) patients received either no antituberculous therapy or inadequate treatment. The median survival of appropriately treated HIV-infected patients was 14.1 months compared with less than 2 months in those not receiving appropriate therapy. Of the 18 patients who completed at least 18 months of therapy, 13 died during the follow-up period. Of these 13 deaths, one died of tuberculosis, nine died of AIDS-related causes and three died from other causes.

Thus, these three reports from New York City demonstrated that early effective treatment of patients with AIDS and MDRTB can have a dramatic impact with the median survival exceeding one year. A subsequent multicenter prospective study has provided additional support that effective treatment for MDRTB among patients with HIV impacts on mortality [28]. Twelve patients with a median CD4 cell count of $51/mm^3$ were enrolled and 11 patients received treatment that included at least three drugs with in vitro activity against the MDRTB isolate. The cumulative probabilities of survival at one year and at 18 months were 75% (95% CI 51-100) and 66% (95%CI 38-93), respectively.

4.   RECOMMENDATIONS FOR EMPIRIC TREATMENT

Despite the above findings for both HIV-infected and HIV-uninfected patients with MDRTB, specific recommendations regarding empiric coverage for patients suspected of having MDRTB are difficult. Obviously, the greater the number of drugs used, the more likely at least two will have in vitro activity. More drugs, however, invariably lead to greater toxicity, drug-drug interactions, and costs. Thus, decisions about initial therapy must take into account individual, institutional and larger geographic factors. While awaiting susceptibility data for both first-line and second-line antituberculosis agents at institutions where outbreaks are ongoing, it is reasonable to initiate empiric therapy for the outbreak strain. This has often meant using six- or seven-drug regimens until susceptibility data are available. Institutions that have adopted this policy have seen improved outcomes [28,29]. At institutions where no known outbreaks have occurred but where drug resistance has been encountered, the CDC-recommended four-drug regimen is appropriate.

Individual patient characteristics must also play a role in selecting empiric treatment. Details of a previous history of tuberculosis including prior treatment and susceptibility data, contact with persons who have documented tuberculosis and the contacts' susceptibility data if available, exposure to MDRTB at an institution (e.g., hospital, prison or shelter) and immigration from a country where MDRTB is endemic all must be considered in optimizing empiric therapy. For individuals deemed to be at high risk for MDRTB, an initial regimen that includes more than the currently recommended four drugs, including at least two new drugs, is reasonable. In general, the optimal drugs for treating MDRTB should include the other first-line antituberculosis agents and the quinolones, when in vitro data support their use [18,19].

5.   CONCLUSION

Evidence has been presented that suggests that the prompt initiation of effective therapy for MDRTB can impact substantially on outcome and greatly reduce mortality, even among HIV-infected patients. Nevertheless, MDRTB remains a devastating illness, especially for those with the most advanced immunosuppression. Treatment regimens are complex, often associated with significant toxicity and can exceed 18 to 24 months. To maximize the likelihood of a beneficial therapeutic response, clinicians must be aggressive in obtaining specimens, treating empirically on the basis of institutional and patient characteristics, accessing culture and susceptibility data so drug regimens can be modified, if necessary, and assuring adherence to the prescribed antituberculosis regimen through a directly observed therapy program.

REFERENCES

1.   Frieden TR, Sterling T, Pablos-Mendez A, Kilburn JO, Cauthen GM, Dooley SW. The emergence of drug-resistant tuberculosis in New York City. N Engl J Med 1993; 328: 521-526.
2.   Sepkowitz KA, Telzak EE, Recalde S, Armstrong D, and the New York City Area Tuberculosis Working Group. Trends in the susceptibility of tuberculosis in New York City, 1987-1991. Clin Infect Dis 1994; 18: 755-759.
3.   Bloch AB, Cauthen GM, Onorato IM, et al. Nationwide survey of drug-resistant tuberculosis in the United States. JAMA 1994; 271: 665-671.
4.   Alland D, Kalkut GE, Moss AR, et al. Transmission of tuberculosis in New York City - an analysis by DNA fingerprinting and conventional epidemiologic methods. N Engl J Med 1994;330: 1710-1716.

5. Small PM, Hopewell PC, Samir P, et al. The epidemiology of tuberculosis in San Francisco - A population-based study using conventional and molecular methods. N Engl J Med 1994; 330: 1703-1709.

6. Edlin BR, Tokars JI, Grieco MH, et al. An outbreak of multidrug resistant tuberculosis among hospitalized patients with the acquired immunodeficiency syndrome. N Engl J Med 1992; 326: 1514-1521.

7. Fischl MA, Daikos GL, Uttanchandani RB, et al. Clinical presentation and outcome of patients with HIV infection and tuberculosis caused by multiple-drug resistant bacilli. Ann Intern Med 1992; 117: 184-190.

8. Centers for Disease Control and Prevention. Nosocomial transmission of multidrug-resistant tuberculosis among HIV-infected persons - Florida and New York, 1988-1991. MMWR 1991; 40: 585-591.

9. Centers for Disease Control and Prevention. Outbreak of multidrug-resistant tuberculosis at a hospital - New York City, 1991. MMWR 1993; 42: 427, 433-434.

10. Centers for Disease Control and Prevention. Transmission of multidrug-resistant tuberculosis among immunocompromised persons in a correctional system - New York, 1991. MMWR 1992; 41: 507-509.

11. Pearson ML, Jereb JA, Frieden TR, et al. Nosocomial transmission of multidrug-resistant Mycobacterium tuberculosis. A risk to patients and health care workers. Ann Intern Med 1992; 117: 191-196.

12. Fujiwara PI, Cook SV, Rutherford CM, et al. A continuous survey of drug-resistant tuberculosis, New York City, April 1994. Arch Intern Med 1997; 157: 531-536.

13. Turett GS, Telzak EE, Torian LV, et al. Improved outcomes for patients with multidrug-resistant tuberculosis. Clin Infect Dis 1995; 21: 1238-1244.

14. Salomon N, Perlman D, Friedman P, Buchstein S, Kreiswirth BN, Mildvan D. Predictors and outcome of multidrug-resistant tuberculosis. Clin Infect Dis 1995; 21: 1245-1252.

15. Park MM, Davis AL, Schluger NW, Cohen H, Rom WN. Outcome of MDR-TB patients, 1983-1993: prolonged survival with appropriate therapy. Am J Respir Crit Care Med 1996; 153: 317-324.

16. Youmans GP, et al. Proceedings of the staff meetings of the Mayo Clinic 1946; 21: 126.

17. Pyle MM. Proceedings of the staff meetings of the Mayo Clinic 1947; 22: 465.

18. Iseman MD, Huitt G. Treatment of multidrug-resistant tuberculosis, Chapter 11,175-190. In: Bastian I, Portaels F (eds.), Multidrug-resistant tuberculosis. Kluwer Academic Publ., The Netherlands, 2000.

19. Crofton J, Van Deun A. Treatment of multidrug-resistant tuberculosis in developing countries, Chapter 12, 191-203. In: Bastian I, Portaels F (eds.), Multidrug-resistant tuberculosis. Kluwer Academic Publ., The Netherlands, 2000.

20. Peloquin CA, Auclair B. Pharmacology of second-line antituberculosis drugs, Chapter 10, 163-174. In: Bastian I, Portaels F (eds.), Multidrug-resistant tuberculosis. Kluwer Academic Publ., The Netherlands, 2000.

21. Farmer PE, Shin SS, Bayona J, et al. Making DOTS-plus work, Chapter 19, 285-306. In: Bastian I, Portaels F (eds.), Multidrug-resistant tuberculosis. Kluwer Academic Publ., The Netherlands, 2000.

22. Mitchison DA, Nunn AJ. Influence of initial drug resistance on the response to short-course chemotherapy of pulmonary tuberculosis. Am Rev Respir Dis 1986; 133: 423-430.

23. Goble M, Iseman MD, Madsen LA, Waite D, Ackerson L, Horsburgh CR. Treatment of 171 patients with pulmonary tuberculosis resistant to isoniazid and rifampin. N Engl J Med 1993; 328: 527-532.

24. Telzak EE, Sepkowitz K, Alpert P, et al. Multidrug-resistant tuberculosis in patients without HIV infection. N Engl J Med 1995; 333: 907-911.

25. Telzak EE, Sepkowita K, Medard F, et al. Durable remission after successful treatment of multidrug-resistant tuberculosis among HIV-negative patients. Abstract in 35th Annual Meeting of the Infectious Diseases Society of America, September 13-16, 1997, San Francisco, CA, USA.

26. Iseman MD, Goble M. Multidrug-resistant tuberculosis (letter). N Engl J Med 1996; 334: 267.

27. Telzak EE, Sepkowitz K, Turett G. Multidrug-resistant tuberculosis (letter). N Engl J Med 1996; 334: 268-269.

28. Edlin BR, Attoe LS, Grieco MH, et al. Recognition and treatment of primary multidrug-resistant tuberculosis (MDRTB) in HIV-infected patients. IXth International Conference on AIDS, 1993, Berlin.

29. Lockhart B, Sharp V, Squires K, et al. Improved outcome of MDRTB in patients receiving a five or more drug initial therapy. IXth International Conference on AIDS, 1993, Berlin.

Chapter 14

Chemoprophylaxis and BCG in contacts of multidrug-resistant tuberculosis

Richard A. Stapledon[1], Richard Lumb[2] and Irene S. Lim[2]
[1]South Australian Tuberculosis Sevices, Department of Thoracic Medicine, Royal Adelaide Hospital, Adelaide SA 5000, Australia
[2]Infectious Diseases Laboratories, Institute of Medical and Vetirinary Science, PO Box 14 Rundle Mall, Adelaide SA 5000, Australia

1. INTRODUCTION

The emerging threat of multi-drug resistant tuberculosis (MDRTB) has many adverse implications. Persons with active disease due to multidrug-resistant *Mycobacterium tuberculosis* represent a major public health problem because they can transmit a disease that is potentially untreatable. The cost to the individual and the community is enormous considering the degree of individual suffering from being chronically diseased, having long-term complex and toxic therapy, prolonged hospitalisation, loss of social contact and possibly the means of livelihood. There is no clear consensus on the most effective regimens in treating those that have the disease and those that are infected. The cost of treatment is excessive and current therapeutic regimens have a high failure rate often resulting in death. The risk of infection to health care workers (HCW) is a major problem and ways to minimise these risks have to be actively pursued. There is the added dilemma of how best to protect the uninfected. There are no easy or certain solutions to these problems.

213

I. Bastian and F. Portaels (eds.), Multidrug-Resistant Tuberculosis, 213-224.

2. PREVENTION AND CONTROL OF TUBERCULOSIS

The likelihood of becoming infected with *M. tuberculosis* depends on (i) the infectiousness of the index case, (ii) environmental factors eg overcrowding, inadequate ventilation, (iii) duration and intensity of exposure, (iv) susceptibility of the contact, and (v) characteristics of the infecting strain [1]. There appears to be no significant difference in the risk of infection among contacts of previously untreated cases regardless of the organism's drug-susceptibility pattern [2,3]. Therefore the fundamental strategies for the prevention and control of tuberculosis (TB) remain crucial in dealing with MDRTB.

The three strategies for minimising the risk for *M. tuberculosis* transmission are described in detail in another chapter [4]. Administrative measures that ensure the early detection and effective treatment of patients with active disease are the most important intervention. The weak link in these measures is the lack of proven effective treatment regimens for MDRTB. The second strategy is the implementation of effective TB infection-control programmes to prevent institutional transmission (eg. in homeless shelters, health care and correctional facilities)[5]. This may require institutional upgrading to provide an appropriate level of ambient ventilation in buildings, availability of rooms with negative pressure ventilation, use of high-efficiency particulate air (HEPA) filtration and ultra-violet air disinfection in crucial areas [6]. These strategies have proven effective in controlling nosocomial outbreaks [7,8]. The final strategy, the use of personal respirators for staff protection, complements the above administrative and environmental control measures for minimising transmission but the need for HEPA respirators is debatable [9].

3. CHEMOPROPHYLAXIS

3.1 Rationale

Treatment to prevent development of active disease in persons with evidence of latent TB infection is supported by numerous animal and human studies [10-13]. Those who will benefit most from this form of treatment are: (i) close contacts of an infectious case, especially infants, children and the immunocompromised; (ii) human immunodeficiency virus (HIV) infected persons with recent or past TB infection; and (iii) persons with evidence of recent tuberculin skin test (TST) conversion (within 2 years). Those with previous, inadequately treated TB or a chest radiograph lesion consistent with inactive TB may also benefit from preventive treatment, especially if they have co-morbidities such as silicosis, poorly controlled diabetes or chronic renal disease [14].

3.2 Treatment of drug susceptible TB infection

Isoniazid (INH) monotherapy administered for a period of 6-12 months has been the most widely recommended and studied drug for this purpose. Treatment for 12 months appears to provide optimal preventive benefit for persons, especially HIV-infected individuals, infected with drug-sensitive organisms. However, a 6-month regimen still affords a high level of efficacy with the associated benefits of better compliance, less drug toxicity and improved cost effectiveness [12,15]. Treatment for less than 6 months is considerably less effective. Recent studies suggest that alternative shorter regimens such as rifampicin (RIF) for 3 months, RIF/pyrazinamide (PYZ) for 2 months, INH/RIF for 3 months or weekly rifapentine for 3 months may be more efficacious than 6 months of INH [16-18].

The use of preventive treatment has been hampered by concerns about the potential risks outweighing the benefits in asymptomatic individuals, inadequate drug compliance, and the possibility of acquired resistance. The latter is more likely if active disease is missed and therefore monotherapy inadvertently used. In developing countries the priorities are improved case finding and effective treatment of cases with active disease. The cost and practical issues relating to reliable diagnosis of infection, exclusion of active disease (especially in HIV-infected persons), and implementation of safe and adequate treatment programmes limit the use of chemoprophylaxis. Furthermore, in areas with high infection rates, the potential for reinfection exists and might negate the benefit of prior preventive treatment.

3.3 HIV and TB co-infection

HIV seropositive individuals co-infected with *M. tuberculosis* have a very high likelihood of progressing to active TB. Following recent infection the risk of progression to disease is approximately 40% within the first 6 months whilst for the previously infected, the chance of reactivation is as much as 8-10% per annum [19,20]. TB can in turn adversely influence the course of HIV disease [21]. Preventive treatment is therefore considered a high priority in these individuals and has proven effective in reducing the incidence of TB [13]. In developing countries where the impact of HIV infection has been the greatest, reservations exist over its use because of the practical issues outlined earlier and the lack of sufficient information as to whether a broad-based preventive treatment strategy should be implemented in TB control programmes [22].

3.4   Chemoprophylaxis for drug-resistant TB

Single-drug resistance to INH is the most common form of resistance in *M. tuberculosis*. When there is a high likelihood of infection with an INH-resistant strain, RIF for a minimum period of 6 months is recommended for those at most risk, sometimes with the addition of ethambutol (ETH) [14]. RIF has been shown to be efficacious [23,24] but acquired drug resistance is a concern [25]. The finding of initial resistance to RIF in HIV-infected individuals developing TB who had previously used rifabutin for *M. avium* complex prophylaxis supports this concern [26].

There is no proven therapeutic regimen for the treatment of infection with a MDR strain. Two approaches have been considered: observation alone or a "trial" of multidrug therapy based on a determination of the likelihood of recent infection with a MDRTB strain and the relative risk to the individual for disease development. The uncertainty surrounding chemoprophylaxis for MDRTB infection has important implications for those at risk, including HCWs and the immunodeficient, and may not be resolved until new drugs with similar efficacy to INH and RIF are discovered.

In 1992, the Centers for Disease Control and Prevention (CDC) issued comprehensive recommendations on the management of contacts with likely MDRTB infection but described the treatment options as problematic [27]. A risk assessment approach was proposed that firstly evaluated contacts to determine the likelihood of recent infection with a MDR strain of *M. tuberculosis*. The evaluation considered the potential infectiousness of the source case, the level and circumstances of exposure, and finally the past history of the individual to indicate whether prior infection with a drug susceptible strain was probable. These criteria were used to rank individuals according to the probability of infection. Observation alone or management as for contacts of a drug susceptible case was recommended for those exposed (positive tuberculin reactors) but with a low probability of MDRTB infection. Those with an intermediate to high probability of infection were further classified according to the risk for subsequent progression to disease. Multidrug preventive treatment was recommended for those with a high likelihood of MDRTB infection and those with risk factors predisposing to disease, particularly HIV co-infection.

The choice of drugs for preventive therapy should logically be based on results of susceptibility tests for first and second line drugs from the presumed source case. In the absence of such information, CDC have suggested the combinations of ETH and PYZ, or PYZ and a fluoroquinolone for a duration of at least 6-12 months. The longer regimen was suggested for HIV-infected contacts. If proportionate drug susceptibility testing demonstrated partial resistance to INH or RIF, then these drugs were to be considered in infected individuals without risk factors that enhance progression to disease [27].

The results of a Delphi survey reported in 1994, where expert panelists were asked to suggest possible preventive therapy regimens in response to three scenarios, further underlined the difficulties (eg. reliance on clinical judgement and limited unproven treatment options) associated with management of MDRTB contacts. The panelists did not limit treatment to those at high risk only, recommending it to all exposed persons. The study did not determine a consensus treatment regimen but the combination most favoured was PYZ and ciprofloxacin (CIP) [28]. The use of ETH and PYZ as proposed by CDC rated poorly and the use of INH or RIF was deemed inappropriate.

A decision analysis by Stevens and Daniel [29] evaluated the potential benefit of PYZ/CIP preventive therapy in HIV-seronegative HCWs exposed to MDRTB. Using probabilities for a range of variables derived from published reports, this analysis marginally favoured treatment. Under such circumstances, patient preference was considered the significant determinant as to whether or not treatment was commenced.

3.5 Drug options

When treatment for persons strongly suspected of infection with an MDR strain is instituted, the present consensus recommendation appears to be at least 2 drugs used daily for a period of 6-12 months based on drug susceptibility testing of the source case [27,28]. Treatment should be directly supervised by health care workers with special TB expertise. While intermittent supervised therapy is suggested as an equally effective option for those infected with a drug susceptible strain, there is no data to support this strategy in infection with a presumed MDR strain.

PYZ, a first line anti-tuberculous drug, together with a fluoroquinolone is the most commonly used preventive regimen. The action of PYZ is not well understood but is considered to have significant sterilising activity against semi-dormant populations of *M. tuberculosis* at low pH and to enhance the effect of a bactericidal drug [30]. Adverse effects include arthralgia, hepatotoxicity, acute gout, rash, fatigue, and photosensitive skin reaction.

Results of a recent study suggest an improved outcome in MDRTB patients treated with a multi-drug regimen that included a quinolone [31]. Of the fluoroquinolones, CIP and ofloxacin have been the most extensively used. While they appear to have early bactericidal activity, a significant sterilising effect has not been shown [32]. Sparfloxacin has a broader spectrum of activity and may offer improved benefits but causes significant photosensitive skin reactions. Side effects from these drugs are uncommon with short or long term use but animal studies suggest the possibility of an adverse effect on growing cartilage and therefore care in pregnant women and children is advised [14].

ETH is regarded as a bacteriostatic agent against actively growing organisms when used at the normally recommended dose (15 mg/kg). The effect may be bactericidal if given in a larger dose (25 mg/kg) but the risk of toxicity, particularly optic neuritis, increases. It is not considered to have significant sterilising activity and hence its use as a preventive agent can be questioned [33].

Most second line anti-tuberculous drugs including cycloserine, para-aminosalicylic acid (PAS) and ethionamide are not recommended because of their poor efficacy and higher rates of toxicity [27]. Other drugs that have also come under consideration such as clarithromycin, clofazimine, amoxycillin/clavulanate and metronidazole do not appear to offer new benefits.

3.6 Limitations

Patient and doctor preference, and drug intolerance are the main impediments to the successful implementation or completion of preventive therapy [34]. These impediments can be due to the diagnostic imprecision in recognising infection in many individuals, the resulting risk of over-treatment, different cultural beliefs and attitudes, and the unproven efficacy of MDRTB treatment regimens. A preventive treatment programme is costly and may result in a disproportionate use of resources but it could be cost effective in the longer term if MDR disease is prevented.

4. BACILLE CALMETTE GUÉRIN

National policies regarding the role of BCG in tuberculosis prevention and control programmes vary widely. In countries with a low-incidence of tuberculosis, there has been a declining interest in BCG vaccination because of conflicting reports regarding vaccine efficacy, vaccine safety and difficulties in interpretation of the TST post-BCG vaccination [35]. The rise of drug resistance as a public health problem has led to a renewed interest in BCG vaccination [35-39].

Two recent meta-analyses have helped to clarify the findings of a number of studies that have reported quite disparate results regarding the efficacy of BCG vaccination. Rodrigues *et al* [40] investigated the protective effect of BCG against meningeal and miliary tuberculosis. They concluded that the protective effect of BCG against these severe forms of tuberculosis was 86% in randomised trials and 76% in case control studies. An attempt to determine the overall protective efficacy of BCG against pulmonary tuberculosis was unsuccessful because of methodological variability. In the second meta-analysis, Colditz *et al* [41] reviewed the results of 14 clinical trials and 12 case control studies. Their evaluation estimated the overall protective effect of BCG to be 51% in clinical trials and 50% in case control studies. They also determined that BCG efficacy was greater in studies where vaccination was conducted in younger populations than in populations where vaccination occurred at older ages.

Some countries have a strategy of ongoing surveillance of contacts for TB patients using regular TST and INH preventive therapy for persons who demonstrate a skin test conversion. However, the strategy may be compromised by inadequacies in the TST sensitivity and specificity, and the failure of persons to present for regular skin testing. The strategy may be further compounded by poor compliance in those receiving INH preventive therapy. Studies have compared the TST/INH chemoprophylaxis strategy with BCG vaccination. Greenberg *et al* [42] found that BCG required an efficacy of only 13.1% to prevent more cases of TB than the TST/INH strategy. However, with perfect TST/INH compliance, which is possible at an individual level, BCG will require a protective efficacy of 46.1% before the benefit exceeds that of TST/INH, suggesting that the potential benefits of TST/INH may be superior. The study was criticised [43] principally for undervaluing the potential effectiveness of annual TST, overstating the risk of INH-associated hepatitis, and ignoring the risks of adverse reactions to BCG vaccination. Marcus and colleagues [38] conducted an analysis designed to overcome the deficiencies of the Greenberg study. They found BCG vaccination resulted in less morbidity and mortality than annual TST for HCWs when the workplace incidence of *M. tuberculosis* infection exceeded 0.06%, or BCG efficacy exceeded 3%.

Homeless persons represent a high-risk group for tuberculosis in low-incidence countries [44]. The mobility of this population makes regular skin testing and compliance with preventive therapy particularly difficult. A decision analysis performed on a hypothetical cohort of homeless persons over 35 years of age found that BCG vaccination of such a group was cost effective when BCG vaccine efficacy reached 50%. However, the argument for BCG vaccination would be eroded if the cost per tuberculosis case decreased [45].

A decision analysis compared the usefulness of BCG vaccination with post-infection preventive therapy for HCWs exposed to MDRTB [37]. The results were so close that the two choices were considered almost equal. Variations in the probabilities that favoured BCG vaccination included a greater protective efficacy for BCG, a decrease in the efficiency of detection of infection, an increased incidence of MDRTB, non-compliance with preventive therapy and an infecting MDRTB strain resistant to both ciprofloxacin and pyrazinamide.

A retrospective study by Kritski *et al* [3] examined the incidence and risk factors associated with tuberculosis among contacts of MDRTB index cases. Of particular interest was that BCG vaccination of the contacts before the index case developed MDRTB had a 69% protective effect in the contact group. Tuberculosis developed in 8/153 (5%) contacts who had received BCG and in 9/65 (14%) of those who had not. Among BCG vaccinated contacts <25 years of age, tuberculosis developed in 5/113 (4.4%) of contacts compared with 4/21 (19%) of contacts who had not received BCG vaccination.

BCG vaccination overcomes the compliance problems of routine TST/INH preventive therapy strategy. It gives partial and variable protection regardless of the drug susceptibility profile of the infecting *M. tuberculosis* strain over an undefined period of time [36,38-41]. However, it renders future interpretation of the TST imprecise. There is also the potential for adverse events (localised subcutaneous abscess, regional lymphadenopathy and disseminated disease) related to the use of a live vaccine, particularly in the immunocompromised [35,46].

Comprehensive infection control strategies properly instituted and maintained are highly effective in protecting persons in contact with patients with suspected or confirmed tuberculosis, but fail, or are less effective when the undiagnosed patient remains at large and untreated [6-8,47]. BCG vaccination should therefore be considered seriously in those with regular risk of exposure to persons with MDRTB. This includes HCWs in settings associated with a high risk of tuberculosis transmission, and close contacts of cases of failed or ineffectively treated MDRTB, especially young children. BCG may be considered in persons exposed to MDRTB, but in whom preventive treatment is contraindicated or has been ceased due to an adverse reaction. When BCG is contraindicated, the only option is to remove that person from the infected environment. Before a MDRTB contact receives BCG, a thorough patient evaluation is mandatory to ensure that the individual does not have a contraindication for BCG vaccination. The person should also be counselled regarding the risks and benefits associated with both BCG vaccination and TB preventive therapy.

For persons in developing countries with a high incidence of tuberculosis and where MDRTB is increasingly common [48], exposure to tuberculosis is likely to occur at an early age, the isolate's susceptibility pattern is usually unknown, and second-line drugs are frequently unobtainable. Under these conditions, neonatal BCG vaccination remains a priority and the only option.

5. SUMMARY

The selection criteria for preventive treatment of individuals exposed to MDRTB are not precise. The choice and duration of treatment regimens is largely empirical, their efficacy unproven but often associated with toxicity that leads to discontinuation of therapy or non-compliance. BCG does offer a degree of protection against TB independent of drug susceptibility of the infecting strain. Despite the potential for adverse events, there is a place for the use of BCG in the uninfected who may be regularly exposed to MDRTB. The dilemmas surrounding the appropriate response to MDRTB infection highlight the fact that the main focus should be on TB prevention and control by minimising the risk of transmission. This requires the full support of health care providers, health administrators and politicians.

ACKNOWLEDGEMENT

The authors gratefully acknowledge the secretarial assistance of Mrs Charli Bayley in the preparation of the manuscript.

REFERENCES

1. Sepkowitz KA. How contagious is tuberculosis? Clin Infect Dis 1996; 23: 954-962.
2. Snider DE Jr, Kelly GD, Cauthen GM, Thompson NJ, Kilburn JO. Infection and disease among contacts of tuberculosis cases with drug-resistant and drug-susceptible bacilli. Am Rev Respir Dis 1985; 132: 125-132.
3. Kritski AL, Marques MJO, Rabahi MF, Vieira MAMS, Werneck-Barroso E, Carvalho CES, Andrade GDN, Bravo-De-Souza R, Andrade LM, Gontijo PP, Riley LW. Transmission of tuberculosis to close contacts of patients with multidrug-resistant tuberculosis. Am J Respir Crit Care Med 1996; 153: 331-335.
4. Jarvis W, Richards C. Administrative, engineering, and personal protective measures for controlling multidrug-resistant tuberculosis, Chapter 18, 269-284. In: Bastian I, Portaels F (eds.), Multidrug resistant tuberculosis. Kluwer Academic Publ., The Netherlands, 2000.
5. Guidelines for preventing the transmission of Mycobacterium tuberculosis in health-care facilities, 1994. Centers for Disease Control and Prevention. MMWR Morb Mortal Wkly Rep 1994; 43(RR-13): 1-132.

6. Institutional control measures for tuberculosis in the era of multiple drug resistance. ACCP/ATS Consensus Conference. Chest 1995; 108: 1690-1710.
7. Blumberg HM, Watkins DL, Berschling JD, Antle A, Moore P, White N, Hunter M, Green B, Ray SM, McGowan Jr JE. Preventing nosocomial transmission of tuberculosis. Ann Intern Med 1995; 122: 658-663.
8. Maloney SA, Pearson ML, Gordon MT, Del Castillo R, Boyle JF, Jarvis WR. Efficacy of control measures in preventing nosocomial transmission of multidrug-resistant tuberculosis to patients and health care workers. Ann Intern Med 1995; 122: 90-95.
9. Adal KA, Anglim AM, Palumbo CL, Titus MG, Coyner BJ, Farr BM. The use of high-efficiency particulate air-filter respirators to protect hospital workers from tuberculosis: a cost-effectiveness analysis. N Engl J Med 1994; 331: 169-173.
10. Ferebee SH, Palmer CE. Prevention of experimental tuberculosis with isoniazid. Am Rev Tuberc Pul Dis 1956; 73: 1-18.
11. Comstock GW, Baum C, Snider DE Jr. Isoniazid prophylaxis among Alaskan Eskimos: a final report of the bethel isoniazid studies. Am Rev Respir Dis 1979; 119: 827-30.
12. Efficacy of various durations of isoniazid preventative therapy for tuberculosis: five years of follow-up in the IUAT trial. International Union Against Tuberculosis Committee on Prophylaxis. Bull World Health Organ 1982; 60: 555-564.
13. Bucher HC, Griffith LE, Guyatt GH, Sudre P, Naef M, Sendi P, Battegay M. Isoniazid prophylaxis for tuberculosis in HIV infection: a meta-analysis of randomized controlled trials. AIDS 1999; 13: 501-507.
14. Bass JB Jr, Farer LS, Hopewell PC, O'Brien R, Jacobs RF, Ruben F, Snider DE Jr, Thornton G. Treatment of tuberculosis and tuberculosis infection in adults and children. American Thoracic Society and the Centers for Disease Control and Prevention. Am J Respir Crit Care Med 1994; 149: 1359-1374.
15. Snider DE Jr, Caras GJ, Koplan JP. Preventive therapy with isoniazid. Cost-effectiveness of different durations of therapy. JAMA 1986; 255: 1579-1583.
16. Lecoeur HF, Truffot-Pernot C, Grosset JH. Experimental short-course preventive therapy of tuberculosis with rifampin and pyrazinamide. Am Rev Respir Dis 1989; 140: 1189-93.
17. A double-blind placebo-controlled clinical trial of three anti-tuberculosis chemoprophylaxis regimens in patients with silicosis in Hong Kong. Hong Kong Chest Service/Tuberculosis Research Centre, Madras/British Medical Research Council. Am Rev Respir Dis 1992; 145:36-41.
18. Ji B, Truffot-Pernot C, Lacroix C, Raviglione MC, O'Brien RJ, Olliaro P, Roscigno G, Grosset J. Effectiveness of rifampin, rifabutin and rifapentine for preventive therapy of tuberculosis in mice. Am Rev Respir Dis 1993; 148: 1541-46.
19. Daley CL, Small PM, Schecter GF, Schoolnik GK, McAdam RA, Jacobs WR Jr, Hopewell PC. An outbreak of tuberculosis with accelerated progression among persons infected with the human immunodeficiency virus. An analysis using restriction-fragment-length polymorphisms. N Engl J Med 1992; 326: 231-235.
20. Narain JP, Raviglione MC, Kochi A. HIV-associated tuberculosis in developing countries: epidemiology and strategies for prevention. Tuber Lung Dis 1992; 73: 311-321.
21. Nakata K, Rom WN, Honda Y, Condos R, Kanegasaki S, CaoY, Weiden M. Mycobacterium tuberculosis enhances human immunodeficiency virus-1 replication in the lung. Am J Respir Crit Care Med 1997; 155: 996-1003.
22. Tuberculosis preventive therapy in HIV-infected individuals. A joint statement of the WHO Tuberculosis Programme and the Global Programme on AIDS, and the International Union Against Tuberculosis and Lung Disease (IUATLD). Wkly Epidemiol Rec 1993; 68: 361-364.

23. Villarino ME, Ridzon R, Weismuller PC, Elcock M, Maxwell RM, Meador J, Smith PJ, Carson ML, Geiter LJ. Rifampin preventive therapy for tuberculosis infection: experience with 157 adolescents. Am J Respir Crit Care Med 1997; 155: 1735-1738.

24. Polesky A, Farber HW, Gottlieb DJ, Park H, Levinson S, O'Connell JJ, McInnis B, Nieves RL, Bernardo J. Rifampin preventive therapy for tuberculosis in Boston's homeless. Am J Respir Crit Care Med 1996; 154: 1473-1477.

25. Livengood JR, Sigler TG, Foster LR, Bobst JG, Snider DE Jr. Isoniazid-resistant tuberculosis. A community outbreak and report of a rifampin prophylaxis failure. JAMA 1985; 253: 2847-2849.

26. Bishai WR, Graham NMH, Harrington S, Page C, Moore-Rice K, Hooper N, Chaisson RE. Brief Report: Rifampin-resistant tuberculosis in a patient receiving rifabutin prophylaxis. N Engl J Med 1996; 334: 1573-76.

27. Management of persons exposed to multidrug-resistant tuberculosis. MMWR Morb Mortal Wkly Rep 1992; 41(RR-11): 61-71.

28. Passannante MR, Gallagher CT, Reichman LB. Preventive therapy for contacts of multidrug-resistant tuberculosis. A Delphi survey. Chest 1994; 106: 431-434.

29. Stevens JP, Daniel TM. Chemoprophylaxis of multidrug-resistant tuberculous infection in HIV-uninfected individuals using ciprofloxacin and pyrazinamide. A decision analysis. Chest 1995; 108: 712-717.

30. Heifets L, Lindholm-Levy P. Pyrazinamide sterilizing activity in vitro against semi dormant Mycobacterium tuberculosis bacterial populations. Am Rev Respir Dis 1992; 145: 1223-25.

31. Telzak EE, Sepkowitz K, Alpert P, Mannheimer S, Medard F, El-Sadr W, Blum S, Gagliardi A, Salomon N, Turett G. Multidrug-resistant tuberculosis in patients without HIV infection. N Engl J Med 1995; 333: 907-911.

32. Sirgel FA, Botha FJ, Parkin DP, Van de Wal BW, Schall R, Donald PR and Mitchison DA. The early bactericidal activity of ciprofloxacin in patients with pulmonary tuberculosis. Am J Respir Crit Care Med 1997; 156: 901-905.

33. Mitchison DA. The action of antituberculosis drugs in short-course chemotherapy. Tubercle 1985; 66: 219-225.

34. Menzies D, Adhikari N, Tannenbaum T. Patient characteristics associated with failure of tuberculosis prevention. Tuber Lung Dis 1996; 77: 308-314.

35. The role of BCG vaccine in the prevention and control of tuberculosis in the United States. MMWR Morb Mortal Wkly Rep 1996; 45(RR-4): 1-18.

36. Brewer TF, Colditz GA. Bacille Calmette-Guérin vaccination for the prevention of tuberculosis in health care workers. Clin Infect Dis 1995; 20: 136-142.

37. Stevens JP, Daniel TM. Bacille Calmette Guérin immunization of health care workers exposed to multidrug-resistant tuberculosis: a decision analysis. Tuber Lung Dis 1996; 77: 315-321.

38. Marcus AM, Rose DN, Sacks HS, Schechter CB. BCG vaccination to prevent tuberculosis in health care workers: a decision analysis. Prev Med 1997; 26: 201-207.

39. Jenney AWJ, Spelman DW. In support of Bacillus of Calmette and Guérin for healthcare workers. Infect Control Hosp Epidemiol 1998; 19: 191-193.

40. Rodrigues LC, Diwan VK, Wheeler JG. Protective effect of BCG against tuberculous meningitis and miliary tuberculosis: a meta-analysis. Int J Epidemiol 1993; 22: 1154-1158.

41. Colditz GA, Brewer TF, Berkey CS, Wilson ME, Burdick E, Fineberg HV, Mosteller F. Efficacy of BCG vaccine in the prevention of tuberculosis. Meta-analysis of the published literature. JAMA 1994; 271: 698-702.

42. Greenberg PD, Lax KG, Schechter CB. Tuberculosis in house staff. A decision analysis comparing the tuberculin screening strategy with the BCG vaccination. Am Rev Respir Dis 1991; 143: 490-495.

43. Reichman LB, Jordan TJ. Decision analysis comparing the tuberculin screening strategy with BCG vaccine. Am Rev Respir Dis (letter) 1992; 145: 732.

44. Nolan CM, Elarth AM, Barr H, Saeed AM, Risser DR. An outbreak of tuberculosis in a shelter for homeless men. A description of its evolution and control. Am Rev Respir Dis 1991; 143: 257-261.

45. Nettleman M. Use of BCG vaccine in shelters for the homeless: A decision analysis. Chest 1993; 103: 1087-1090.

46. Lotte A, Wasz-Hockert O, Poisson N, Engbaek H, Landmann H, Quast U, Andrasofszky B, Lugosi L, Vadasz Mihailescu P, Pal D, Sudic D. Second IUATLD study on complications induced by intradermal BCG-vaccination. Bull Int Union Tuber Lung Dis 1988; 63: 47-59.

47. Menzies D, Fanning A, Yuan L, Fitzgerald M. Tuberculosis among health care workers. N Engl J Med 1995; 332: 92-98.

48. Cohn DL, Bustreo F, Raviglione MC. Drug-resistant tuberculosis: Review of the worldwide situation and the WHO/IUATLD global surveillance project. Clin Infect Dis 1997; 24 (Suppl 1): S121-130.

Chapter 15

Multidrug-resistant tuberculosis and the health care worker

David M. Weinstock and Kent A. Sepkowitz
Memorial Sloan-Kettering Cancer Center and Weill Medical College of Cornell University

1. INTRODUCTION

The continued resurgence of tuberculosis (TB) and the increasing prevalence of multidrug resistant strains have placed a burden on urban health care facilities across the globe [1]. Because of their ongoing contact with patients, health care workers (HCWs) are at risk of contracting and spreading multidrug resistant tuberculosis (MDRTB). To date, hundreds of HCWs in the United States have developed tuberculin skin test (TST) conversions during outbreaks of MDRTB. Based on current reports, at least 20 HCWs have acquired active MDRTB from an occupational exposure and several have died [2,3]. Numerous other HCWs with both latent and active MDRTB have undoubtedly gone unreported.

Several reviews of TB and the HCW have been published emphasizing the potential risk of nosocomial spread [2,4-12]. In general, the risk of TB infection and disease is increased 2-10 fold among HCWs compared to the general population [11,13,14]. During hospital outbreaks, TST conversion rates have ranged from 0-77% with an average between 20-50% [4,7,12,15-17]. TB is the sixth most common occupationally acquired infection among HCWs [5], and HCWs comprised >3% of all TB cases reported to the United States' Centers for Disease Control and Prevention (CDC) in 1993 [18]. Specific health care occupations with the highest risk of TST conversion

I. Bastian and F. Portaels (eds.), Multidrug-Resistant Tuberculosis, 225-239.
© 2000 *Kluwer Academic Publishers. Printed in the Netherlands.*

include nurses, laboratory workers, housekeepers, security personnel and, perhaps, pulmonary specialists and pathologists [19-26].

Over the past decade, CDC released a series of guidelines to help institutions prevent the nosocomial spread of TB [27-36]. Many health care facilities across the United States achieved reductions in nosocomial transmission of both sensitive- and MDR-TB after implementing some or all of these guidelines (Table 1)[3,19,21,23,37-44]. However, many questions remain regarding the management of a HCW exposed recently or remotely to a patient with MDRTB. We therefore will review the problem of occupationally acquired MDRTB with specific attention to risk assessment, post-exposure evaluation and prophylactic therapy. A complementary chapter in this book describes in more detail the issues surrounding chemoprophylaxis and BCG vaccination for MDRTB contacts [45].

2.   OUTBREAKS OF NOSOCOMIAL MDRTB INVOLVING HCWS: WHAT IS KNOWN

During the urban TB outbreaks of the 1980s and early 1990s, the majority of MDRTB cases encountered in patients and HCWs were the result of nosocomial spread. The stories were similar in most outbreaks: a patient with HIV is admitted to a regular room with what appears to be a case of bacterial pneumonia. Failure to improve after 7-10 days on routine antibacterial antibiotics leads to the delayed consideration of tuberculosis as the diagnosis. During the period prior to diagnosis, dozens of HCWs are exposed.

The precise number of HCWs infected with MDRTB in this fashion is difficult to estimate because of incomplete routine TST programs in many outbreak hospitals during this time. Further compounding the problem is the fact that many HCWs developed a TST conversion while caring for numerous patients with tuberculosis, some of whom have had drug-sensitive disease and others MDRTB. No available test can distinguish latent infection with drug-susceptible versus drug-resistant disease. Confusing matters still further, many cases may have been reported in more than one publication.

All published outbreaks of MDRTB involving HCWs are listed in Table 2 [4,17,22,46-52]. As many as 150 HCWs with MDRTB have been reported, although, as noted, several individuals may have been included in more than one publication. Eight of 25 HIV-negative patients with active MDRTB reported by Telzak et al were HCWs [47]. Of the eight, five were physicians, two were nurses, and one was a hospital administrator. Frieden et al reported 357 patients infected from 1990-1993 with the highly resistant "W" strain of MDRTB during a multi-institutional outbreak in New York

Table 1. Studies of healthcare worker tuberculin skin test conversion rates after implementation of CDC's "Guidelines for preventing the transmission of TB in health-care settings, 1990"[27]

Authors	Study Period	N	Location	Annual TST Conversion Rate			Description
				Before (%)	After (%)	Reduction (%)	
Bangsberg et al.[38]	1992-1993	89	New York, NY	6.4	0.0	100	Study of medical house staff.
Holzman et al.[21]	1992-1994	2132	New York, NY	4.2	1.2	71.4	Performed at public hospital with >200 new TB patients annually and a rate of MDRTB > 15%.
Blumberg et al.[44]	1992-1997	2144	Atlanta, GA	6.0	1.1	81.8	Prospective study of all house staff at an urban medical center with >200 new TB patients annually.
Maloney et al.[3]	1990-1992	90	New York, NY	16.7	5.1	69.5	Retrospective cohort study of HCWs on wards housing patients with TB.
Louther et al.[23]	1991-1994	1303	New York, NY	7.2	3.3	54.2	Housekeeping, laundry, security, and physician-nurse groups had the highest conversion rates.
Wurtz et al.[43]	1991-1993	23	Chicago, IL	26.1	6.3	75.3	Prospective study of medical house staff.
Wenger et al.[42]	1990-1992	25	Miami, FL	28.0	0.0	100	Prospective study of HCWs on wards housing HIV patients with TB. MDRTB among HIV patients also fell from 80% to 45% of TB cases.
Blumberg et al.[37]	1992-1994	5153	Atlanta, GA	6.6	0.8	87.9	Number of TB exposure episodes decreased from 4.4 to 0.6 per month. Number of patient days per month that a TB patient was not in isolation decreased from 35.4 to 3.3.
Fella et al.[39]	1991-1993	249	New York, NY	41.4	11.6	72.0	Prospective study at inner-city hospital with large HIV and methadone populations.

Table 2. Studies of MDRTB with reports of either tuberculin skin test conversions or active MDRTB among health care workers. Individual health care workers may be included in more than one report.

Authors	Study Period	Location	HCWs with Active MDRTB	TST Conversions (% of exposed HCWs)	Comments
Telzak, et al.[47]	1991 - 1994	New York, NY	8		Study of 25 HIV negative patients from 7 hospitals.
Beck-Sague, et al.[4]	1988 - 1990	Miami, FL		13 (33%)	HCWs exposed to HIV positive patients in the hospital and outpatient clinic.
Coronado, et al.[48]	1990 – 1991	New York, NY	1		HCW among 16 patients with an identical MDRTB strain.
Hewlett, et al.[46]	1991 – 1992	New York, NY		12 (57%)	HCWs on an HIV ward during an outbreak of 32 cases of MDRTB.
Ridzon, et al.[51]	1995	Atlanta, GA	1		HCW with nosocomially acquired HIV and a history of drug susceptible TB exposed during an MDRTB outbreak.
Frieden, et al.[49]	1990 – 1993	New York, NY	20		Among 357 patients infected with "strain W" resistant to seven drugs. Thirteen of 20 HCWs were HIV positive.
Ikeda, et al.[50]	1991	Albany, NY		46 (6.6%)	All HCWs were exposed to a single patient with MDRTB resistant to seven drugs.
Pearson, et al.[17]	1989 – 1991	New York, NY		11 (34%)	Six of 12 HCWs working on HIV ward TST converted.
CDC[52]	1988 - 1991	Miami, FL New York, NY	8	19 (37%)	Reports from outbreaks at 4 hospitals. Only 2 of 8 HCWs had known exposures.
Jereb, et al.[22]	1989 - 1992	New York, NY	6		All HCWs had an identical strain resistant to seven drugs. Two of six HCWs were HIV positive.

City [49]. Over 95% of cases were believed to have acquired MDRTB through nosocomial spread at one of eleven hospitals. Twenty of the 357 patients were HCWs, of whom thirteen were HIV positive. Included among these twenty were six nurse's aides, five physicians, and four nurses. Ikeda et al documented TST conversion in 46 HCWs after exposure to a single patient with MDRTB [50]. No active cases of MDRTB were noted. During another outbreak involving 52 patients, six HCWs developed active MDRTB with a strain resistant to seven drugs [22]. Of the six HCWs, two were physicians, two were nurses, and two worked in ancillary services. Ridzon et al reported MDRTB in a HCW who TST converted in 1988 after exposure to two patients with drug sensitive TB [51]. A course of isoniazid prophylaxis was discontinued due to gastrointestinal distress. Two years later, she acquired HIV through a needlestick injury. In 1995, she presented with fever, night sweats, and weight loss and was found to have TB resistant to both isoniazid and rifampin.

Table 3. Factors associated with an increased likelihood of nosocomial spread of MDRTB to HCWs

Longer period of smear positivity and infectiousness
Higher rates of treatment failure
Available therapies less efficacious and poorly tolerated
Longer hospitalization
Progressive inanition may require intense HCW involvement
Association with HIV positive patients
Atypical presentation
Multiple hospital admissions
Poor response to treatment

For several reasons, drug resistant TB may be more likely than drug susceptible disease to undergo nosocomial spread (Table 3)[2,4,17,48,49,53-55]. First, because of delays in instituting proper therapy and second-line medication side effects, patients with MDRTB often are sicker than other tuberculosis patients and therefore may require more frequent and intense HCW involvement [4]. Second, once appropriate therapy is instituted, response may be slow, meaning the period of infectiousness may persist. Because of concerns about continued contagion, placement of such patients into an out-patient or long-term care environment may be delayed by the receiving health care institution.

As a result of this and other factors, patients with MDRTB may remain hospitalized longer than other TB patients, again extending the period of potential transmissibility to hospital staff [53]. Pearson et al. reported that HCWs working on wards with MDRTB patients were more likely to TST convert than HCWs on other wards (34% vs. 2%)[17]. Fourteen of the 16 MDRTB isolates from that outbreak had identical DNA fingerprints using restriction fragment length polymorphism (RFLP) analysis, while each of the drug-sensitive isolates had different fingerprints. In a study by Coronado et al. [48], patients with MDRTB were more likely to have been hospitalized within three rooms of an infectious patient than patients with drug-sensitive TB. Six of the 8 patients with MDRTB had identical RFLP fingerprints.

The majority of patients involved in the nosocomial outbreaks of MDRTB in the 1980s and early 1990s were HIV infected (Table 3)[4,27,34,48,49,52,55-64]. According to studies utilizing molecular typing techniques, among patients with HIV, up to 60% of active TB results from recently acquired infection [54]. Therefore, the risk of contracting and developing active MDRTB is increased in areas with high community and institutional rates of TB drug resistance [34,56,57,62]. HIV-positive patients may have multiple hospital admissions, often have atypical clinical and radiographic presentations of active TB [63,65], and may respond poorly to therapy, thereby increasing and prolonging the possibility of spreading nosocomial strains of TB.

3.   PREVENTING ACTIVE MDRTB AMONG HCWS: BCG VERSUS TST SCREENING AND PROPHYLACTIC THERAPY

The Bacillus Calmette-Guerin vaccine (BCG) and the strategy of TST testing with isoniazid prophylaxis are the two cornerstones of tuberculosis control programs worldwide and in the US. The relative effectiveness of each approach has been frequently compared. The potential utility of BCG has been established in numerous field trails and, more recently, in various health care models and meta-analyses. In 1965, Springett used a mathematical analysis to support BCG vaccine for HCWs whenever the nosocomial conversion rate exceeded 1% per year [66]. In a 1979 survey of United States physicians, Barrett-Connor showed an 80% reduction in the incidence of active TB among BCG recipients [11]. Nettleman et al. used a Markov model to demonstrate the superior cost-effectiveness of a TB vaccine with 50% efficacy over infection control practices using the TST [67]. A meta-analysis of available trials using BCG for prevention of TB showed an efficacy of approximately 50% with a 71% reduction in TB deaths [68]. Greenberg et al. used decision analysis to compare TST screening to BCG vaccination among house staff [69]. At their institution, where only 63% of residents are compliant with annual TST screening and only 45% of residents who became TST positive began isoniazid, BCG required an efficacy of only 13.1% to prevent more cases of TB than TST screening and isoniazid prophylaxis [69].

Reports from the Occupational Safety and Health Administration, the CDC and independent authors show poor HCW compliance with TST screening and prophylactic therapy [2,69-73] On average, less than 25% of HCWs identified by TST screening complete at least six months of therapy [74]. One study showed increased HCW compliance with prophylactic therapy when included within a comprehensive TST program that facilitated early referral to a physician for evaluation [75]. This suggests that the increasing concern and increasing awareness of nosocomial disease have effectively been translated into improved compliance. No matter the rising optimism for adherence with simple single drug prophylaxis, reports of adherence with multidrug regimens given for possible latent MDRTB are dismal: HCWs have typically been unable to complete such courses, due to significant side effects and questionable benefit [76].

The potential benefit for HCWs of BCG vaccination over TST screening may be increased in the setting of high rates of MDRTB. Kritski et al. followed close contacts of patients in Brazil with MDRTB [77]. Those contacts who had previously received BCG were 3.1 times less likely to develop active MDRTB than those contacts who had not received BCG. In an outbreak of isoniazid-resistant TB among adolescents at a school in Ireland, subjects who had not received neonatal BCG were over five times more likely to develop active TB than those who had (3.6% vs. 0.7%)[78]. Therefore, the efficacy of BCG may be unaffected by drug resistance while the value of post-exposure prophylaxis for TST converters is unknown [32].

Two concerns about BCG have been raised. First, the loss of the TST as a sign of TB infection compromises outbreak detection and investigation, and the efforts of infection control personnel to evaluate and prevent nosocomial exposure [28]. Second, universal vaccination of HCWs with BCG could change the routine evaluation of HCWs after TB exposure or when presenting with nonspecific complaints like cough, fever, weight loss, and malaise.

Because of these and other concerns, in 1988 the United States Advisory Committee on Immunization Practices (ACIP) removed HCWs from the list of persons for whom BCG should be considered. Revised recommendations from the ACIP, the Advisory Council for the Elimination of Tuberculosis and the Hospital Infection Control Practices Advisory Committee support the initial recommendations [30,36]. However, in certain situations, BCG "may contribute to the prevention and control of TB when other strategies are inadequate" [30]. BCG should be considered in settings where a high percentage of TB is MDRTB, transmission of TB to HCWs is "likely", and comprehensive TB control programs are implemented but are not "successful" [30,36]. BCG vaccination is not recommended for HCWs infected with HIV and, according to the CDC, should not be required for employment [30].

4.   MANAGING THE HCW AFTER EXPOSURE TO MDRTB

In the publications, "Management of Persons Exposed to Multidrug Resistant Tuberculosis" [32], and "Guidelines for Preventing the Transmission of *Mycobacterium tuberculosis* in Health-Care Facilities" [28], the CDC recommends that, after exposure to a patient with potential MDRTB, all HCWs without a prior positive TST should undergo TST testing immediately and, if negative, twelve weeks later. Those HCWs with a prior positive TST and no evidence of immunosuppression need no further evaluation.   Those who TST convert and those who are anergic or immunocompromised should be considered for prophylactic therapy based on the likelihood of both infection with MDRTB and progression to active disease. To assess the former, several factors should be considered including the infectiousness of the source MDRTB case, the closeness and intensity of the exposure and the HCW's likelihood of additional exposure to other cases with drug susceptible TB. Patients with TB and either a cough, positive sputum smear, and/or multiple contacts who have recently TST converted should be considered highly infective [32]. Transmission has been described following medical procedures including bronchoscopy, endoscopy, endotracheal intubation, sputum collection, administration of aerosol therapy, and performance of autopsies.

Active TB will develop in 3.3% of immunocompetent persons in the first year after a TST conversion [65], while up to 37% of persons with HIV who are newly infected with TB progress to active disease in the first six months [54,79-82]. Therefore, the presence of HIV or other immunodeficiency in the HCW is the most important factor in assessing the likelihood of progression to active TB [32]. Multidrug prophylactic therapy should be strongly considered for all HCWs with HIV after prolonged or intense exposure to MDRTB regardless of TST status or CD4 cell count.

5.   PROPHYLAXIS OF THE HCW EXPOSED TO MDRTB

Prophylactic regimens for MDRTB exposed patients are of unproven efficacy. Furthermore, no clinical data exists on the risks and benefits of regimens that do not include isoniazid or rifampin [32]. Therefore, the CDC recommends that all HCWs exposed to MDRTB isolates with less than 100% resistance to isoniazid should be treated with isoniazid. Similarly, those with 100% resistance to isoniazid but less than 100% resistance to rifampin should receive a course of rifampin [32].

In a recent Delphi survey, 31 experts evaluated options for prophylaxis after MDRTB exposure [83]. None of the proposed drug regimens were considered "appropriate" by the panel, including regimens using isoniazid or rifampin for strains with less than 100% resistance. Two drug regimens containing pyrazinamide and ethambutol have been advocated by the CDC [32,33], but were poorly regarded in the Delphi survey for a scenario involving a nurse who was exposed to MDRTB [83]. A regimen of pyrazinamide and ofloxacin has also been advocated by the CDC [32,33], but is poorly tolerated [76,84]. In the Delphi survey, a similar regimen of pyrazinamide 1500mg daily and ciprofloxacin 750mg twice a day for four months was deemed "somewhat appropriate" by over 50% of the TB experts [83]. Considering the potential toxicity and questionable efficacy of available prophylactic therapy, careful observation remains a reasonable alternative for the immunocompetent HCW exposed to MDRTB. This approach, although unsettling for newly infected workers, has become more accepted by many experts, particularly because it preserves drug options should the HCW eventually develop active MDRTB.

6. FURLOUGHING THE HCW WITH ACTIVE MDRTB

According to CDC guidelines, HCWs with active pulmonary or laryngeal TB can return to the workplace once they are being treated with adequate therapy and have documentation of three negative sputum smears [28]. At that point, the HCW is considered "noninfectious." Because of the difficulties in treating MDRTB, a more conservative approach may be appropriate regarding when to allow a HCW with MDRTB to return to work. Some experts prefer to furlough HCWs with active MDRTB until they are culture negative [27,28]. The basis of this conservative approach includes the fact that, in animal studies, inhalation of a single airborne droplet with 1-3 viable tuberculous bacilli can cause infection [85]. Based on evidence using drug sensitive TB, nearly all smear negative, culture positive patients will no longer be culture positive after two weeks of appropriate therapy [85]. However, treatment failure occurs more often with MDRTB than drug sensitive TB and resistance to all of the highly bactericidal, first-line agents is common. The smear negative HCW with MDRTB may still present potential risk for transmission even after two weeks of appropriate therapy.

Thus, use of smear status may underestimate the potential for transmission in patients with MDRTB.

Risk should be minimized for HCWs who are in contact with ill and debilitated patients. Telzak et al. reported a mean time of three months from diagnosis to microbiologic response (date of obtaining first negative culture specimen) in 24 HIV-negative patients with MDRTB [47]. An additional 1-2 months would be necessary before negative cultures could be finalized. Thus, a furlough of 4-5 months or longer may be necessary for HCWs with active MDRTB. Immunocompromised HCWs are likely to respond less rapidly and may require even longer furloughs.

7.   ADDRESSING HCW CONCERNS OVER MDRTB

In 1930, Baldwin, Director of the Trudeau Foundation, recognized the perceived danger of working among TB patients and coined the term "phthisiophobia" [86]. A similar HCW fear of caring for patients with MDRTB may exist today. In a 1995 survey of 544 HCWs at an urban medical center [87], 11% of nurses felt they should be able to refuse to care for patients with MDRTB. One-third of doctors and nurses thought that patients with MDRTB should be cared for in a special hospital. No consistent professional ethic or tradition has been established to guide HCWs in the treatment of patients with communicable diseases [88]. The conflict between HCW beneficence, altruism, rights, and duties is complex. The HCW with significant concerns has unclear ethical and legal obligations to care for patients with suspected or proven MDRTB. The quality of care that such HCWs provide may also be compromised by their fear of nosocomial disease.

Immunocompromised HCWs are at particular risk for acquiring and spreading MDRTB. The employ of immunocompromised HCWs in settings with a high risk for nosocomial MDRTB creates ethical, legal, and practical problems with no simple solutions. The CDC recommends that, if requested by the employee, employers should offer but not compel a work assignment in which an immunocompromised HCW could avoid TB exposure [30]. Therefore, the HIV infected HCW and his or her primary physician should address decisions about exposure, risk and safety.

8. CONCLUSIONS

By the late 1980s, increases in drug resistant TB, the AIDS epidemic, and poor compliance with infection control measures combined to create a very real risk of both nosocomial drug-susceptible and multidrug-resistant TB infection. The publication and implementation of CDC guidelines for preventing the transmission, assessing the risk, and evaluating an outbreak of MDRTB have helped control the morbidity and mortality of this disease in HCWs. However, hundreds of HCWs have already been infected with MDRTB and constitute a formidable reservoir of potential future disease. More efficacious and less toxic therapies are necessary to help infected HCWs avoid reactivation and its sequelae. Further reduction of risk for the uninfected HCW awaits a dramatically more rapid means of diagnosing drug resistant TB. Only with the development of such techniques will the risk for nosocomial spread of MDRTB truly be minimized.

REFERENCES

1. Snider DE, Roper WL. The new tuberculosis. N Engl J Med 1992; 326: 703-705.
2. Menzies D, Fanning A, Yuan L, Fitzgerald M. Tuberculosis among health care workers. N Engl J Med 1995; 332: 92-98
3. Maloney SA, Pearson ML, Gordon MT, Del Castillo R, Boyle JF, Jarvis WR. Efficacy of control measures in preventing nosocomial transmission of multidrug-resistant tuberculosis to patients and health care workers. Ann Intern Med 1995; 122: 90-95.
4. Sepkowitz KA. Tuberculosis and the health care worker: A historical perspective. Ann Intern Med 1994; 120: 71-79.
5. Sepkowitz KA. AIDS, tuberculosis and the health care worker. Clin Infect Dis 1995; 20: 232-242.
6. Sepkowitz KA. Occupationally acquired infections in health care workers: part I. Ann Intern Med 1996; 125: 826-834.
7. Bowden KM, McDiarmid MA. Occupationally acquired tuberculosis: what's known. J Occup Med 1994; 36: 320-325.
8. Markowitz SB. Epidemiology of tuberculosis among health care workers. Occup Med 1994; 9: 589-608.
9. Farer LS, Atkinson ML. Tuberculosis and the health worker. Am J Public Health 1981; 71: 1200-1201.
10. Goldman KP. Tuberculosis in hospital doctors. Tubercle 1988; 69: 237-240.
11. Barrett-Connor E. The epidemiology of tuberculosis in physicians. JAMA 1979; 241: 33-38.
12. Catanzaro A. Nosocomial tuberculosis. Am Rev Respir Dis 1982; 125: 559-562.
13. Sepkowitz KA, Friedman CR, Hafner A, et al. Tuberculosis among urban health care workers: a study using restriction fragment length polymorphism typing. Clin Infect Dis 1995; 21: 1098-1102.
14. Meredith S, Watson JM, Citron KM, Cockcroft A, Darbyshire JH. Are health care workers in England and Wales at increased risk of tuberculosis? BMJ 1995; 313: 522-525.

15. Griffith DE, Hardeman JL, Zhang Y, Wallace RJ, Mazurek GH. Tuberculosis outbreak among health care workers in a community hospital. Am J Respir Crit Care Med. 1995; 152: 808-811.
16. Haley CE, et al. Tuberculosis epidemic among hospital personnel. Infect Control Hosp Epidemiol 1989; 10: 204-210.
17. Pearson ML, Jereb JA, Frieden TR, et al. Nosocomial transmission of multi-drug resistant *Mycobacterium tuberculosis*: a risk to patients and health care workers. Ann Intern Med 1992; 117: 191-196.
18. Expanded tuberculosis surveillance and tuberculosis morbidity – United States, 1993. MMWR Morb Mortal Wkly Rep 1994; 43: 361-366.
19. Fridkin SK, Manangan L, Bolyard E, Jarvis WR. SHEA-CDC TB survey, part I: status of TB infection control programs at member hospitals, 1989-1992. Infect Control Hosp Epidemiol 1995; 16: 129-134.
20. Malasky C, et al. Occupational tuberculosis infections among pulmonary physicians in training. Am Rev Respir Dis 1990; 142: 505-507.
21. Holzman RS. A comprehensive control program reduces transmission of tuberculosis (TB) to hospital staff [Abstract]. Clin Infect Dis 1995; 21: 733.
22. Jereb JA, Klevens M, Privett TD, et al. Tuberculosis in health care workers at a hospital with an outbreak of multidrug-resistant *Mycobacterium tuberculosis*. Arch Intern Med 1995; 155: 854-859.
23. Louther J, Rivera P, Feldman J, Villa N, DeHovitz J, Sepkowitz KA. Risk of tuberculin conversion according to occupation among health care workers at a New York City hospital. Am J Respir Crit Care Med 1997; 156: 201-205.
24. Louther J, et al. Employee TST conversion rates according to occupation at a New York City hospital [Abstract]. Am J Infect Control 1995; 23: 114.
25. Sepkowitz KA. Tuberculin skin testing and the health care worker: lessons of the Prophit survey. Tuber Lung Dis 1996; 77: 81-85.
26. Daniels M, Ridehalgh F, Springett VH, Hall IM. In: Tuberculosis in young adults: report on the Prophit Tuberculosis Survey, 1936-1944. HK Lewis and Co. Ltd, London, 1948.
27. Guidelines for preventing the transmission of tuberculosis in health-care settings, with special focus on HIV-related issues. MMWR Morb Mortal Wkly Rep 1990; 39 Suppl RR-17.
28. Guidelines for preventing the transmission of *Mycobacterium tuberculosis* in health-care facilities, 1994. MMWR Morb Mortal Wkly Rep 1994; 43:(RR-13): 1-132.
29. Bolyard EA, Tablan EC, Williams WW, et al. Guideline for infection control in health care personnel, 1998. Infect Control Hosp Epidemiol 1998; 19: 407-463.
30. Immunization of health-care workers: recommendations of the Advisory Committee on Immunization Practices (ACIP) and the Hospital Infection Control Practices Advisory Committee (HICPAC). MMWR Morb Mortal Wkly Rep 1997; 46(RR-18): 1-42.
31. Jarvis WR, Bolyard EA, Bozzi CJ, et al. Respirators, recommendations, and regulations: the controversy surrounding protection of health care workers from tuberculosis. Ann Intern Med 1995; 122: 142-146.
32. Management of persons exposed to multidrug-resistant tuberculosis. MMWR Morb Mortal Wkly Rep 1992; 41(RR-11): 61-71.
33. National action plan to combat multidrug-resistant tuberculosis. MMWR Morb Mortal Wkly Rep 1992; 41(RR-11): 5-48.
34. Prevention and treatment of tuberculosis among patients infected with Human Immunodeficiency Virus: principles of therapy and revised recommendations. MMWR Morb Mortal Wkly Rep 1998; 47(RR-20): 1-51.

35. Recommendations for prevention and control of tuberculosis among foreign-born persons: report of the working group on tuberculosis among foreign-born persons. MMWR Morb Mortal Wkly Rep 1998; 47(RR-16): 1-26.

36. The role of BCG vaccine in the prevention and control of tuberculosis in the United States. A joint statement by the Advisory Council for the Elimination of Tuberculosis and the Advisory Committee on Immunization Practices. MMWR Morb Mortal Wkly Rep 1996; 45(RR-4): 1-18.

37. Blumberg HM, Watkins DL, Berschling JD, et al. Preventing the nosocomial transmission of tuberculosis. Ann Intern Med 1995: 122: 658-661.

38. Bangsberg DR, Crowley K, Knirsch C, et al. Declining TST conversion rates among medical housestaff during the New York City tubercuolosis epidemic: facilities and policies for isolating HIV-related pneumonia. Infect Control Hosp Epidemiol 1994; 15(Suppl): 40.

39. Fella P, Rivera P, Hale M, Squires K, Sepkowitz K. Dramatic decrease in tuberculin skin test conversion rate among employees at a hospital in New York City. Am J Infect Control 1985; 23: 352-356.

40. Beck-Sague C, Dooley SW, Hutton MD, et al. Hospital outbreak of multi-drug rsistant *Mycobacterium tuberculosis* infections: factors in transmission to staff and HIV-infected patients. JAMA 1992; 268: 1280-1286.

41. Stroud LA, Tokars JI, Grieco MH, et al. Evaluation of infection control measures in preventing the nosocomial transmission of multidrug-resistant *Mycobacterium tuberculosis* in a New York City hospital. Infect Control Hosp Epidemiol 1995; 16: 141-147.

42. Wenger PN, Otten J, Breeden A, Orfas D, Beck-Sague CM, Jarvis WM. Control of nosocomial transmission of multidrug-resistant *Mycobacterium tuberculosis* among health care workers and HIV-infected patients. Lancet 1995; 345: 235-240.

43. Wurtz R, Cocchiaerlla L, Cohen R. Efficacy of routine infection control measures to limit occupational tuberculosis infection [Abstract M31]. Infect Control Hosp Epidemiol 1994; 15: 40.

44. Blumberg HM , Sotir M , Erwin M , Bachman R , Shulman JA. Risk of house staff tuberculin skin test conversion in an area with a high incidence of tuberculosis. Clin Infect Dis 1998; 27: 826-33.

45. Stapledon RA, Lumb R, Lim IS. Chemoprophylaxis and BCG in contacts of multidrug-resistant tuberculosis, Chapter 14, 213-224. In: Bastian I, Portaels F (eds.), Multidrug-resistant tuberculosis. Kluwer Academic Publ., The Netherlands, 2000.

46. Hewlett D, et al. Outbreak of mutidrug-resistant tuberculosis at a hospital – New York City, 1991. MMWR Morb Mortal Wkly Rep 1993; 42: 427, 433-434.

47. Telzak EE, Sepkowitz K, Alpert P, et al. Multidrug-resistant tuberculosis in patients without HIV infection. N Engl J Med 1995; 333: 907-911.

48. Coronado VG, Beck-Sague CM, Hutton MD, et al. Transmission of multi-drug resistant *Mycobacterium tuberculosis* among patients with human immunodeficiency virus infection in an urban hospital: epidemiologic and restriction fragment length polymorphism analysis. J Infect Dis 1993; 168: 1052-1055.

49. Frieden TR, Sherman LF, Maw KL, et al. A multi-institutional outbreak of highly drug-resistant tuberculosis: epidemiology and clinical outcomes. JAMA 1996; 276: 1229-1235.

50. Ikeda RM, Birkhead GS, DiFerdinando GT, et al. Nosocomial tuberculosis: an outbreak of a strain resistant to seven drugs. Infect Control Hosp Epidemiol 1995; 16: 152-159.

51. Ridzon R, Kenyon T, Luskin-Hawk R, Schultz C, Walway S, Onorato IM. Nosocomial transmission of human immunodeficiency virus and subsequent transmission of

multidrug-resistant tuberculosis in a health care worker. Infect Cont Hosp Epidemiol 1997; 18: 422-423.

52. Nosocomial transmission of multidrug-resistant tuberculosis among HIV-infected persons – Florida and New York, 1988-1991. MMWR Morb Mortal Wkly Rep 1991; 40: 585-591.

53. Goble M, Iseman MD, Madsen LA, Waite D, Ackerson L, Horsburgh CR. Treatment of 171 patients with pulmonary tuberculosis resistant to isoniazid and rifampin. N Engl J Med 1993; 328: 527-532.

54. Alland D, Kalkut GE, Moss AR, et al. Transmission of tuberculosis in New York City: an analysis by DNA fingerprinting and conventional epidemiologic methods. N Engl J Med 1994; 330: 1710-1716.

55. Edlin BR, Tokars JI, Grieco MH, et al. An outbreak of multidrug-resistant tuberculosis among hospitalized patients with the acquired immunodeficiency syndrome. N Engl J Med 1992; 326: 1514-1521.

56. Moore M, Onorato IM, McCray E, Castro KG. Trends in drug-resistant tuberculosis in the United States, 1993-1996. JAMA 1997; 278: 833-837.

57. Small PM, Hopewell PC, Singh SP, et al. The epidemiology of tuberculosis in San Francisco: a population-based study using conventional and molecular methods. N Engl J Med 1994; 330: 1703-1709.

58. Di Perri G, Cadeo G, Castelli F, et al. Transmission of HIV-associated tuberculosis to health care workers. Infect Control Hosp Epidemiol 1993; 14: 67-72.

59. Dooley SW, Villarino ME, Lawrence M, et al. Nosocomial transmission of tuberculosis in a hospital unit for HIV-infected patients. JAMA 1992; 267: 2632-2634.

60. Nosocomial transmission of multidrug-resistant tuberculosis to health-care workers and HIV-infected patients in an urban hospital – Florida. MMWR Morb Mortal Wkly Rep 1990; 39: 718-722.

61. Barnes PF, et al. Tuberculosis in patients with human immunodeficiency virus infection. N Engl J Med 1991; 324: 1644-1650.

62. Fischl MA, Uttamchandani RB, Daikos GL, et al. An outbreak of tuberculosis caused by multiple drug resistant tubercle bacilli among patients with HIV infection. Ann Intern Med 1992; 117: 177-183.

63. Fischl MA, Daikos GL, Uttamchandani RB, et al. Clinical presentation and outcome of patients with HIV infection and tuberculosis caused by multiple drug-resistant bacilli. Ann Intern Med 1992; 117: 184-190.

64. Havlir DV, Barnes PF. Tuberculosis in patients with human immunodeficiency virus infection. N Engl J Med 1999; 340: 367-373.

65. DesPrez RM, Heim CR. *Mycobacterium tuberculosis.* In: Mandell GL, Douglas RG Jr., Bennett JE (eds), Principles and practices of infectious diseases. 3rd ed. Churchill Livingstone, New York, 1990.

66. Springett VH. The value of BCG vaccination. Tubercle 1965; 46: 76-84

67. Nettleman MD, Geerdes H, Roy MC. The cost-effectiveness of preventing tuberculosis in physicians using tuberculin skin testing or a hypothetical vaccine. Arch Intern Med 1997; 157: 1121-1127.

68. Colditz GA, et al. Efficacy of BCG vaccine in the prevention of tuberculosis: meta-analysis of the published literature. JAMA 1994; 271: 698-702.

69. Greenberg PD, Lax KG, Schecter CB. Tuberculosis in house staff. Am Rev Respir Dis 1991; 143: 490-495.

70. Fagan MJ, Poland GA. Tuberculin skin testing in medical students: a survey of US medical schools. Ann Intern Med 1994; 120: 930-931.

71. Lane NE, Paul RI, Bratcher DF, Stover BH. A survey of policies at children's hospitals regarding immunity of health care workers: are physicians protected? Infect Control Hosp Epidemiol 1997; 400-404.
72. Nolan CM. Tuberculosis in health care professionals: assessing and accepting the risk. Ann Intern Med 1994; 120: 964-965.
73. Raad I, Cusick J, Sheretz RJ, Sabbagh M, Howell N. Annual tuberculin skin testing of employees at a university hospital: a cost-benefit analysis. Infect Control Hosp Epidemiol 1989; 10: 465-469.
74. Roy M, Fredrickson M, Good NL, Hunter SA, Nettleman MD. Correlation between frequency of tuberculosis and compliance with control strategies. Infect Control Hosp Epidemiol 1997; 18: 28-31.
75. Camins BC, Bock N, Watkins DL, Blumberg HM. Acceptance of isoniazid preventive therapy by health care workers after tuberculin skin test conversion. JAMA 1996; 275: 1013-1015.
76. Horn DL, Hewlett D Jr, Alfalla C, Peterson S, Opal SM. Limited tolerance of ofloxacin and pyrazinamide prophylaxis against tuberculosis [Letter]. N Engl J Med 1994; 330: 1241.
77. Kritski AL, Ozorio Marques MJ, Rabahi MF, et al. Transmission of tuberculosis to close contacts of patients with multidrug-resistant tuberculosis. Am J Respir Crit Care Med 1996; 153: 331-335.
78. Shannon A, Kelly P, Lucey M, Cooney M, Corcoran P, Clancy L. Isoniazid resistant tuberculosis in a school outbreak: the protective effect of BCG. Eur Respir J 1991; 4: 778-782.
79. Di Perri G, et al. Nosocomial epidemic of active tuberculosis among HIV-infected patients. Lancet 1989; 2: 1502-1504.
80. Daley CL, Smalk PM, Schecter GF, et al. An outbreak of tuberculosis with accelerated progression among persons infected with the human immunodeficiency virus: an analysis using restriction-fragment-length polymorphisms. N Engl J Med 1992; 326: 231-235.
81. Sepkowitz KA, Raffalli J, Riley L, Kiehn TE, Armstrong D. Tuberculosis in the AIDS era. Clin Microbiol Rev 1995; 8: 180-199.
82. Small PM, Shafer RW, Hopewell PC, et al. Exogenous reinfection with multidrug-resistant *Mycobacterium tuberculosis* in patients with advanced HIV infection. N Engl J Med 1993; 328: 1137-1144.
83. Passannante MR, Gallagher CT, Reichman LB. Preventive therapy for contacts of multidrug-resistant tuberculosis. A Delphi survey. Chest. 1994; 106: 431-434.
84. Sepkowitz KA, Telzak EE, Recaide S, Armstrong D. Trends in the susceptibility of tuberculosis in New York City, 1987-1991. Clin Infect Dis 1994; 18: 755-759.
85. Menzies D. Effect of treatment on contagiousness of patients with active pulmonary tuberculosis. Infect Control Hosp Epidemiol 1997; 18: 582-586.
86. Baldwin ER. The danger of tuberculosis infection in hospitals and sanatoria. United States Veterans' Bureau Medical Bulletin 1930; 6: 1-4.
87. Sugarman J, Terry P, Faden RR, Holmes DE, Fogarty L, Pyeritz RE. Professional health care workers' attitudes toward treating patients with mutlidrug-resistant tuberculosis. J Clin Ethics 1995; 7: 222-227.
88. Zuger A, et al. Physicians, AIDS, and occupational risk: historic traditions and ethical obligations. JAMA 1987; 258: 1924-1928.

Chapter 16

The development of new chemotherapeutics for multidrug-resistant tuberculosis

Clifton E. Barry, III
Tuberculosis Research Section, Laboratory of Host Defenses, NIAID, NIH, Rockville, Maryland

1. INTRODUCTION

Despite massive recent public attention for the development of new and improved vaccines for tuberculosis the development of new chemotherapeutic interventions has, by comparison, languished [1,2]. This is largely due to a lack of private sector interest in what is commonly perceived as a low profit potential market. The widely quoted figure that one-third of the population of the planet has already been infected with the bacillus that causes tuberculosis highlights the folly of a vaccine-only approach [3]. Counting on the private sector to undertake lead molecule identification and optimization, preclinical testing, and clinical evaluation of new antituberculars without significant public sector involvement and support is simply not a realistic option given the demographics of tuberculosis. Unfortunately, the emergence and spread of strains resistant to the front-line therapies of isoniazid and rifampicin is rapidly rendering the current arsenal of drugs obsolete and without new therapies there is a high likelihood of a return to pre-antibiotic mortality rates. Even directly observed therapy with existing antituberculosis drugs is ineffective in the face of existing levels of drug resistance [4,5].

The situation is all the more disturbing because our ability to identify, optimize, and develop new preclinical candidates has never looked so promising. Our understanding of basic mycobacterial physiology has never

I. Bastian and F. Portaels (eds.), Multidrug-Resistant Tuberculosis, 241-252.

been greater now that the complete genome sequence is in hand [6]. With this understanding and the tools being developed for monitoring whole-organism transcriptional and translational responses, we are in a position to confidently identify good drug targets through the development of *in vitro* and *in vivo* assays. Simultaneously, organic chemistry has undergone a revolution in the ability to create fantastically diverse libraries of small molecules as potential new therapeutics for disabling these critical targets through the use of combinatorial chemistry [7,8]. This revolution promises a new age of antibiotics of high specificity, good pharmacokinetics, and low toxicity. The major remaining question is who will pick up and utilize these tools to develop and deliver new antituberculosis drugs? This review will attempt to illuminate the drug development pipeline from compounds recently introduced into the clinic to concepts recently introduced into the laboratory.

2. THE NEAR END OF THE PIPELINE: SEMISYNTHETIC DERIVATIVES OF RIFAMYCIN FOR THE TREATMENT OF MULTIDRUG-RESISTANT TUBERCULOSIS

Probably the major recent efforts in preclinical TB drug development have focussed on semisynthetic derivatives of rifampicin, a critical component of current tuberculosis therapy that inhibits RNA polymerase [9,10]. Rifabutin, a spiropiperidyl derivative of rifampicin, has been demonstrated to have superior *in vitro* and *in vivo* activity to its parent compound [11-14]. Rifabutin shows activity against a subset of rifampicin-resistant strains making it a viable option for treatment of multidrug-resistant tuberculosis (MDRTB) in some cases [15]. The molecular determinants of the subset that retains rifabutin sensitivity despite rifampicin resistance have been carefully determined. Specific alterations in *rpoB* are associated with resistance to all rifamycin derivatives while other alterations are associated with resistance to rifampin and rifapentine but not rifabutin and another new derivative, KRM-1648 [16-18]. These results suggest that rapid identification of the genetic alterations that result in rifampin resistance may be of substantial value in predicting efficacy of rifabutin treatment.

The long duration of therapy (with resulting poor compliance) is one of the primary obstacles to TB control and one of the instigating factors in the development of drug resistance. Shortening this therapy therefore represents a significant goal for the development of new agents [19]. An improved therapeutic with either an extended serum half-life or an exceptionally tight binding constant for its target would allow the possibility of significantly decreasing the duration of therapy. An alternative to shortening the total duration of therapy that would simplify direct observation would be a drug that could be administered on a less frequent dosing schedule. This was, in part, the rationale for the preclinical development of rifamycin analogs with altered pharmacokinetic properties such as rifapentine [20]. Rifapentine has been shown to have a significantly extended serum half-life compared with rifampicin [21]. For this reason clinical trials of rifapentine given once weekly in combination with isoniazid were undertaken [22]. Unfortunately patients enrolled in this study developed rifamycin monoresistance more frequently than patients treated with rifampicin and isoniazid twice weekly. These studies make the future contribution of rifapentine to tuberculosis therapy unclear.

The most recent entries into this area are the benzoxazinorifamycins such as KRM-1648 [23]. This compound has been shown to have a better MIC than the parent compound in combination therapy *in vitro* and in murine models of tuberculosis [24-30]. Although small-scale clinical trials aimed at safety evaluation have been initiated this compound has not yet been assessed for efficacy in humans.

3. TARGETING LATENT ORGANISMS – METRONIDAZOLE AND BEYOND

Another opportunity for new antimycobacterials arises because of the relatively poor efficacy of many existing antimycobacterials against so-called "latent" organisms (Figure 1). These ostensibly non-replicating organisms are thought to constitute a reservoir of infection in patients that have mounted a successful immune response to TB infection [31,32]. Because of their metabolic inactivity, or the biochemical details of their physiology, these organisms are known to be resistant to the existing front-line antimycobacterial agents, isoniazid and rifampicin [33,34]. This resistance is thought to be responsible for the large discrepancy in the length of time required to treat patients (months) as compared with the length of time required to sterilize an *in vitro* culture of the bacilli (days). Pyrazinamide, another component of the front-line anti-tuberculosis regimen, has been thought to exert activity against this special population of bacilli since it can be used to achieve sterility in animal models of tuberculosis persistence [35,36]. These organisms have many distinctive metabolic features, some of which may give rise to a unique sensitivity to nitroimidazoles such as metronidazole [34]. This sensitivity may be due to productive reduction of the nitro group under the microaerophilic or anaerobic conditions that are used to replicate the dormant state *in vitro*.

Unfortunately this observation has not been extended to animal models of infection or latency where metronidazole has been shown to have little effect on either actively replicating or latent organisms [37-39]. However, other nitroimidazoles have been shown to have good antitubercular activity [40]. In some cases these compounds have been further developed and preliminary *in vitro* and animal studies have demonstrated efficacy of particular derivatives against both actively replicating and dormant bacilli (D.R. Sherman, M.J. Hickey, A. Towell, Y. Yuan, C.E. Barry, III, C.K. Stover, unpublished results). Obviously these compounds deserve further preclinical evaluation as activity against non-replicating organisms offers the hope of substantially shortening the duration of therapy.

A more basic approach to drug development has involved the identification of enzyme activities that are suspected of being important to survival during non-replicating persistence. These enzymes have been recognised in an *in vitro* model in which tubercle bacilli adapt to microaerophilic conditions (which may replicate the conditions that occur during granuloma formation) [31]. For example, enzymes of the glyoxylate shunt such as isocitrate lyase have been the subject of recent research as novel targets for directly attacking nonreplicating bacilli [41].

4.   THE TROUBLE WITH PRODRUGS

Many antimycobacterial agents are prodrugs that require cellular activation by which they are converted into an active form that then interacts with their cellular target. The problem with prodrugs lies in their dependence upon a microbial enzyme for activation. This dependence offers an escape route for the organism in the event that the activating enzyme's activity is not essential or can be compensated for by another activity. Thus prodrugs are, in general, associated with higher mutational frequencies engendering resistance than are drugs that interact specifically with a cellular target.

Isoniazid is the prototypical prodrug, as it requires activation by the catalase-peroxidase KatG to a poorly defined active form before it can exert a lethal effect on targets involved in mycolic acid biosynthesis [42,43]. KatG also plays a role as an important enzyme involved in the mycobacterial strategy for resisting oxidative damage from the host cell [44]. Nonetheless, this function can be adequately performed by other enzymes within the tubercle bacillus so loss of KatG function is the single most common mechanism utilized by the bacterium to acquire isoniazid resistance [45-47]. Resistance frequencies for isoniazid thus range to as high as 1 in 10^5 organisms [48]. Other antimycobacterial drugs have been proposed as

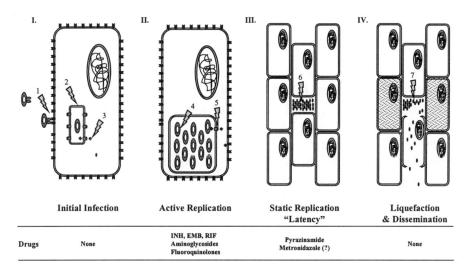

	Initial Infection	Active Replication	Static Replication "Latency"	Liquefaction & Dissemination
Drugs	None	INH, EMB, RIF Aminoglycosides Fluoroquinolones	Pyrazinamide Metronidazole (?)	None

Figure 1. Potential points of intervention in the disease progression of pulmonary tuberculosis. Stage I represents the initial infection including the process of internalization and phagosome re-modelling. Possible sites of intervention include interfering with: (1) a receptor involved in cell entry, (2) proteins involved in phagosome construction and function, and (3) peptides, glycolipids or other small molecules that mediate specific interactions with the host cell to modify host response. Stage II represents the period of active intracellular growth of the organism targeted by many current therapies. Potential intervention sites represented by (4) include interference with enzymes essential for *in vivo* growth of the bacilli, including cell wall biosynthetic targets, proteins involved in DNA/RNA synthesis and central metabolism. Enzymes involved in the biosynthesis of small molecules required for acquisition of nutrients such as siderophores required for iron acquisition might also be valuable targets (5). Stage III represents the static state of bacterial replication matched by death following containment in a granuloma of activated lymphocytes. Potential targets in this stage (6) are much more speculative but include enzymes involved in anaerobic or microaerophilic adaptation as well as enzymes involved in caseum or lipid metabolism. Other targets might include growth- promoting factors or regulatory molecules involved in growth phase regulation produced by the bacteria and possibly also cytokine therapy to modulate the host immune response. Stage IV represents the breakdown of the metastable granuloma and release of the organisms into the lungs. Targets worth considering in this stage (7) would include those involved in tissue destruction and lysis of the cell as well as enzymes involved in the production of specific molecules required for transmission.

prodrugs, including important front-line therapies such as pyrazinamide and second-line therapies such as ethionamide [49].

The problem of prodrugs is addressed by the modern methods of developing new chemotherapeutics. For example, three-dimensional space scanning using combinatorial chemistry to optimize direct binding of molecules will avoid the selection of prodrugs as preclinical candidates for the next generation of antituberculosis drugs.

5.   THE DEEP END OF THE DREAM POOL; A NEW PARADIGM FOR DRUG DEVELOPMENT

There are many strategies for antimicrobial drug development. In increasing order of sophistication they can be characterized as:
1. screening random compound collections for antimicrobial activity against whole organisms,
2. screening random compound collections against a particular enzyme target, and
3. optimizing a known, but weakly active, lead compound for activity and pharmacokinetics.

In many ways some of the first and second-line antituberculars can be seen as weakly active lead compounds. Although, in general, derivatives that build upon a pre-existing pharmacophore and result only in an improved version of an existing drug make risky starting points (as the rifamycin saga illustrates), the underlying rationale for selecting a known antibiotic is extremely compelling. They offer proven antibacterial activity, known pharmacokinetic and toxicology profiles and often a substantial history of structure-activity relationships from the original development work. In addition such lead compounds sometimes come complete with a known target and mechanism of inhibition and details of the cellular regulation of pathways involving the target enzyme. It is possible to preserve some of these advantages by using a known antituberculosis drug to guide target selection to the level of the biochemical pathway to be inhibited but then altering the enzyme selected for inhibition through the development of a new pharmacophore. This can be done effectively once a detailed understanding of the regulatory mechanisms involved in control of certain biochemical pathways are elucidated and understood. This is where drug design intersects convincingly with genomics.

There are many potential targets in the natural progression of pulmonary tuberculosis as Figure 1 illustrates. Exploring interference with some other aspect than normal bacterial replication is an attractive possibility because so many of the current therapies target only one phase of the life cycle. The recent completion of the genomic DNA sequence of *Mycobacterium tuberculosis* H37Rv will allow us to undertake such target identification and lead optimization with a precision and speed that has not been previously possible. There are about 4000 open reading frames in the genome of *M.*

tuberculosis and recent advances in immobilized DNA microarray techniques have allowed the construction of arrays that reflect 97% of these genes [50]. Using these arrays it has been possible to define the transcriptional response of the cell to treatment with front-line antituberculosis drugs such as isoniazid [51]. These studies as well as studies with other antibiotics are revealing multiple overlapping control mechanisms, some specific for inhibition of a particular enzyme in a biosynthetic pathway, others responsive to more global stresses such as the complete shutdown of metabolism. Between these two extremes lie regulatory networks that reflect transcriptionally-controlled groups of genes involved in units of metabolism, for example in cell wall structure and function. Therefore in an array experiment as a function of time and concentration it is possible to elucidate the various steps that led to actual cell death beginning with very specific transcriptional responses to inhibition of particular enzymes and ending with very general patterns reflecting complete cellular collapse. This set of molecular "fingerprints" offer valuable clues allowing the complete dissection of the mode of action of a drug in considerable detail.

Specific control units can also be exploited by linking their promoter to an easy to read reporter such as luciferase. Luciferase, both the enzyme from firefly and the enzyme from bacteria, has been used to monitor the number of viable mycobacteria during infection models *in vitro* and *in vivo* [52-56]. Luciferase reporter assays have also been applied to antimycobacterial drug discovery using constitutive promoters because of the dependence of the activity upon intracellular ATP levels [57,58]. Using fusions to induced operons reflecting units of co-transcriptionally controlled genes allows for a positive reporter readout. Positive readouts offer a significant advantage for high-throughput screening because they minimize the importance of errors in sample manipulation and therefore reduce follow-up time for false actives. Such reporter strains offer extremely rapid readouts of the efficacy of a potential inhibitor because transcriptional responses tend to be very rapid. They also allow the simultaneous screening of compound libraries against multiple enzymatic activities and they do so in the context of the whole cell, allowing pre-screening for impermeable lead compounds.

We have created such a promoter fusion from an INH-induced gene cluster, originally identified by screening proteins whose synthesis was up-regulated by drug treatment as assessed by ^{35}S-methionine incorporation [59]. This result was subsequently confirmed by DNA microarray hybridization suggesting that the regulation was at the level of the RNA transcript [51]. This operon was shown to encode a group of five proteins whose transcription was upregulated coordinately upon INH treatment (Rv2243-Rv2247). The promoter region for the most upstream of these

(Rv2243, *fabD*) was amplified by PCR and cloned behind the *luc* gene from firefly. Light production from this reporter is specifically induced upon INH treatment as well as upon treatment with other inhibitors of mycolic acid synthesis such as ethionamide, but not by other slightly more generic inhibitors of cell wall synthesis such as ethambutol (R.E. Lee, C.E. Barry, III, unpublished results). This strain has been used to develop and implement a high-throughput 96-well plate-based screen for inhibitors of mycolic acid synthesis.

Using techniques of solid-phase split-and-pool chemistry it is now possible to make hundreds of thousands of analogs of a pharmacophore where previously only hundreds or thousands could be sampled. This expansion of the sampling of the three-dimensional fit of an inhibitor with an enzyme has facilitated the development of some extremely potent drugs with inhibition constants that very typically run into the single digit nanomolar range – one hundred to a thousand times better than existing front-line antimycobacterials [60,61]. Obviously this sort of improvement in MIC will not only affect the drug dosage for therapy but also stands a chance of reducing the time required for effective treatment. This technology is important for optimization of an existing lead series as well as for discovery of new lead molecules. The steps toward an improved lead molecule can be checked by array fingerprint to confirm that the desired mode of toxicity is being optimized and that this optimization is limited to the desired pathway.

6.   CONCLUSION

In addition to all the normal requirements for a new antimicrobial agent (nanomolar MIC, low toxicity, good pharmacokinetics and oral bioavailability, stability, specificity, etc), there is one peculiar requirement for a new antimycobacterial agent: it must be inexpensive. MDRTB is a disease of the urban poor of the developed world and the critically impoverished of the developing world. Development of an expensive therapeutic will result in the same pattern of restricted misuse and abuse that spawned MDRTB in the first place. Thus price has to be a critical component of the drug development pathway from the beginning. Expensive multistep synthetic modifications of difficult-to-isolate natural products are not acceptable solutions nor are expensive monomers acceptable in combinatorial library generation. The conquest of MDRTB requires development of an inexpensive drug (or drugs) that is also distributed appropriately to patients so that they will benefit from it without the potential for the emergence of resistance regardless of their socioeconomic status. To do so will probably require the introduction of new clinical candidates in pairs or under very controlled circumstances to avoid unintentional and ineffective monotherapy. These interventions will require significant public sector involvement and investment in tools for the rapid diagnosis of drug resistance and in the development of new antibiotics. The technology to accomplish these goals is at our fingertips, only the will and the commitment are at issue.

REFERENCES

1. Anonymous. *Blueprint for tuberculosis vaccine development [Report of a workshop]*, (National Institute of Allergy and Infectious Diseases, National Institutes of Health, Rockville, MD, 1998).
2. Advisory Council for the Elimination of Tuberculosis (ACET). Tuberculosis elimination revisited: obstacles, opportunities, and a renewed commitment. MMWR 1999; 48: 1-14.
3. WHO *TB-a global emergency. WHO report on the TB epidemic.* WHO, Geneva, 1994.
4. Coninx R, Mathieu C, Debacker M, Mirzoev F, Ismaelov A, de Haller R, Meddings DR. First-line tuberculosis therapy and drug-resistant Mycobacterium tuberculosis in prisons. Lancet 1999; 353: 969-973.
5. Farmer P, Bayona J, Becerra M, Furin J, Henry C, Hiatt H, Kim JY, Mitnick C, Nardell E, Shin S. The dilemma of MDR-TB in the global era. Int J Tuberc Lung Dis 1998; 2: 869-876.
6. Cole ST, Brosch R, Parkhill J, Garnier T, Churcher C, Harris D, Gordon SV, Eiglmeier K, Gas S, Barry CE, 3rd, Tekaia F, Badcock K, Basham D, Brown D, Chillingworth T, Connor R, Davies R, Devlin K, Feltwell T, Gentles S, Hamlin N, Holroyd S, Hornsby T, Jagels K, Barrell BG. Deciphering the biology of *Mycobacterium tuberculosis* from the complete genome sequence. Nature 1998; 393: 537-544.
7. Bailey DS, Bondar A, Furness LM. Pharmacogenomics - it's not just pharmacogenetics. Curr Opin Biotechnol 1998; 9: 595-601.
8. Veber DF, Drake FH, Gowen M. The new partnership of genomics and chemistry for accelerated drug development. Curr Opin Chem Biol 1997; 1: 151-156.
9. Chopra I, Brennan P. Molecular action of anti-mycobacterial agents. Tuber Lung Dis 1997; 78: 89-98.
10. Winder FG. Mode of action of antimycobacterial agents and associated aspects of the molecular biology of the mycobacteria, p. 353-438. In: Ratledge C, Standford J (eds.), The Biology of the Mycobacteria, Vol. 1. Academic Press, London, 1982.
11. Jabes D, Della Bruna C, Rossi R, Olliaro P. Effectiveness of rifabutin alone or in combination with isoniazid in preventive therapy of mouse tuberculosis. Antimicrob Agents Chemother 1994; 38: 2346-2350.
12. Ungheri D, Della Bruna C, Sanfilippo A. Activity of the spiropiperidyl rifamycin LM 427 on rifampicin resistant Mycobacterium tuberculosis. G Ital Chemioter 1984; 31: 211-214.
13. Della Bruna C, Schioppacassi G, Ungheri D, Jabes D, Morvillo E, Sanfilippo A. LM 427, a new spiropiperidylrifamycin: in vitro and in vivo studies. J Antibiot (Tokyo) 1983; 36: 1502-1506.
14. Sanfilippo A, Della Bruna C, Marsili L, Morvillo E, Pasqualucci CR, Schioppacassi G, Ungheri D. Biological activity of a new class of rifamycins. Spiro-piperidyl- rifamycins. J Antibiot (Tokyo) 1980; 33: 1193-1198.

15. Sato K, Tomioka H, Saito H, Kawahara S, Hidaka T. In vitro activities of benzoxazinorifamycin KRM-1648 against Mycobacterium tuberculosis. Kekkaku 1996; 71: 459-464.

16. Williams DL, Spring L, Collins L, Miller LP, Heifets LB, Gangadharam PR, Gillis TP. Contribution of rpoB mutations to development of rifamycin cross- resistance in Mycobacterium tuberculosis. Antimicrob Agents Chemother 1998; 42: 1853-1857.

17. Yang B, Koga H, Ohno H, Ogawa K, Fukuda M, Hirakata Y, Maesaki S, Tomono K, Tashiro T, Kohno S. Relationship between antimycobacterial activities of rifampicin, rifabutin and KRM-1648 and rpoB mutations of Mycobacterium tuberculosis. J Antimicrob Chemother 1998; 42: 621-628.

18. Moghazeh SL, Pan X, Arain T, Stover CK, Musser JM, Kreiswirth BN. Comparative antimycobacterial activities of rifampin, rifapentine, and KRM-1648 against a collection of rifampin-resistant *Mycobacterium tuberculosis* isolates with known *rpoB* mutations. Antimicrob Agents Chemother 1996; 40: 2655-2657.

19. Mitchison DA. How drug resistance emerges as a result of poor compliance during short course chemotherapy for tuberculosis. Int J Tuberc Lung Dis 1998; 2: 10-15.

20. Jarvis B, Lamb HM. Rifapentine. Drugs 1998; 56: 607-616.

21. Keung A, Eller MG, McKenzie KA, Weir SJ. Single and multiple dose pharmacokinetics of rifapentine in man: part II. Int J Tuberc Lung Dis 1999; 3: 437-444.

22. Vernon A, Burman W, Benator D, Khan A, Bozeman L. Acquired rifamycin monoresistance in patients with HIV-related tuberculosis treated with once-weekly rifapentine and isoniazid. Tuberculosis Trials Consortium. Lancet 1999; 353: 1843-1847.

23. Saito H, Tomioka H, Sato K, Emori M, Yamane T, Yamashita K, Hosoe K, Hidaka T. In vitro antimycobacterial activities of newly synthesized benzoxazinorifamycins. Antimicrob Agents Chemother 1991; 35: 542-547.

24. Yamamoto T, Amitani R, Suzuki K, Tanaka E, Murayama T, Kuze F. In vitro bactericidal and in vivo therapeutic activities of a new rifamycin derivative, KRM-1648, against *Mycobacterium tuberculosis*. Antimicrob Agents Chemother 1996; 40: 426-428.

25. Mor N, Simon B, Heifets L. Bacteriostatic and bactericidal activities of benzoxazinorifamycin KRM- 1648 against Mycobacterium tuberculosis and Mycobacterium avium in human macrophages. Antimicrob Agents Chemother 1996; 40: 1482-1485.

26. Doi N. Therapeutic efficacy of benzoxazinorifamycin KRM-1648 against experimental murine tuberculosis: (1). A study on the efficacy of short course treatment with the intratracheal and intravenous infection model. Kekkaku 1998; 73: 53-64.

27. Kelly BP, Furney SK, Jessen MT, Orme IM. Low-dose aerosol infection model for testing drugs for efficacy against Mycobacterium tuberculosis. Antimicrob Agents Chemother 1996; 40: 2809-2812.

28. Klemens SP, Cynamon MH. Activity of KRM-1648 in combination with isoniazid against *Mycobacterium tuberculosis* in a murine model. Antimicrob Agents Chemother 1996; 40: 298-301.

29. Klemens SP, Grossi MA, Cynamon MH. Activity of KRM-1648, a new benzoxazinorifamycin, against *Mycobacterium tuberculosis* in a murine model. Antimicrob Agents Chemother 1994; 38: 2245-2248.

30. Reddy MV, Luna-Herrera J, Daneluzzi D, Gangadharam PR. Chemotherapeutic activity of benzoxazinorifamycin, KRM-1648, against Mycobacterium tuberculosis in C57BL/6 mice. Tuber Lung Dis 1996; 77: 154-9.

31. Wayne LG. Dormancy of *Mycobacterium tuberculosis* and latency of disease. Eur J Clin Microbiol Infect Dis 1994; 13: 908-914.

32. Parrish NM, Dick JD, Bishai WR. Mechanisms of latency in Mycobacterium tuberculosis. Trends Microbiol 1998; 6: 107-112.
33. McCune R, Lee SH, Deuschle K, McDermott W. Ineffectiveness of isoniazid in modifying the phenomenon of microbial persistence. Am Rev Tuberculosis Pulm Dis 1957; 76: 1106-1109.
34. Wayne LG, Sramek HA. Metronidazole is bactericidal to dormant cells of *Mycobacterium tuberculosis*. Antimicrob Agents Chemother 1994; 38: 2054-2058.
35. McDermott W, Tomsett R. Activation of pyrazinamide and nicotinamide in acidic environments in vitro. Am Rev Tuberc 1954; 70: 748-754.
36. McCune RM, Tompsett R, McDermott W. The fate of *Mycobacterium tuberculosis* in mouse tissues as determined by the microbial enumeration technique. J Exp Med 1956; 104: 763-803.
37. Brooks JV, Furney SK, Orme IM. Metronidazole therapy in mice infected with tuberculosis. Antimicrob Agents Chemother 1999; 43: 1285-1288.
38. Paramasivan CN, Kubendiran G, Herbert D. Action of metronidazole in combination with isoniazid & rifampicin on persisting organisms in experimental murine tuberculosis. Indian J Med Res 1998; 108: 115-119.
39. Dhillon J, Allen BW, Hu YM, Coates AR, Mitchison DA. Metronidazole has no antibacterial effect in Cornell model murine tuberculosis. Int J Tuberc Lung Dis 1998; 2: 736-742.
40. Ashtekar DR, Costa-Perira R, Nagrajan K, Vishvanathan N, Bhatt AD, Rittel W. In vitro and in vivo activities of the nitroimidazole CGI 17341 against Mycobacterium tuberculosis. Antimicrob Agents Chemother 1993; 37: 183-186.
41. Wayne LG, Lin K-Y. Glyoxylate metabolism and adaptation of *Mycobacterium tuberculosis* to survival under anaerobic conditions. Infect Immun 1982; 37: 1042-1049.
42. Slayden RA, Barry CE, III. The genetics and biochemistry of isoniazid resistance in *Mycobacterium tuberculosis*. Microbes and Infection (in press).
43. Zhang Y, Heym B, Allen B, Young D, Cole S. The catalase-peroxidase gene and isoniazid resistance of *Mycobacterium tuberculosis*. Nature 1992; 358: 591-593.
44. Sherman DR, Mdluli K, Hickey MJ, Arain TM, Morris SL, Barry CE, 3rd, Stover CK. Compensatory *ahpC* gene expression in isoniazid-resistant *Mycobacterium tuberculosis*. Science 1996; 272: 1641-1643.
45. Musser JM, Kapur V, Williams DL, Kreiswirth BN, van Soolingen D, van Embden JD. Characterization of the catalase-peroxidase gene (*katG*) and *inhA* locus in isoniazid-resistant and -susceptible strains of *Mycobacterium tuberculosis* by automated DNA sequencing: restricted array of mutations associated with drug resistance. J Infect Dis 1996; 173: 196-202.
46. Marttila HJ, Soini H, Eerola E, Vyshnevskaya E, Vyshnevskiy BI, Otten TF, Vasilyef AV, Viljanen MK. A Ser315Thr substitution in KatG is predominant in genetically heterogeneous multidrug-resistant *Mycobacterium tuberculosis* isolates originating from the St. Petersburg area in Russia. Antimicrob Agents Chemother 1998; 42: 2443-2445.
47. Marttila HJ, Soini H, Huovinen P, Viljanen MK. *katG* mutations in isoniazid-resistant *Mycobacterium tuberculosis* isolates recovered from Finnish patients. Antimicrob Agents Chemother 1996; 40: 2187-2189.
48. Mdluli K, Swanson J, Fischer E, Lee RE, Barry CE, 3rd. Mechanisms involved in the intrinsic isoniazid resistance of *Mycobacterium avium*. Mol Microbiol 1998; 27: 1223-1233.
49. Konno K, Feldmann FM, McDermott W. Pyrazinamide susceptibility and amidase activity of tubercle bacilli. Am Rev Respir Dis 1967; 95: 461-469.

50. Behr MA, Wilson MA, Gill WP, Salamon H, Schoolnik GK, Rane S, Small PM. Comparative genomics of BCG vaccines by whole-genome DNA microarray. Science 1999; 284: 1520-1523.

51. Wilson M, DeRisi J, Kristensen H-K, Imboden P, Rane S, Brown PO, Schoolnik GK. Exploring drug-induced alterations in gene expression in *Mycobacterium tuberculosis* by microarray hybridization. Proc Natl Acad Sci USA 1999; 96: 12833-8.

52. Snewin VA, Gares MP, Gaora PO, Hasan Z, Brown IN, Young DB. Assessment of immunity to mycobacterial infection with luciferase reporter constructs. Infect Immun 1999; 67: 4586-4593.

53. Bonay M, Bouchonnet F, Pelicic V, Lagier B, Grandsaigne M, Lecossier D, Grodet A, Vokurka M, Gicquel B, Hance AJ. Effect of stimulation of human macrophages on intracellular survival of Mycobacterium bovis Bacillus Calmette-Guerin. Evaluation with a mycobacterial reporter strain. Am J Respir Crit Care Med 1999; 159: 1629-1637.

54. Riska PF, Su Y, Bardarov S, Freundlich L, Sarkis G, Hatfull G, Carriere C, Kumar V, Chan J, Jacobs WR, Jr. Rapid film-based determination of antibiotic susceptibilities of Mycobacterium tuberculosis strains by using a luciferase reporter phage and the Bronx Box. J Clin Microbiol 1999; 37: 1144-1149.

55. Michele TM, Ko C, Bishai WR. Exposure to antibiotics induces expression of the Mycobacterium tuberculosis sigF gene: implications for chemotherapy against mycobacterial persistors. Antimicrob Agents Chemother 1999; 43: 218-225.

56. Shawar RM, Humble DJ, Van Dalfsen JM, Stover CK, Hickey MJ, Steele S, Mitscher LA, Baker W. Rapid screening of natural products for antimycobacterial activity by using luciferase-expressing strains of Mycobacterium bovis BCG and Mycobacterium intracellulare. Antimicrob Agents Chemother 1997; 41: 570-574.

57. Arain TM, Resconi AE, Hickey MJ, Stover CK. Bioluminescence screening in vitro (Bio-Siv) assays for high-volume antimycobacterial drug discovery. Antimicrob Agents Chemother 1996; 40: 1536-1541.

58. Arain TM, Resconi AE, Singh DC, Stover CK. Reporter gene technology to assess activity of antimycobacterial agents in macrophages. Antimicrob Agents Chemother 1996; 40: 1542-1544.

59. Mdluli K, Slayden RA, Zhu Y, Ramaswamy S, Pan X, Mead D, Crane DD, Musser JM, Barry CE, 3rd. Inhibition of a *Mycobacterium tuberculosis* beta-ketoacyl ACP synthase by isoniazid. Science 1998; 280: 1607-1610.

60. Dolle RE. Comprehensive survey of chemical libraries yielding enzyme inhibitors, receptor agonists and antagonists, and other biologically active agents: 1992 through 1997. Mol Diversity 1998; 3: 199-233.

61. Barry CE, III, Slayden RA, Sampson AE, Lee RE. The use of genomics and combinatorial chemistry in the development of new antimycobacterial drugs. Biochem Pharmacol 2000; 59: 221-231.

Chapter 17

Population dynamics and control of multidrug-resistant tuberculosis

Christopher Dye[1] and Brian G. Williams[2]
[1]*Communicable Diseases Prevention and Control, World Health Organization, Geneva, Switzerland*
[2]*CSIR, Johannesburg, South Africa*

1.   INTRODUCTION

Threshold theory in infectious disease epidemiology states that there is some combination of case detection and cure rates above which tuberculosis, including multidrug-resistant tuberculosis (MDR; resistance to at least isoniazid and rifampicin) cannot spread through a population. The analytical challenge in MDR control is to identify which combinations of case detection and cure rates ensure that the number of MDR cases will decline, and to calculate the rate of decline.

The central, relevant epidemiological concept is the basic case reproduction number, $\bar{R}_0$, defined as the number of secondary cases produced when one infectious case is introduced into a fully susceptible population [1]. An infectious disease has the greatest potential for spread at the start of an epidemic, fuelled by the maximum number of susceptible hosts. As more people acquire infection, infectious individuals are increasingly likely to contact those who are already (at least partially) immune, and who cannot therefore be reinfected. When $\bar{R}_0 < 1$ an outbreak is unlikely or, if the disease is already present, incidence is likely to fall towards elimination.

I. Bastian and F. Portaels (eds.), Multidrug-Resistant Tuberculosis, 253-267.
© 2000 *Kluwer Academic Publishers. Printed in the Netherlands.*

Drug-resistant tuberculosis can never be completely eliminated so long as drug-susceptible disease persists. Because of the large reservoir of human infection (about 1 in 3 people are infected; [2]) and the slow progression to disease, drug-susceptible tuberculosis will persist for decades to come in highly endemic areas. Resistant strains will continue to arise from susceptible strains by mutation, and these resistant strains will sometimes be transmitted because treatment and drug action are always delayed, and because cure rates are always less than 100%. In short, $\bar{R}_0$ will never be zero; the question is whether it can be kept below its threshold value of 1. The further below threshold, the quicker will be the decline towards elimination. Provided case detection is prompt and treatment efficacious, the incidence of MDR can in principle be kept to insignificant levels.

But how prompt must the detection of MDR cases be? And what treatment efficacy of MDR cases is needed? The goal of this chapter is to provide some answers from epidemiological models, and then to match the predictions with observations on MDR treatment outcomes in national control programmes.

2.   A MATHEMATICAL MODEL FOR MDR

We assume that the natural history of MDR is qualitatively the same as drug-susceptible TB; the essential differences are quantitative. A guiding principle in mathematical epidemiology is to make the simplest model capable of answering the question at hand. The compartmental model in Figure 1 is closely related to an earlier tuberculosis model [3], but with some structural adjustments appropriate to the MDR problem. What follows is a sketch of how the model works; full mathematical details will appear elsewhere [4].

By using a compartmental model, in which individuals in a population are put into mutually exclusive groups, we presume that there is a clear distinction between drug-susceptible and drug-resistant disease. If either isoniazid (INH) or rifampicin (RMP) resistance is under the control of several gene mutations (a quantitative trait) which are found together, then we might expect a variable response to treatment. However, the consistency of sample classification between reference laboratories (98% or better; [5]) indicates that the separation can be reliably made in the face of any variability in drug sensitivity.

We imagine a strain of MDR spreading through a population, in which some individuals are uninfected, and some are already infected with drug-susceptible *Mycobacterium tuberculosis* (MTB) or with a strain that is resistant to only one drug (INH or RMP). Prior infection with any strain of

MTB provides partial protection against re-infection with a MDR strain, and will therefore hinder the spread of MDR. In the long run, drug-resistant strains will replace drug-susceptible ones as a result of differential selection. But we are mainly concerned here with the dynamics of MDR before it becomes very common (say, less than 5% of cases). Under these limited circumstances, the pool of individuals carrying latent, drug-susceptible or mono-resistant infections will be relatively large and approximately constant.

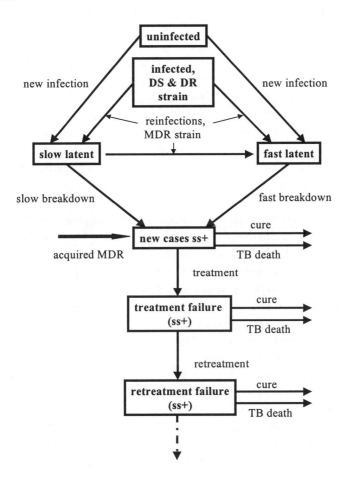

Figure 1. Flow chart of mathematical model for MDR, from [4]; ss+, sputum smear-positive.

In previous work, we have made the distinction between fast and slow breakdown from latent to infectious TB [as in 6,7], but ignored the distribution of breakdown times for fast TB [unlike 8]. In this analysis, we are interested in the short-term and long-term dynamic responses of MDR to increased control effort, and so have allowed for both.

Because our focus is on the dynamics of MDR – whether it can be eliminated and over what period – our model deals only with infectious TB, and not with the total tuberculosis burden. Infectiousness is often equated with smear-positive disease; we adopt that equivalence in this analysis when comparing model predictions with observations on the treatment outcomes of smear-positive MDR patients.

Case finding removes infectious cases from the prevalent pool. If cases are not detected and treated they will either die, become "chronic excretors", or cure naturally (not shown in Figure 1). Of those treated, a proportion is cured, with a very low chance of relapse. That chance is assumed here to be zero based on what is known about drug-susceptible cases; future work may show that it is significantly higher for MDR cases. Treatment failures include all cases that are not permanently cured. Failures may be identified as those persistently smear-positive after five months of treatment. Or they may become temporarily smear-negative, and relapse some time later (usually within months, or at most a few years). Together these two possibilities imply that failures will be less infectious on average than new smear-positive cases.

We distinguish between patients seeking first treatment or retreatment, because the success of chemotherapy is often different. New MDR cases are not usually known to be multidrug-resistant, and are therefore given a standard short-course regimen. They are much more likely to fail on such a regimen than patients carrying susceptible strains of MTB are. After failure, most will seek a second course of treatment. As known failures, they may be tested for drug resistance and given a regimen that might include second-line drugs, if such drugs are available. The cure rate is typically higher with regimens including second-line drugs.

Our model does not identify patients by age or sex. Because children are less likely to develop smear-positive disease, we assume that some fraction of the population (< 100%) is capable of developing infectious TB, and estimate that fraction as the proportion of person 15 years and older. This fraction varies from country to country. By ignoring gender, we do not assume that MDR epidemiology is the same in men and women; rather, that we aim for the right results for men and women on average.

This is a model both of "primary" MDR (cases that arise by transmission) and "acquired" MDR (cases that become both INH and RMP resistant during a course of treatment). Acquired MDR cases arise most often by the addition of RMP resistance to INH resistance, rather than the other way round (Figure 2).

How is MDR different from drug-susceptible tuberculosis? First, since MDR does not generally become common without drug pressure, MDR strains must have lower relative fitness on average than susceptible ones. That is, there is a cost of resistance, though that cost may be temporary [9,10] and small [11]. They are differentially selected, and spread through the population, because the typical MDR case remains infectious for longer than a drug-susceptible case. Analysis of the distribution of drug sensitive and resistant strains in clusters of Dutch TB cases indicated that INH-resistant strains are 30% (10-50%) less transmissible from active cases than INH-susceptible strains [12]. However, there are no comparable data for MDR strains. We do not know yet whether MDR strains are reproductively less successful on average because resistant bacteria cannot compete within hosts, because transmitted bacteria are less infective, or because individuals infected with MDR strains are less likely to breakdown to active TB. In this analysis, we assume that MDR strains come to predominate within some hosts because treatment is sufficient to kill susceptible strains only. The cost of resistance is expressed as a reduction in the infective contact rate, rather than by assuming a reduced progression to disease, but our conclusions are not sensitive to this assumption about mechanism.

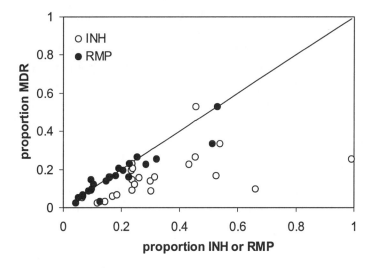

Figure 2. Correlations between the proportions of TB cases that are MDR and the proportions that are either rifampicin (RMP) or isoniazid (INH) resistant in patients that have previously been treated (acquired resistance). The correlation between MDR and RMP is stronger ($r^2 = 0.84$, slope = 0.73) than the correlation between MDR and INH ($r^2 = 0.67$, slope = 0.60), indicating that MDR mostly arises when RMP resistance is added to INH resistance. Data from 23 countries [5].

Second, MDR is often transmitted under different circumstances than drug-susceptible disease, for example in prisons. Here the contact rate between infectious cases and susceptibles (i.e. more than the typical 10-14 contacts/year; [13]) may be higher, with an increase pro rata in the basic case reproduction number. In this paper, we have used a per capita contact rate of 14/year, ranging from 10/year to 18/year.

We want to use the model to determine what case detection and cure rates are required for elimination, and how long it will take to eliminate MDR. To do this, we need to know whether the basic case reproduction number is less than 1, and how much less than 1. Some care is needed in the interpretation of reproduction numbers for diseases with serial intervals lasting many years (like TB) because of partial immunity and changing age structures [14]. Allowing for both acquired (prior infection) and innate (age-related) immunity and all the processes depicted in Figure 1, we calculate a modified basic case reproduction number, $\bar{R}_0$. Although the full formula for $\bar{R}_0$ is algebraically complex (and will be derived elsewhere), it can be condensed to:

$\bar{R}_0$ = average duration of infectiousness

x per capita contact rate

x probability that infection leads to infectious TB

$\bar{R}_0$ measures the capacity for MDR to spread through a population in which some people are already infected with susceptible or mono-resistant strains of MTB (but not MDR), and where infectiousness is limited by case finding and treatment of varying efficiency. $\bar{R}_0$ is therefore not a constant for MDR, but varies from one population to another.

To carry out the analysis below, we use the full algebraic formula to calculate $\bar{R}_0$, incorporating best estimates of all model parameters. To allow for uncertainty in parameter values, we also calculate by Monte Carlo simulation the probability that $\bar{R}_0 < 1$ for any combination of treatment interval and cure rate. Although MDR cannot be eliminated completely (as already noted), we equate this with the "probability of elimination", which is to be interpreted as the chance that MDR incidence will decline towards extinction.

3.   DYNAMICS AND CONTROL OF MDR

First we distinguish the epidemiological effects of mutation and selection ("acquired" MDR) on the one hand, and transmission ("primary" MDR) on the other. The higher the mutation rate, and the higher the selection pressure, the sooner we expect to see MDR emerge (Figure 3). The incidence of acquired MDR does not influence, per se, the rate of spread of the epidemic after emergence. Two of the epidemics in Figure 3 clearly have the same shape and can be superimposed on one another by shifting along the horizontal time axis. The third slower epidemic was generated by applying case detection and cure rates that reduce the value of $\bar{R}_0$. In this case, the transmission rate of MDR is lower because the average duration of infectiousness is shorter.

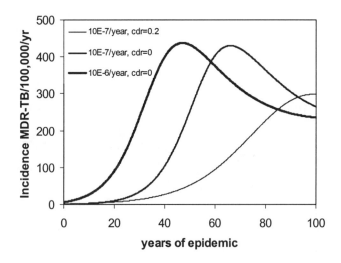

Figure 3. Hypothetical epidemics of MDR generated with the model depicted in Figure 1. The incidence of acquired MDR and case detection rates for the 3 curves are, from left to right, 10^{-6}/yr and 0, 10^{-7}/yr and 0, 10^{-7}/yr and 0.2. Lowering the incidence of acquired MDR delays the emergence of MDR without affecting the rate of spread (compare left and middle curves). Lowering the basic case reproduction number slows the rate of spread (compare middle and right curves).

Current best estimates of model parameters give $\bar{R}_0 = 1.60$ (5th, 95th centiles 1.02, 2.67) in the absence of chemotherapy, and when MDR is invading a population where 30% of the population is already infected with susceptible or mono-resistant bacilli. We use these parameter values throughout this paper. With a reproduction number of this magnitude, MDR incidence doubles every 5.3 years while the epidemic is growing exponentially (Figure 4). A ten-fold increase takes 18.6 years. $\bar{R}_0$ would rise to 1.98 if MDR were spreading through a fully susceptible population (i.e. almost no-one infected with drug-susceptible or other resistant strains).

Case detection and cure rates that ensure $\bar{R}_0 < 1$ will force the incidence of MDR to decrease. Figure 4 shows the consequences of three different interventions from year 10 onwards: with a MDR case detection rate of 0.5 (50% of prevalent infectious cases detected and treated annually) and a cure rate of 0.25 (25% infectious cases become permanently non-infectious), $\bar{R}_0$ remains just above 1. After a short period of adjustment to the intervention, MDR incidence therefore continues its long-term increase, albeit at a slower rate than before the intervention. When the cure rate is raised to 0.5, incidence declines, and it does so even more quickly when the cure rate is 0.75. For any combination of case detection and cure rates that ensure $\bar{R}_0 < 1$, the rate of decline in incidence is fastest immediately after the intervention is introduced (the lines in Figure 4 are concave when incidence is plotted on a log scale). The rate of decline in MDR incidence is insensitive to the initial MDR incidence rate.

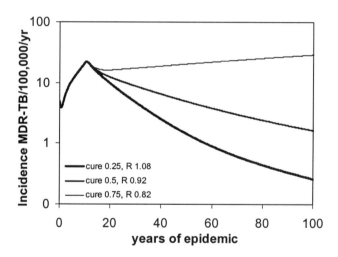

Figure 4. Impact of different cure rates on the dynamics of MDR incidence. The cure rates and consequent $\bar{R}_0$ s for the 3 curves are, from top to bottom, 0.25 and 1.08, 0.5 and 0.92, 0.75 and 0.82. Incidence declines in the long term when $\bar{R}_0 < 1$, and the rate of decline is fastest immediately after the intervention is introduced in year 10. Note that the vertical axis is a log scale.

The point estimate of $\bar{R}_0$ over a much wider range of MDR case detection and cure rates is shown in Figure 5, where case detection is expressed more intuitively as its reciprocal, the number of months to treatment or re-treatment or, more precisely, the duration of infectiousness. The right-hand axis indicates the cure rate of new, infectious MDR cases; the cure rates of re-treatment cases were assumed to be 38% lower, based on a review of treatment outcomes in six countries [15]. The contours on this map join points of equal $\bar{R}_0$, and the contours become flatter as $\bar{R}_0$ increases. This means that good case finding is less effective when the cure rate is low. Under poor treatment, many people remain persistently infectious, even if they are treated quickly [3,16]. $\bar{R}_0 = 1$ is the most important contour: any combination of treatment interval and cure rate lying above that line will lead to MDR elimination; any combination below it will allow persistence.

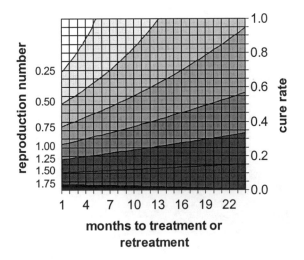

Figure 5. Basic case reproduction numbers for various combinations of treatment interval and cure rate. Contours join lines of equal $\bar{R}_0$. The contour for $\bar{R}_0 = 1$ separates MDR persistence from decline [4].

Figure 6 presents a more cautious assessment of the impact of control. Here we incorporate all uncertainty in model parameter values in calculating, not point estimates of $\bar{R}_0$, but the probability that $\bar{R}_0 < 1$, or the probability of elimination. Elimination of MDR is most likely in the upper left-hand corner of the graph. The vertical line on this map marks the treatment interval (16 months) corresponding with an annual detection rate of 70% of prevalent infectious MDR cases. The horizontal lines mark the range of cure rates for MDR patients observed under standard short-course chemotherapy in six countries [15], from Ivanovo Oblast in Russia (cure rate 11%) to Hong Kong (cure rate 60%). The wide gap between these lines indicates that the quality of case management varies enormously between countries. In the best case, Hong Kong, the probability of elimination would be 80%, assuming an annual case detection rate of 70%.

The cure rates of patients carrying fully susceptible bacilli, or bacilli that are resistant to either rifampicin or isoniazid, are much higher than 60% - at least 80% in Hong Kong and Peru [15]. Accordingly, the probability of eliminating mono-resistant disease, or of preventing an outbreak in the first place, is expected to be better than 90%, again assuming a 70% annual case detection (Figure 6).

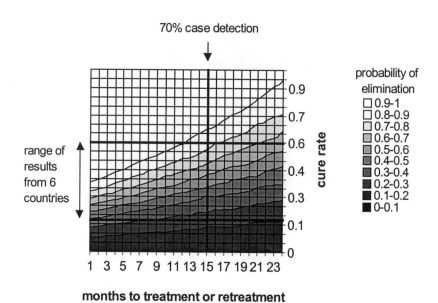

Figure 6. Probability that $\bar{R}_0$ <1 (= "probability of elimination") for various combinations of treatment interval and cure rate. Contours join lines of equal probability. Horizontal lines mark the best (Hong Kong) and worst (Ivanovo) outcomes of treatment for MDR cases using short-course chemotherapy [15]. The vertical line marks the interval between treatment corresponding to an annual detection rate of 70% of prevalent cases [4].

If the incidence of MDR is likely to decline, we need to know how long it will take to achieve a significant reduction. Figure 7 charts the number of years needed to reduce MDR incidence by 90%, a 10-fold reduction. These results are insensitive to the initial incidence rate. Even for Hong Kong this would be as long as 40 years with 70% case detection. Moreover, the gradient of the surface is very steep in this region of the graph, indicating that small changes in the treatment interval and especially the cure rate would dramatically affect the rate of decline of MDR. Thus, MDR would essentially never be eliminated if the cure rate fell just 10% from 60% to 50%, with case detection remaining at 70%. Figure 7 suggests that the cure rate needs to be as high as 85% to be confident that the incidence of primary MDR will decline significantly (by a factor of 10) on a reasonable time-scale (20 years, the same as for a 10-fold expansion during the exponential growth phase).

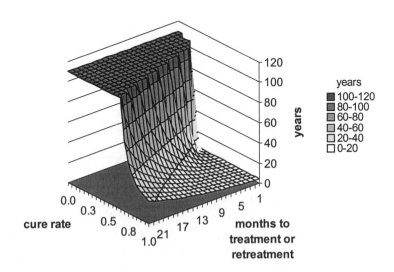

Figure 7. Three-dimensional surface showing the number of years required to cut the incidence of primary MDR by 90%, for combinations of treatment interval and cure rate.

A ten-fold reduction in 20 years is an average fall of 12% per year, which is about the maximum rate of reduction in incidence of primary disease that has been achieved operationally in good national TB control programmes [3,13]. It is strikingly less than the 42% per year observed in New York City under intense control between 1992 and 1997 (Figure 8; [17], T. Frieden and P. Fujiwara, personal communication). This sharp rate of decline in MDR incidence in New York was possible because a high proportion of cases represented recent, nosocomial transmission to individuals co-infected with HIV [18, 19]. Institution of effective control measures rapidly prevented the further spread of infection. Where a smaller proportion of MDR cases arises from recent infection (i.e. among HIV-negatives), and where transmission is less easily prevented (i.e. outside institutions like hospitals and prisons), we would not expect to achieve such a precipitous fall in MDR incidence.

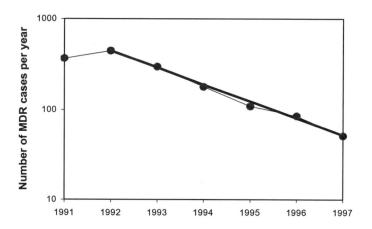

Figure 8. Number of MDR cases reported in New York City, 1991-97, plotted on a logarithmic scale. Data from [17] and T. Frieden and P. Fujiwara, personal communication

4.   CONCLUSIONS

Calculations with our mathematical model show that, to be at least 90% certain of achieving a 10-fold reduction in the incidence of primary MDR in 20 years, programmes should achieve a MDR cure rate of 85% and an annual MDR case detection rate of 70%. Best practice short-course chemotherapy cannot apparently cure more than 60% of MDR cases (as seen in Hong Kong and Peru), and there is a big gap between the best and worst performers [15].

We draw two conclusions about MDR control from this comparison of model and data. First, programmes which are curing less than 60% of MDR cases (e.g. Ivanovo Oblast in Russia) are probably failing to exploit the full potential of short-course chemotherapy with first-line drugs. If such programmes also achieve low cure rates of drug-susceptible cases (e.g. less than 80% treatment success), they need to verify that essential elements of the DOTS strategy are in place – an uninterrupted drug supply, sputum smear microscopy for diagnosis, directly-observed therapy, and standardized short-course therapy, at least for drug-susceptible patients.

Second, a new strategy is needed to bridge the gap between the achievable 60% and desirable 85% cure rates for MDR cases, and to shorten the average duration of infectiousness of these cases. We make no attempt here to propose what that new strategy should be, merely remarking that the analytical framework we have developed can be used to explore a variety of options for control. Four methods are available for shortening the duration of infectiousness and improving the cure rate: (1) active rather than passive detection of infectious cases, (2) isolation of infectious cases, (3) earlier testing for drug-resistance, e.g. without waiting for a potentially drug-resistant, new smear-positive case to fail treatment, (4) use of more costly second-line drugs. The goal is to identify the strategy – combining these four tools - which minimizes the number of future cases or deaths due to TB (including MDR), given available resources [20].

It is not surprising that our proposed criteria for MDR control are essentially the same as WHO's targets for the control of susceptible tuberculosis, though the WHO targets have not previously been derived in this way. To be cautious, we used a best estimate of the fitness of MDR as compared with susceptible TB of 1 (average 0.9), so the natural history of MDR is not very different from that of susceptible TB. (If relative fitness turns out to be lower than supposed here, then it will be easier to solve the MDR problem, e.g. elimination would require a lower average cure rate.) Indeed, we can use Figure 6 to argue that it should be possible to eliminate susceptible or mono-resistant disease, or prevent outbreaks of these strains, by virtue of the high cure rates (80% or greater) that can be achieved with short-course chemotherapy. It is crucial to make best use of cheap first-line drugs to minimize the incidence of acquired MDR. Prevention is the easier part of the MDR problem; the difficult part will be to bring under control established MDR epidemics.

In summary, we have used mathematical modelling, together with treatment results from six countries, to investigate whether passive case detection and standard short-course chemotherapy (SSCC) can prevent and reverse the spread of multidrug-resistant tuberculosis (MDRTB). We have found that best-practice SSCC (achieving cure rates of 80% or more) is highly likely to bring strains resistant to isoniazid or rifampicin under control, and to prevent the emergence of MDR-TB. However, SSCC is not certain to contain MDRTB once it has emerged because the cure rate is unlikely to exceed 60% with first-line drugs. Our calculations suggest that, to be at least 90% certain of achieving a 10-fold reduction in primary MDR incidence within 20 years, programmes should achieve a cure rate of 85% with an annual case detection rate of 70%. Further analysis (which could be done with the framework developed here) is needed to identify the strategy that minimizes the number of future cases or deaths due to TB (including MDRTB), given available resources. That strategy is likely to combine active case detection, patient isolation, earlier testing for drug-resistance, and the use of second-line drugs.

ACKNOWLEDGEMENTS

We thank M Espinal, T Frieden, A Laszlo, N Nagelkerke and M Raviglione for helpful comments on various aspects of this work.

REFERENCES

1. Anderson RM, May RM. Infectious Diseases of Humans: Dynamics and Control. Oxford University Press, Oxford, 1991.
2. Dye C, Scheele S, Dolin P, Pathania V, Raviglione, M.C. Global burden of tuberculosis: estimated incidence, prevalence and mortality by country. JAMA 1999; 282: 677-686.
3. Dye C, Garnett GP, Sleeman K, Williams B. Prospects for global tuberculosis control under the WHO DOTS strategy. Lancet 1998; 352: 1886-1891.
4. Dye C and Williams BG. Criteria for the control of drug-resistant tuberculosis. Manuscript in preparation.
5. WHO/IUATLD. Anti-Tuberculosis Drug Resistance in the World. World Health Organizaiton, Geneva, 1997 (WHO/TB/97.22).
6. Blower S, Small PM, Hopewell PC. Control strategies for tuberculosis epidemics: new models for old problems. Science 1996; 73: 497-500.
7. Blower SM, Gerberding, JL. Understanding, predicting and controlling the emergence of drug-resistant tuberculosis: a theoretical framework. J Mol Med 1998; 76: 624-636.
8. Vynnycky E & Fine PEM. The natural history of tuberculosis: the implications of age-dependent risks of disease and the role of reinfection. Epidemiol Infect 1997; 119: 183-201.
9. Schrag SJ, Perrot V. Reducing antibiotic resistance. Nature 1996; 381: 120-121.
10. Bjorkman J, Hughes D, Andersson DI. Virulence of antibiotic-resistant Salmonella typhimurium. Proc Natl Acad Sci USA 1998; 95: 3949-3963.
11. Bottger EC, Springer B, Pletschette M, Sander P. Fitness of antibiotic-resistant microorganisms and compensatory mutations. Nature Med 1998; 4: 1343-1344.
12. Soolingen D van, Borgdorff MW, Hass P de, Sebek MMGG, Veen J, Dessens M, Kremer K, Embden JDA van. Molecular epidemiology in the Netherlands: a nation-wide study from 1993 through 1997. Tub Surv Res Unit Prog Rep 1999; 10, 107-144.
13. Styblo K. Epidemiology of Tuberculosis. Selected papers, volume 24. Royal Netherlands Tuberculosis Association, The Hague 1991.
14. Vynnycky E & Fine PEM. The long-term dynamics of tuberculosis and other disease with long serial intervals: implications of and for changing reproduction numbers. Epidemiol Infect 1998; 121: 309-324.
15. Espinal MA, Kim SJ, Suarez PG, Kam KM, Khomenko AG, Migliori GB, Baez J, Kochi A, Dye C, Raviglione MC. Standard short-course chemotherapy for drug-resistant tuberculosis: treatment outcomes in six countries. Submitted.
16. Styblo K, Bumgarner R. Tuberculosis can be controlled with existing technologies: evidence. Tub Surv Res Unit Prog Rep 1991; 2, 60-72.
17. Frieden TR, Fujiwara PI, Washko RM, Hamburg MA. Tuberculosis in New York City – turning the tide. New Engl J Med 1995; 333: 229-233.

18. Frieden TR, Woodley CL, Crawford JT, Lew D, Dooley, SM. The molecular epidemiology of tuberculosis in New York City: the importance of nosocomial transmission and laboratory error. Tub Lung Dis 1996; 77: 407-413.
19. Frieden TR, sherman LF, Maw KL, Fujiwara PI, Crawford JT, Nivin B, Sharp V, Hewlett D Jr, Brudney K, Alland D, Kreiswirth BN. A multi-institutional outbreak of highly drug-resistant tuberculosis. Epidemiology and clinical outcomes. JAMA 1996; 276: 1229-1235.
20. Espinal MA, Dye C, Raviglione MC, Kochi A. Rational "DOTS Plus" for the control of MDR-TB. Int J Tuberc Lung Dis 1999; 3: 561-563.

Chapter 18

Administrative, engineering, and personal protective measures for controlling *Mycobacterium tuberculosis*

Chesley Richards and William R. Jarvis
Hospital Infections Program, Centers for Disease Control and Prevention. Atlanta, Georgia

1. INTRODUCTION

Multidrug-resistant *Mycobacterium tuberculosis* (MDRTB) is defined as *Mycobacterium tuberculosis* (MTB) with resistance to at least isoniazid and rifampin. Prevention and control of MDRTB represent an important growing challenge to public health in industrialized countries and in countries with limited resources. The worldwide upsurge of MDRTB in the 1990's was associated with multiple factors, including the human immunodeficiency virus (HIV) epidemic, sub-optimal patient adherence with curative therapy, and transmission of MDRTB in healthcare and other institutional settings. One important component of the overall control of MDRTB is the prevention of transmission of *Mycobacterium tuberculosis* (MTB) in health care settings, or nosocomial transmission. Although there is no ongoing surveillance system for nosocomial or occupational MTB infections or disease, recent studies suggest annual tuberculin skin test (TST) conversion rates among health care workers (HCWs) range from 0.3 to 5.5% [1-5]. Similarly, studies suggest that the risk of developing active tuberculosis (TB) is higher among HCWs than the general population in the United States, especially in areas where TB prevalence is high [5-8]. The centerpiece of any effort to prevent nosocomial transmission of MTB is the development of

I. Bastian and F. Portaels (eds.), Multidrug-Resistant Tuberculosis, 269-284.
© 2000 *Kluwer Academic Publishers. Printed in the Netherlands.*

an effective TB control program within the healthcare facility. In this chapter, we will review administrative, engineering, and personal respiratory protective measures that form the core of an effective TB control program. Such measures also reduce the nosocomial transmission of MDRTB. Recommendations for these measures are based on guidelines published by the Centers for Disease Control and Prevention (CDC), which are primarily aimed towards developed countries [9]. In addition, we discuss measures for prevention of MTB transmission that can be undertaken in countries and regions with limited resources.

2.   HEALTH CARE FACILITY RISK ASSESSMENT

Before the TB control program can be developed, healthcare facility personnel should assign primary responsibility for TB control to one individual and then conduct a risk assessment to determine the institutional or unit/ward level of risk of nosocomial transmission of MTB to HCWs, or patients (Table 1). The risk assessment should start with a review of the community or regional MTB profile and the number of patients or HCWs with MTB infection or disease at the health care facility. In addition to the number of inpatients or outpatients treated for TB, a review of antituberculous drug susceptibility patterns of MTB isolates is especially important to assess the number and distribution of susceptibility patterns of MDRTB strains. Such a review provides an estimate of the amount of MDRTB in both the community and the healthcare facility. Next, the risk assessment should include a review of HCW TST conversion rates and a review of current facility TB infection control practices. After the assessment is completed, the facility's risk is classified in one of five risk categories. These categories are minimal risk, very low risk, low risk, intermediate risk, or high risk (Table 2). The design of and resource allocation for the TB infection control program will vary depending on the level of risk identified through the assessment.

3.   ADMINISTRATIVE MEASURES

Administrative measures are those activities aimed at expeditiously identifying and treating patients with TB, while protecting HCWs and patients. These measures include the development of a written TB infection control plan that promotes the early identification, diagnosis, isolation, and treatment of TB patients in addition to HCW education, training, and screening for MTB. Administrative measures represent the first and most important tier of a TB control program; they are the least costly, and should be implemented in all facilities. Administrative measures are not static, but require ongoing evaluation to monitor both compliance with and effectiveness of the measures, as well as modification to minimize nosocomial MTB transmission.

Table 1. Healthcare facility MTB risk assessment

1.	Review the community TB profile
2.	Review the number, location, and drug susceptibility profile for TB patients treated in the facility, including outpatient and inpatient areas
3.	Review tuberculin skin test results for health care workers
4.	Sample medical records of TB patients to determine:
	• Interval from admission to screening and diagnosis
	• Interval from diagnosis to treatment initiation
	• Interval from admission to initiation of isolation for suspected TB patients
	• Duration of isolation and therapy
5.	Observe facility MTB infection control practices
6.	Review recent environmental evolution and maintenance procedures

3.1   Infection control plan

After the risk assessment is completed, the first step for the TB control practitioner or team should be the development of a written TB infection control plan (Table 3). The plan should contain specific policies regarding the identification, diagnosis, and clinical management of patients suspected of having TB along with patient isolation procedures and policies. The plan should outline education and training of HCWs about TB in combination with individualized counselling and screening for latent TB infection. A protocol for evaluating HCW TST conversions should be included in the plan together with plans for coordination with public health departments or the ministry of health.

3.2   Early identification and diagnosis

Maintaining a high index of suspicion of MTB and enhancing early identification of suspected TB patients are the first steps in preventing transmission. To identify patients suspected of having TB, each facility should develop clinical prediction rules based on previous experience and overall TB burden. The prediction rules may vary depending on the prevalence of TB in the community and on clinical, radiographic, and laboratory characteristics of TB patients in the healthcare facility. Furthermore, the expected predictive value of patient screening tests in the health care facility should be known and should be used to guide decisions.

Once screening tests are positive, the recommended diagnostic tests should be available and dependable.

Table 2. Facility risk categories for nosocomial TB transmission

Category	Description
Minimal	No TB patients in facility or community
Very low risk	No TB in-patients in the facility in the last year; suspected TB patients are referred to another facility
Low risk	1-5 TB patients in the last year AND No excess healthcare worker conversions or evidence of person-to-person transmission
Intermediate	6 or more TB patients in the last year AND No excess healthcare worker conversions or evidence of person-to-person transmission
High	TB in-patients AND Excess healthcare worker conversions or evidence of person-to-person transmission

3.2.1   Specimen collection

An important part of the initial evaluation of patients suspected of having TB is the collection of an adequate sputum specimen for microscopic evaluation and culture. Although generally to be avoided for patients with suspected TB, cough-inducing procedures (e.g., for sputum induction) may sometimes be necessary for adequate patient evaluation. Where feasible, cough-inducing procedures should be performed in areas with local exhaust ventilation devices. If this is not feasible, the procedures should be done at a minimum in a room that meets TB isolation room requirements. A protocol for specimen processing and culture should include measures to minimize risk of nosocomial transmission to HCWs who obtain or process the specimen.

3.2.2   Ambulatory Settings

Patients in ambulatory care settings, including emergency departments, pose a special challenge for TB control programs. Minimizing the time of exposure to patients who have infectious TB by shortening waiting times is an important yet simple intervention in most ambulatory care facilities. In areas with limited resources, waiting areas outside the hospital may be an option to minimize TB exposure. In addition to minimizing waiting room times, the TB control plan should outline procedures to rapidly identify patients who have clinical signs and symptoms suggestive of active TB (chronic cough of > 3 weeks duration, weight loss, or hemoptysis). Patients on TB therapy or who were recently treated for TB should be presumed to be infectious until active disease is ruled out.

Table 3. Elements of a TB infection control plan

Element	Risk category				
	Minimal	Very low	Low	Intermediate	High
Assign responsibility for TB control within the facility	R	R	R	R	R
Conduct a risk assessment	Y	Y	Y	6-12 months	3 months
Develop a TB control plan	R	R	R	R	R
Periodically reassess risk	Y	Y	Y	6-12 months	3 months
Identify, evaluate, and initiate treatment for patients who may have active TB	N/A	R	R	R	R
Manage patients with TB in ambulatory and emergency care settings	R	R	R	R	R
Manage hospitalized patients with TB, including isolation protocols and policies	N/A	N/A	R	R	R
Engineering controls	O	O	R	R	R
Personal respiratory protection	N/A	V	R	R	R
Cough-inducing and aerosol-generating procedures	O	O	R	R	R
Healthcare worker education and training	R	R	R	R	R
Healthcare counselling and TST screening	B	V	Y	6-12 months	3 months
Problem evaluation	R	R	R	R	R
Coordination with public health departments or agencies	R	R	R	R	R

R=recommended; Y=yearly; N/A=not applicable; O=optional; V=variable

Patients suspected to have infectious TB should be triaged to other areas such as separate waiting rooms or TB isolation rooms. The initial healthcare facility risk assessment should guide the development of a triage protocol for ambulatory settings. In clinical areas where large numbers of TB patients are seen, a TB isolation room in the ambulatory area is optimal. For ambulatory care settings that do not have a large number of TB patients, a TB isolation room may not be necessary. Patients suspected to have infectious TB should wear a surgical mask to minimize droplet aerosolization to reduce the risk of transmission to non-infected individuals in the area. Likewise, tissues to contain secretions from coughing or sneezing should be used.

3.3   Patient isolation

A crucial component of TB control is the implementation of a protocol for infectious TB patient isolation. This protocol should specify the number and types of TB isolation rooms available, when TB isolation should be initiated and discontinued, and who is responsible for instituting and discontinuing TB isolation. Also crucial to the TB isolation protocol are the methods used to monitor TB isolation practices and manage patients who do not follow TB isolation procedures. Especially for children with TB, policies regarding screening of family members should be outlined along with the use of masks by visitors. Isolation discontinuation should occur only if TB has been definitively ruled out or after three consecutive negative acid fast bacilli (AFB) specimens have been obtained from patients on antituberculous therapy.

3.4   Healthcare worker education and training

Policies regarding HCW education and training should be clearly defined in the infection control plan. Ideally, HCWs, including physicians, should receive basic training about TB before starting their assignment. Although the specific components may vary, important elements of the program include basic concepts about the epidemiology, diagnosis, and treatment of TB; potential for occupational exposure; and infection control principles and practices to reduce MTB transmission. HCWs should understand the purpose of TST testing for latent TB and the principles of preventive therapy. HCWs should understand their responsibility to seek medical evaluation if they suspect they have TB (e.g., cough >3 weeks, weight loss) and should know whom to notify in the employee health, occupational health, or infection control program. Finally, healthcare facility personnel should ensure that HCW health/medical information is maintained in a confidential manner and that a nonpunitive work policy exists for leave for medical treatment until the HCW is noninfectious. The level and detail of the education program may vary depending on the level of involvement different HCWs have with TB patients.

3.5   Health care worker counselling and screening

In addition to education and training, the infection control plan should establish an HCW TB counselling, screening, and evaluation program. The program should provide for counselling that includes individualized risk assessment and reiteration of TB control guidelines as described in the education program. All HCWs who are at risk of exposure to TB patients should participate in the TST screening program, unless they have documentation of previously treated TB and have no signs or symptoms of active TB. The program also should include an evaluation protocol for HCWs who have signs and symptoms of active TB. HCW should not return to work until TB has been excluded or they have received therapy and are determined to not be infectious.

Bacille Calmette-Guerin (BCG) vaccination to prevent tuberculosis is not widely used in the United States but is part of routine immunization practice globally, especially in countries with limited resources. In the United States, BCG has been considered for use in exceptional situations involving HCWs, but currently is not routinely recommended [10]. In countries where routine BCG vaccination occurs in childhood, the most important consideration is whether to revaccinate healthcare workers. At present, no benefit has been demonstrated for revaccination, and it is not recommended [11].

3.6   Cough induction

As previously discussed, procedures that induce cough from patients with active TB should be done in areas with local exhaust ventilation (see section 4.1) or in patient isolation rooms. An alternative for areas with limited resources is outdoor sputum collection. For sputum collection in patient rooms, HCWs should wear respiratory protective devices (see section 5.1).

3.7   Discharge planning

Before discharge, all patients should have a discharge plan developed that includes arrangements for outpatient follow-up and medications. This is especially important because an incomplete course of therapy increases the risk of treatment failure and subsequent multidrug resistance. Optimally, short course directly observed therapy (DOTS) should be used to maximize compliance with therapy. Such therapy should be promptly modified upon the identification of drug-resistant MTB strains.

3.8   Program evaluation

Periodic evaluation of the TB infection control program is key to assessing its effectiveness. Evaluation should include reassessment of the risk profile for the healthcare facility and include an assessment of compliance with recommended TB infection control policies and practices.

4.   ENGINEERING CONTROLS

The second tier of the TB control program is the use of engineering controls in the healthcare facility to minimize transmission of airborne droplet nuclei that carry viable MTB. In general, engineering controls are more costly than administrative measures. The engineering controls discussed here include ventilation systems and the use of ultraviolet germicidal irradiation (UVGI).

4.1   Ventilation

An important part of a TB control program is the healthcare facility's ventilation system. With respect to TB control, there are two major types of ventilation systems: local exhaust ventilation and general ventilation.

4.1.1   Local exhaust ventilation

Local exhaust ventilation removes airborne contaminants near their source so that persons in the area are not exposed. Two types of devices can be used for this purpose: enclosing devices and exterior devices.

Enclosing devices include laboratory hoods, sputum induction booths, and tents or hoods that completely enclose the patient. These devices should have the capability to remove 99% of airborne particles during the interval between patients.

In comparison, exterior devices do not completely enclose the patient but should have sufficient airflow to prevent cross-currents of airborne droplet nuclei near the patient's face from escaping and exposing other patients and HCWs. The device should maintain an air velocity of ≥ 200 feet per minute at the patient's breathing zone.

The discharge of air from these devices can be either in the room or directly to the outside. If air is discharged in the room, the exhaust fan should be located close to a high-efficiency particulate air (HEPA) filter. If a HEPA filter is not available, the air should be vented to the outside.

4.1.2   General ventilation

The plan for general ventilation in the healthcare facility must be incorporated into any TB control plan. There are three factors in general ventilation for TB control: the dilution and removal of contaminated air, airflow control in patient rooms, and airflow control in the facility.

Two types of general ventilation systems are used for dilution and removal of contaminated air: single-pass and recirculating. In single-pass systems, air comes in from the outside or from a central system and then 100% passes to the outside. In recirculating systems, only a small portion of exhaust air is vented to the outside. The air mixture, still containing potentially infectious droplet nuclei, could potentially circulate into previously uncontaminated areas or may be limited to a single room or group of rooms. The ventilation rate needed is a function of exhaust airflow and room volume and is expressed as air changes per hour (ACH).

Proper airflow patterns within rooms are important to prevent air stagnation or short-circuiting of air from the exhaust. As one would expect, airflow patterns may vary within a room depending on furniture, location of supply and exhausts, temperature differentials within the room, physical movement of HCW and patients, and physical configuration of the space. For example, outside air coming into a room should be vented near the ceiling and exhausted near the floor if the outside air is cooler than the room air. The process is reversed if outside air is warmer than room air. New (clean) air should be directed toward areas in which HCWs are likely to be in order to prevent placing HCWs between the infectious source and exhaust. In order to visualize complex air-mixing patterns, smoke tubes may be used. Air-mixing patterns must be evaluated to detect areas of air stagnation.

In addition to patterns within patient rooms, airflow patterns in the facility are important for preventing contamination of other areas. Directional airflow from less contaminated areas to more contaminated areas is generally accomplished through the creation of negative pressure in contaminated areas. The minimum pressure necessary to achieve directional airflow is very small (approximately 0.001 inch of water pressure) and is affected by how well the room is sealed. This pressure differential can be achieved with exhaust flow of 10%. However, operating characteristics of the negative pressure ventilation system may be significantly affected by opening and closing of doors and windows in the room and to outside areas. If the existing ventilation system is such that it is incapable of achieving negative pressure, alternatives include the use of fixed-room air recirculation systems, portable room-air recirculation units, and centrifugal blowers.

Positive pressurization of the corridor also can be used to drive air into the isolation room.

Once negative pressure is established, monitoring becomes an important part of overall maintenance and a specific schedule should be included in the TB infection control plan. Smoke from smoketubes can be used to monitor airflow directions visually.

4.2   HEPA filtration

HEPA filters are air-cleaning devices that at a minimum remove 99.7% of particles >0.3 µm in diameter. HEPA filters may be used in a variety of ways to reduce the concentration of contaminated particles. HEPA filters may be used to clean air before discharge to the outside, before recirculating in the room, or before recirculating in the facility. HEPA filters can be placed in exhaust ducts, ducts discharging air into the ventilation system, or in exhaust ducts or vents that discharge air from booths or enclosures into the surrounding room or in portable room-air cleaners.

Proper installation, testing, and maintenance are crucial if an HEPA filtration system is used, especially for recirculating systems.

4.3   Ultraviolet germicidal irradiation

Experimentally, UVGI is effective in killing or inactivating tubercle bacilli. UV radiation is that portion of the electromagnetic spectrum spanning 100 to 400 nm. Commercially available UVGI lamps with germicidal activity are typically low-pressure vapor lamps that emit radiant energy predominantly at a wavelength of 253.7 nm. UVGI can be used to supplement other engineering controls primarily as a duct irradiation system or in upper-room air irradiation. The clinical effectiveness of UVGI varies depending on configuration and maintenance. It should not replace negative pressure or other infection control practices. Although UV radiation is relatively safe, short-term overexposure can cause erythema and keratoconjunctivitis. Broad-spectrum UV radiation has been associated with increased risk for skin cancer. The National Institute for Occupational Safety and Health (NIOSH) has issued a recommended exposure limit. If UVGI is used, health care facility personnel should consult a competent UVGI systems designer for assistance in developing and implementing the system and developing a monitoring program.

5. PERSONAL RESPIRATORY PROTECTIVE DEVICES

Personal respiratory protective devices are the third tier of the overall TB infection control program. Personal respiratory protective devices are expensive and should be reserved for use by HCWs with high risk of exposure and subsequent infection with TB.

5.1 Respirator's performance criteria

Respirators used in healthcare settings should filter one-micron particles in the unloaded state with a filter efficiency of 95% and a flow rate of up to 50 liters per minute. Furthermore, they should have a face-seal leakage rate of less than 10%, fit different facial sizes and shapes (usually met by having three sizes), and have a facepiece fit check on each use by an HCW.

5.2 Specific respirators

In the United States, the Occupational Safety and Health Administration (OSHA) requires that HCWs needing respirators for protection use devices certified by the National Institute of Occupational Safety and Health (NIOSH). Based on the 1994 TB prevention guideline, these devices should contain filter materials that have 95% or greater efficiency for particles 1 micron or larger in diameter at a flow rate of 85 L/min. In circumstances with a very high risk of transmission to HCWs, a level of respiratory protection exceeding standard criteria may be appropriate and could include the use of negative-pressure respirators that are more protective, such as powered air-purifying particulate respirators, or positive-pressure airline, half-mask respirators.

In 1996, NIOSH implemented a certification process for testing respirators. The process classifies respirators based on their ability to filter 99.95%, 99%, or 95% of particles ≥ 0.3 microns in size. These respirators meet or exceed recommendations made in the 1994 CDC TB prevention guideline. By specifying a range of respirators that would be acceptable for prevention of TB transmission, this certification process allows flexibility in the respiratory device program, both in terms of the type of device used and the costs incurred [12].

5.3 Effectiveness

The two major parameters used to assess personal respiratory protective device effectiveness are face-seal efficacy and filter efficacy.

A proper seal between the HCW's face and the respirator's sealing surface is essential for effective and reliable performance of any negative pressure respirator. Face-seal leakage occurs for a number reasons, including incorrect face-piece size, shape, or sealing lip. Beard growth, perspiration, or facial oils also can cause face-piece slippage. Failure to use all head straps or incorrect positioning of the face-piece on the face can cause slippage. A head strap may be incorrectly positioned or have incorrect tension. Finally, improper respirator maintenance and respirator damage can result in improper face-seal.

If personal respiratory protective devices are used in a healthcare facility, they should be clearly incorporated into the TB infection control plan. Important topics to be addressed include the assignment of responsibility for the respiratory protection program and the development of standard operating procedures. HCWs should receive medical screening to ensure that they are physically capable of wearing the respirators. Further, they should be educated about respirator wear and operation. Face-seal fit testing and fit checking should be performed before repeating use. Respirator maintenance and periodic evaluation also should be incorporated into the respiratory protection program.

A recent evaluation of N95 respirators found that they filtered 95% of particles between 0.1 and 0.3 microns in size. More importantly, 99.5% or more of TB-size particles (0.8 microns) were filtered and no bacteria were re-aerosolized by normal exhalation [13].

6.   EFFECTIVENESS AND ADOPTION OF TB CONTROL PRACTICES

Few studies have assessed the effectiveness of implementing TB control practices in response to the emergence of MDRTB in the United States. In New York City, improved TB infection control practices in hospitals played an important role in reducing the total city-wide number of MDRTB cases from 115 in 1991 to less than 30 in 1993 [14]. TST conversion rates were reduced in one New York hospital from 17% to 5% following implementation of improved TB infection control practices [15]. Similarly, on an HIV ward in a hospital in Miami, Florida, reductions in exposure of HCWs to infectious MDRTB patients (80% to 45%) and HCW TST conversion rates (28% to 18%) occurred following the implementation of primarily administrative measures for TB control [16]. A New York City hospital with an MDRTB outbreak reduced the percentage of acquired immunodeficiency syndrome patients with probable nosocomial MDRTB (8.8 % to 2.6%) following implementation of administrative and engineering measures. However, HCW TST conversion rates remained higher for HCWs on wards with TB patients compared to those on wards without TB patients [17]. Little is known, however, about the incremental impact of each tier of TB control practices or about the effectiveness of TB control practices in other countries, especially in areas with limited resources.

U.S. hospitals have widely adopted all three tiers of TB infection control practices. In 1996, a survey of U.S. hospitals found that 99% had TB isolation rooms meeting CDC recommendations and most had N95 type respirators for HCWs [18]. In contrast, a survey of Belgian hospitals in 1995 revealed that only 24% used masks for HCWs that were capable of filtering one-micron particles [19]. The Belgian hospitals also reported low use of engineering measures such as UVGI (12%) and HEPA filters in ventilation systems (2%).

7. COSTS OF TB CONTROL PRACTICES

Cost estimates for the implementation of TB control practices vary depending upon the study method. In five U.S. hospitals (4 with MDRTB outbreaks) with infection control departments, Kellerman and colleagues reported the additional costs of administrative measures such as TB skin testing program (median cost: $5,568, range $2,393 to $44,902) and of extra infection control personnel for the TB program (median cost: $125,000, range $63,000 to $228,000) [20]. New construction or equipment to implement engineering controls was more expensive (median cost: $163,000, range $45,000 to $524,000). Personal respiratory protective measures including new HEPA respirators (median cost: $83,900, range $2,000 to $223,000), a HEPA respirator fit testing program (median cost: $17,187, range $8,736 to $26,175), and the annual cost of N95 respirators (median cost: $62,023, range $270 to $422,526) also were reported [21]. In contrast, Nettleman and colleagues estimate that mandatory use of HEPA respirators in 159 Veterans Affairs hospitals in the United States would cost $7 million to prevent a case of TB and $100 million to prevent a death from TB [22]. Farr and colleagues estimate that at the University of Virginia, use of HEPA respirators would cost $1.3 million to $18.5 million to prevent one case of occupationally acquired TB [23].

The cost estimates for preventing one episode of occupationally acquired TB given above are from hospitals in the United States where the incidence of TB is relatively low and consequently may overestimate costs to prevent TB cases in areas with higher TB incidence, such as sub-Saharan Africa. Unfortunately, the costs of environmental and personal respiratory protective devices are prohibitive for areas with high TB incidence and limited resources. In comparison, administrative controls should be used in all settings and are less costly than the other tiers of TB control.

8.   SPECIAL CHALLENGES IN LIMITED RESOURCE REGIONS AND COUNTRIES

As discussed previously, little work has been done to assess the incremental impact of each tier of TB infection control practices. In regions or countries with limited resources, costs of most engineering and personal respiratory protective measures are prohibitive [24]. The World Health Organization estimates that 80% of the world's new episodes of MDRTB occur in approximately 20 countries, most of which have limited resources [25]. Although most TB control measures in these countries have concentrated on efforts to increase and improve directly observed therapy (DOT), reduction of HCW exposure and nosocomial/occupational transmission also are important goals. In these regions, efforts should concentrate on administrative measures, especially the early identification of patients with TB. Simple measures also can be used such as ventilation though open windows and outdoor sputum collection to reduce general exposure of other patients and HCWs. Some facilities may be able to improve the rapidity with which AFB smears and culture results are available to clinicians so that appropriate therapy is instituted earlier. A ward "cough officer" can be designated with responsibility to expedite the prompt collection of sputum specimens for diagnostic testing from suspected TB patients thereby reducing the delay in AFB testing [24]. However, substantial resource limitations remain in these countries and focused efforts to increase TB prevention resources in these countries are urgently needed [26,27].

9.   SUMMARY AND CONCLUSIONS

In summary, the control of TB, including MDRTB, in healthcare facilities must be a multifaceted program built on risk assessment, a written TB infection control plan, and periodic re-evaluation. Central to the program is a detailed, written infection control plan that clearly delineates roles, responsibilities, and resources for each of the components of the plan. Administrative controls (which are the least costly) are essential and should be provided in all locations, developed and developing countries alike. Where resources permit, additional measures, such as use of ventilation systems and HCW personal respiratory protective devices, should be used to maximize both patient and HCW protection from TB. In all areas of the world, HCWs are a valuable resource. Occupational acquisition of MTB should be unacceptable. Implementation of CDC or WHO TB guideline recommendations should decrease the risk of occupational exposure and reduce nosocomial MTB transmission.

REFERENCES

1.   Fridkin SK, Manangan L, Bolyard E, SHEA, Jarvis WR. SHEA-CDC TB survey: part I. Status of TB infection control programs at member hospitals, 1989-1992. Infect Control Hosp Epidemiol 1995; 16: 129-134.
2.   Fridkin SK, Manangan L, Bolyard E, SHEA, Jarvis WR. SHEA-CDC TB survey: part II. Efficacy of TB infection control programs at member hospitals, 1992. Infect Control Hosp Epidemiol 1995; 16: 135-140.
3.   Sinkowitz R, Fridkin S, Manangan L, Wenger P, APIC, Jarvis WR. Status of tuberculosis infection control programs at U.S. hospitals, 1989-1992. Am J Infect Control 1996; 24: 226-234.
4.   Malasky C, Jordan T, Potulski F, Reichman LB. Occcupational tuberculosis infections among pulmonary physicians in training. Am Rev Respir Dis 1990; 142: 505-507.
5.   Weinstock DM, Sepkowitz KA. Multidrug-resistant tuberculosis and the health care worker, Chapter 15, 225-239. In: Bastian I, Portaels F (eds.), Multidrug-resistant tuberculosis. Kluwer Academic Publ., The Netherlands, 2000.
6.   Menzies D, Fanning A, Yuan L, Fitzgerald M. Tuberculosis among healthcare workers. N Engl J Med 1995; 332: 92-98.
7.   Barrett-Connor E. The epidemiology of tuberculosis in physicians. JAMA 1979; 241: 133-138.
8.   Weinstein RS, Oshins J, Sacks HS. Tuberculosis infection in Mount Sinai medical students:1974-1982. Mt Sinai J Med 1984; 51: 283-286.
9.   Centers for Disease Control and Prevention. Guidelines for preventing transmission of *Mycobacterium tuberculosis* in healthcare facilities, 1994. MMWR 1994; 43(RR-13): 1-132.
10. Centers for Disease Control and Prevention. The role of BCG in the prevention and control of tuberculosis in the United States. A joint statement by the Advisory Council for the Elimination of Tuberculosis and the Advisory Committee on Immunization Practices. MMWR 1996; 45(RR-4): 1-18.
11. World Health Organization. Statement on BCG revaccination for the prevention of tuberculosis. Weekly Epidemiological Record. 1995; 70: 229-231.
12. U.S. Department of Health and Human Services. NIOSH Guide to the selection and use of particulate respirators certified under 42 CFR Part 84. NIOSH No. 96-101. January, 1996.
13. Willeke K, Qian Y. Tuberculosis control through respirator wear: performance of National Institute for Occupational Safety and Health-regulated respirators. Am J Infect Control 1998; 26: 139-142.
14. Frieden TR, Fujiwara PI, Washko RM, Hamburg MA. Tuberculosis in New York City-- Turning the tide. N Engl J Med 1995; 333: 229-233.

15. Maloney SA, Pearson ML, Gordon MT, Castillo R, Boyle JF, Jarvis WR. Efficacy of control measures in preventing nosocomial transmission of multidrug-resistant tuberculosis to patients and health care workers. Ann Intern Med 1995; 122: 90-95.

16. Wenger PN, Otten J, Breeden A, Orfas D, Beck-Sague CM, Jarvis WR. Control of nosocomial transmission of multidrug-resistant *Mycobacterium tuberculosis* among healthcare workers and HIV-infected patients. Lancet 1995; 345: 235-240.

17. Stroud L, Tokars JI, Grieco MH, Crawford JT, Culver DH, Edlin BR, et al. Evaluation of infection control measures in preventing the nosocomial transmission of multidrug-resistant *Mycobacterium tuberculosis* in a New York City hospital. Infect Control Hosp Epidemiol 1995; 16: 141-147.

18. Manangan L, Simonds DN, Pugliese G, Kroc K, Banerjee SN, Rudnick JR, et al. Are US hospitals making progress in implementing guidelines for prevention of *Mycobacterium tuberculosis* transmission? Arch Intern Med 1998; 158: 1440-1444.

19. Ronveaux O, Jans B, Wanlin M, Uydeboruck M. Prevention of transmission of tuberculosis in hospitals; a survey of practices in Belgium, 1995. J Hosp Infect 1999; 37: 207-215.

20. Kellerman S, Tokars JI, Jarvis W. The cost of selected tuberculosis control measures at hospitals with a history of *Mycobacterium tuberculosis* outbreaks. Infect Control Hosp Epidemiol 1997; 18: 542-547.

21. Kellerman S, Tokars JI, Jarvis WR. The costs of healthcare worker respiratory protection and fit-testing programs. Infect Control Hosp Epidemiol 1999; 19: 629-634.

22. Nettleman MD Fredrickson M, Good NL, Hunter SA. Tuberculosis control strategies: the cost of particulate respirators. Ann Intern Med 1994; 121: 37-40.

23. Adal KA, Anglim AM, Palumbo CL, Titus MG, Goyner BJ, Farr BM. The use of high-efficiency particulate air-filter respirators to protect hospital workers from tuberculosis. A cost-effectiveness analysis. N Engl J Med 1994; 331: 169-173.

24. Harries AD, Maher D, Nunn P. Practical and affordable measures for the protection of health care workers from tuberculosis in low-income countries. Bull World Health Organ 1997; 75: 477-489.

25. World Health Organization. Global tuberculosis control—WHO Report 1999. WHO, Geneva, Switzerland, 1999.

26. Heymann SJ, Brewer TF, Wilson ME, Fineberg HV. The need for global action against multidrug-resistant tuberculosis. JAMA 1999; 281: 2138-2139.

27. Centers for Disease Control and Prevention. Tuberculosis Elimination Revisted: Obstacles, Opportunities, and a Renewed Commitment. MMWR 1999; 48(RR-9): 1-12.

Chapter 19

Making DOTS-Plus work

Paul E. Farmer, Sonya S. Shin, Jaime Bayona, Jim Y. Kim, Jennifer J. Furin
and Joel G. Brenner
Program in Infectious Disease and Social Change, Harvard Medical School, Boston, MA

1.   INTRODUCTION

"We have to think about MDR-TB in a new way. In the past, we have seen it as a virtual
death sentence for people in developing countries, but now we can give people hope of a
cure."
Arata Kochi, WHO Global TB Program, April 5, 1998

The persistent generation and transmission of strains of *Mycobacterium tuberculosis* resistant to the first-line antituberculosis agents have been documented in a large number of settings [1]. In these regions, effective strategies for both the prevention and the treatment of drug-resistant tuberculosis (TB) are required, and delays in their implementation will likely prove costly. Such a strategy must successfully prevent further transmission of new infections through rendering individual patients first, non-infectious, and eventually, cured. Indeed, MDRTB control can only be achieved when all the sources currently fuelling this quietly advancing epidemic are quelled. A central tenet of modern TB control is that *treatment is prevention* [2]. As with drug-susceptible TB, effective therapy for infectious cases is the only acceptable strategy to curtail further spread of drug-resistant strains of *M. tuberculosis*, and the only likely way to defuse what some have termed a "time-bomb" [3,4].

285

I. Bastian and F. Portaels (eds.), Multidrug-Resistant Tuberculosis, 285-306.
© 2000 *Kluwer Academic Publishers. Printed in the Netherlands.*

Can a single strategy potentially fulfil these requirements? Routine application of "directly observed treatment, short-course" (DOTS), the TB control strategy endorsed by the World Health Organization (WHO), is inadequate alone. It is increasingly clear that short-course chemotherapy— the S in DOTS—will fail to cure a substantial majority of patients with MDRTB [5,6]. At the same time, the rest of the strategy might provide an effective framework for the treatment and control of MDRTB. For these reasons, DOTS-based strategies which include provisions for the treatment of patients with drug-resistant TB constitute a timely response to a growing public-health threat. As its name suggests, DOTS-Plus is an extension of the WHO's well-established DOTS strategy [7,8]. As results of operational studies from DOTS-Plus projects for MDRTB are lacking, WHO has announced its support for pilot projects to explore the feasibility and cost efficacy of DOTS-Plus programs [9]. The WHO position on MDRTB has been summarised [10]:

1. to achieve TB control worldwide and to prevent the emergence of antituberculosis drug resistance, the WHO considers implementation of sound TB control based on the DOTS strategy as a top priority;
2. recognizing that MDRTB is a considerable threat to the effectiveness of DOTS in some areas of the world, WHO strongly supports pilot projects to assess the feasibility of DOTS-Plus interventions in a variety of settings, provided DOTS is in place; and
3. based on the results of these pilot projects, WHO and its partners in the newly established Working Group on "DOTS-Plus for MDRTB" will formulate international policy recommendations on MDRTB management.

2.   WHAT IS DOTS-PLUS?

DOTS-Plus is a case-management strategy under the aegis of DOTS designed to manage MDRTB using second-line drugs and infection-control measures. A pilot DOTS-Plus program has been running in urban Peru since 1996 under the auspices of the Peruvian National Tuberculosis Program. A WHO working group was subsequently established in April 1999 to design program protocols and oversee implementation of other DOTS-Plus pilot projects. These additional operational studies are now underway in Peru, South Africa, Haiti, and the former Soviet Union.

Within the DOTS-Plus initiative, two basic models have been proposed for the management of MDRTB: individualized treatment regimens (ITRs) based on drug susceptibility testing (DST) to a full panel of first- and second-line drugs, and a standardized MDRTB treatment regimen [8]. The strengths and weaknesses of each of these models are compared in Table 1. The ITR model has already been piloted in Peru and is described elsewhere in detail [8]. The advantages of ITRs include:

1. a greater likelihood of treatment success, since DST allows clinicians to design regimens comprised of an adequate number of antituberculous medications;
2. a decreased likelihood of inadvertent amplification of drug resistance, since patients will not receive drugs to which their infecting strains have documented resistance;
3. a decreased likelihood of exposing patients to unnecessary toxicity, since no patient receives medications to which his or her infecting strain has documented resistance; and
4. a greater level of flexibility in adjusting regimens based on the clinical course of individual patients [11].

Table 1. Attributes of the two DOTS-Plus models [8]

Attribute	Individualized treatment	Standardized treatment
Efficacy	Maximum	Moderate-high
Cost	High	Moderate-high
Risk of amplifying resistance	Very low	Low-moderate
Toxicity	Moderate	Moderate
Technical capacity required	High	Moderate

The use of ITRs for MDRTB also has potential drawbacks, especially on a program level. This model requires initial laboratory testing, adjustments of treatment regimens based on laboratory results and on changing clinical parameters, and often, non-standardized dosing of antituberculous agents. These features of ITRs may render them initially more expensive and less straightforward than fully standardized regimens. The long-term costs of ITRs, however, may well prove lower if they can achieve high cure rates and avoid the recruitment of additional resistance. Furthermore, training of health personnel, while initially intensive, can lead to long-term benefits for the communities they serve. Operational research addressing these questions is currently underway in a number of DOTS-Plus pilot projects.

Two approaches have been proposed for implementing the standardized model of MDRTB treatment. In the first approach, patients failing empiric short-course chemotherapy regimens are presumed to have MDRTB. Once identified as treatment failures, they then receive a re-treatment regimen including second-line drugs [12]. A second standardized approach relies on knowledge of local epidemiology to design an empiric MDRTB treatment regimen appropriate to the setting in question. This second approach is perhaps most suitable for settings in which an epidemic strain accounts for the majority of incident MDRTB cases. For example, empiric MDRTB regimens were used in New York City during an outbreak of strain "W," although definitive, individualized regimens were subsequently designed upon receiving results of DST [13,14].

There are potential benefits and risks with the standardized models for MDRTB treatment (Table 1). Potential advantages include lower initial costs, since DST is not required for each patient, and greater ease of administration and management, since all patients receive standardized doses of the same antituberculosis drugs. Potential disadvantages include the fact that individual patients with strains susceptible to powerful first-line drugs may fail to receive these drugs in their standardized regimen. Conversely, patients may receive second-line drugs to which their strains are resistant, thus exposing them to unnecessary toxicity and increasing the risk of resistance amplification. In addition to these important drawbacks, there is also a lower likelihood of treatment success, since not all patients will be receiving three or more drugs to which their infecting strain is susceptible. Finally, treatment options may be limited for patients who fail empiric MDRTB treatment regimens and in the process recruit resistance to second-line drugs.

The Peruvian National TB Program is currently piloting a standardized MDRTB treatment regimen in urban Lima. Preliminary results of this 18-month treatment protocol on a small proportion of patients (28 of 174) show a 75% smear-conversion [15]. Preliminary data from South Africa also suggest that cure rates of over 70% can be expected if empiric regimens include an adequate number of drugs [16].

Whether DOTS-Plus programs use ITRs or standardized regimens, several common elements are necessary to ensure their success. Most of these elements are familiar to those who advocate DOTS-based approaches for TB control. DOTS-Plus programs require political will; participation of reference laboratories for DST; uninterrupted access to first- and second-line drugs; strict enforcement of directly observed therapy; and uniform approaches to data collection and outcome evaluation, including standardized cohort analysis and operational research. Each of these will be discussed in detail in the sections that follow.

3.   POLITICAL COMMITMENT

Political commitment is an essential component of any DOTS-based strategy. According to the WHO [17], "Governments must support the DOTS strategy emphatically and make TB control a high political priority. Governments and non-government organizations (NGOs) must be financially committed to long-term TB control, ensuring that all TB patients can have free access to treatment. TB control should be integrated into the existing health system, and supported with leadership from a central TB unit. A well-supported National TB Program will have a program manual, a training program in place, a plan of supervision, and a development plan." Political commitment— local, regional, national, and transnational— will be at least as important to the success of DOTS-Plus programs, for several reasons.

3.1   The additional costs of treating MDRTB

Drug-resistant TB is a new problem; it requires new resources. Although in theory the potential for diversion of funds slated for the treatment of drug-susceptible disease exists, in actuality, the threat of potentially untreatable TB has led in some settings to increases in public funding for TB control. This was the case in New York, for example [18,19] and more recently in Peru [20]. But political will is required in order to bring new resources to bear on this emerging problem. In some settings, such as the former Soviet Union, a higher burden of MDRTB exists within the penitentiary system [21-26]. Accordingly, public monies must be directed to interventions designed to improve the care of patients whose health needs are regarded by many as a low priority — hence the chronic problem of under-funded prison health systems. Sufficient political support can, however, alter funding priorities. In Russia, for example, several oblast governors have declared their commitment to DOTS-Plus programs being launched in Western Siberia, facilitating the procurement of increased international funding for these efforts.

3.2   Strict control of second-line drugs

Strict control of second-line drugs is critical to building and sustaining effective DOTS-Plus programs. Only political will can enforce the strict control of antituberculosis drugs, since international organizations such as the WHO do not have in-country regulatory capacity. In Russia, the Public Health Research Institute and other non-governmental organizations have worked with Russian civilian and prison authorities to develop a legal framework for the control of second-line drugs [27-29]. Although the pharmaceutical industry may baulk at such regulations, strict control may in fact protect the long-term efficacy of their products. Streptomycin is a case in point: due to its haphazard and unmonitored use in the past, the drug currently has limited utility within the former Soviet Union, where in some cohorts a majority of patients are sick from strains of *M. tuberculosis* resistant to this drug [1,28,30].

3.3   Expansion of TB control initiatives

Political will is necessary to expand TB-control strategies. Implementation of DOTS-Plus, a novel strategy, will at times meet with opposition. If pilot projects show DOTS-Plus to be an effective TB-control measure, political commitment will likely be a critical component of a successful campaign to replicate these projects in MDRTB "hot spots". Such endeavours will require intensive technical and human-resource development, including training and re-training of personnel necessary to implement and evaluate DOTS-Plus efforts. The nature and extent of such training will vary from site to site. In parts of the former Soviet Union, for example, an extant TB-control infrastructure must be reinvigorated and updated, whereas in other MDRTB "hot spots" a solid TB infrastructure needs to be developed where there is none. In both types of settings, improved infection-control measures will also require new resources and political will. But one of the most significant expenditures is likely to be the expansion of laboratory capacity. Because MDRTB treatment requires extensive laboratory support, we now examine the role of reference laboratories in making DOTS-Plus projects effective.

4.   THE ROLE OF REFERENCE LABORATORIES

Heifets and Cangelosi have stated [31], "We believe the spread of primary drug resistance calls for immediate action to prevent the real threat in a number of countries of an epidemic of incurable, polyresistant tuberculosis. One step in this direction, among other necessary measures, is implementation of a system for timely detection of drug resistance in new patients." As resistance to antituberculosis drugs becomes an increasing concern, it is becoming ever more clear that only through the rapid identification and effective treatment of MDRTB will this epidemic be controlled. Unfortunately, the diagnosis of MDRTB cannot be made by smear microscopy. Culture of *M. tuberculosis* is required in order to perform DST. Thus, mycobacteriology laboratories have a crucial role to play in halting the transmission of MDRTB [25,31,32]. Properly equipped reference laboratories perform several key tasks, including quality control, surveillance of resistance to first- and second-line drugs, DST to guide patient management, and development of novel technologies for more rapid diagnosis of drug-resistant strains of TB [31,33,34]. Several of these issues are discussed below.

4.1 Drug resistance surveillance

Reference laboratories are critical to the study of trends in antituberculosis drug resistance. That a multinational network of reference laboratories can document such trends has been made clear by the WHO/IUATLD Global Project on Anti-tuberculosis Drug Resistance Surveillance [1], the goal of which was "to ascertain the global magnitude of the problem of anti-tuberculosis drug resistance." To this end, selected reputable laboratories from around the world were asked to join a network of supranational reference laboratories (SRLs). At this writing, more than twenty laboratories constitute the SRL network. The SRLs conduct testing for susceptibility to, at a minimum, four of the first-line antituberculosis drugs: isoniazid (INH), rifampicin (RIF), ethambutol (EMB), and streptomycin (SM); many have the capacity to test for susceptibility to pyrazinamide (PZA) and second-line drugs as well. The SRLs provide data on the levels of drug resistance in both new and previously treated patients.

While surveillance on a global level is key to monitoring national and international trends, these results are too rarely translated into clinically meaningful data for individual patients. As partners in DOTS-Plus programs, SRLs must take on a critical second role: that of providing DST results that can be used to guide the treatment of individuals with MDRTB. The provision of clinically useful data is part of the central mandate of almost all of these laboratories, which means that few changes would be required to bring them into a supranational DOTS-Plus laboratory network. At this writing, a number of prominent mycobacteriologists from Europe, Canada, and the United States have already established a laboratory subgroup of the DOTS-Plus Working Group of the WHO [9].

The importance of DST in the management of patients with MDRTB has been reviewed [8,31,35]. Basing treatment regimens on the results of *in vitro* susceptibility testing is the gold standard of TB therapy in the United States and Europe [31,36,37]. Such clinically relevant testing differs from surveillance in that testing and communication of test results must be performed in as timely a manner as is possible. These results permit clinicians to avoid drugs to which resistance has been documented, and to base a treatment regimen on a firm foundation of four or five drugs to which the patient's infecting isolate demonstrates susceptibility. Culture and susceptibility results can also be used to guide patient management during the course of therapy. In most settings in which resistance to INH and RIF are widespread, susceptibility to second-line agents should also be documented. It should be noted that there is significantly less international standardization of susceptibility testing methods to the second-line drugs: kanamycin (KM), amikacin (AMK), capreomycin (CM), ethionamide

(THA), prothionamide, fluoroquinolones, cycloserine (CS), and para-aminosalicylic acid (PAS). Furthermore, there is less experience correlating the results of *in vitro* testing with the clinical activity of these agents [38].

If DOTS-Plus projects are to be effective, it is clear that more laboratories will need to acquire the infrastructure and skills to conduct DST. Ideally, such laboratories would be located within countries in which MDRTB "hot spots" have been identified. As Heifets and Cangelosi note [31], "the list of such countries may be much longer than is thought by some opponents of laboratory services... we argue that the lack of proper laboratory support for tuberculosis control is not a matter of affordability but rather an underestimation of its importance." It must also be noted, however, that currently designated SRLs have the capacity not only to carry out more testing but also to provide training to colleagues in high TB-incidence settings.

Transnational cooperation involving SRLs, non-governmental organizations, and national TB programs has already demonstrated its utility in implementing one DOTS-Plus Project in a resource-poor "hot spot" of MDRTB transmission [20,39]. Since 1996, the Massachusetts State Laboratory Institute (MSLI), a member of the WHO/IUATLD SRL network, has worked closely with the Peruvian National TB Program, Harvard Medical School, and Partners In Health to provide state-of-the-art DST for the DOTS-Plus program in the northern cone of Lima. Patients with suspected MDRTB submit a sputum specimen, and the MSLI tests the resulting isolates for resistance to INH, RIF, PZA, EMB, SM, KM, CM, ciprofloxacin (CPX), THA, and CS. Additional testing for susceptibility to AMK, PAS, clarithromycin (CLR) and rifabutin (RFB) is provided on a case-by-case basis in conjunction with the National Jewish Hospital in Denver. The MSLI has worked closely with Partners In Health and Harvard Medical School to establish a system for rapid communication of test results. To date, over 500 samples from Peruvian patients have been tested at the MSLI, guiding the individualized treatment of more than 100 patients under the care of the Harvard/Partners team. The MSLI also performs RFLP testing on confirmed MDRTB strains. In addition, MSLI personnel have provided on-site training to their Peruvian colleagues, and other technical exchanges are planned for the coming years. The MSLI is currently in the process of expanding its testing capabilities, and it is hoped that a greater number of samples will be processed in the next phase of the project.

Can MDRTB be treated in the absence of culture and susceptibility data? Preliminary research suggests that in a carefully administered DOTS program based on strictly supervised short-course chemotherapy, over 85% of patients who remain smear positive at the end of treatment will be found to have MDRTB [25,40,41]. If DOTS failure signals MDRTB and resistance to SM is rare, then an empiric regimen based on SM, a fluoroquinolone,

PAS, and two or three other drugs could be formulated. Cure rates may be high if polyresistance— that is resistance to multiple drugs other than the combination of INH plus RIF— is low among patients receiving directly observed empiric MDRTB treatment. Unfortunately, resistance to SM and other first-line drugs is high in many of the "hot spots" identified by the WHO/IUATLD survey. In these settings, CM or KM will often be the injectable drug of choice, and EMB and PZA may be less useful. Standardized regimens should thus incorporate knowledge of the local epidemiology of drug resistance in the design and implementation of treatment programs. SRLs could play a key role in describing such community epidemiology and ensuring that appropriate standardized regimens are used. Nationwide surveys—such as the WHO/IUATLD project discussed above—may not accurately reflect smaller community epidemics. In Peru, for example, data from the National TB Program suggests that resistance to INH and RIF alone is the most common pattern of MDRTB seen in a national sample of patients with a history of treatment [1]. Yet, in a group of previously treated MDRTB patients in northern Lima identified as treatment failures, we found that the most common pattern was combined resistance to INH, RIF, EMB, and SM [42].

The following summary points and recommendations could therefore be made about laboratories and their role in DOTS-Plus programs:

1. mycobacteriology laboratories should be considered an integral component of an effective response to MDRTB, providing essential data for surveillance and treatment decisions on both individual and community levels;
2. the WHO/IUATLD SRL network should be developed to facilitate laboratory-clinician communication of clinically-relevant data;
3. the role of the SRL network should be extended to include DST for second-line drugs, as soon as international standards are set;
4. information systems for accurate management of DST data should be established on local and national levels;
5. the development and dissemination of new technologies for rapid identification of drug resistance must be supported; and
6. new transnational partnerships must be created to provide DST and training for resource-poor areas with large MDRTB burdens; transnational collaboration may prove critical to building capacity in countries with large MDRTB burdens and limited laboratory resources.

5.   PROCUREMENT OF SECOND-LINE ANTITUBERCULOUS DRUGS

"Let's stop waiting for a perfect strategy that will assure universal access to
all drugs in the future. Rather, let us do what we can to improve access today,
even as we commit ourselves to do better tomorrow", Peter Piot, *Access to
Drugs: UNAIDS Technical Update,* 1998 [43].

In order to ensure the success of DOTS-Plus programs, an uninterrupted
supply of affordable, high-quality second-line drugs must be secured. Strict
control of these second-line agents will be essential: inappropriate use of
these medications will generate additional resistance and render these
drugs— our last resort— ineffective [10,12,44]. Furthermore, since our
therapeutic armamentarium is currently limited, new and more effective
antituberculosis drugs will be critical to future TB control. This section will
address some of these issues.

It has been estimated that the treatment regimen cost for MDRTB
patients requiring capreomycin or cycloserine is 215 to 444 times greater
than the treatment regimen cost for standard, drug-susceptible patients [45].
Although experience in Peru suggests that these regimens can be provided
much less expensively, it is nonetheless true that most second-line
antituberculous agents are characterized by exorbitant prices and irrational
price differentials, despite the fact that the majority are currently off-patent
(see Figure 1).

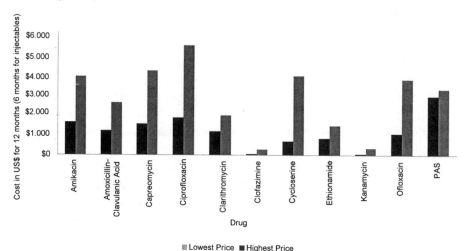

Figure 1. Drug cost comparisons for second-line antituberculosis drugs [8]. The minimum
and maximum prices for treatment for one year with a range of second-line drugs are shown
(cost of treatment for only six months is shown for injectable agents). PAS, para-
aminosalicylic acid.

5.1   Inclusion of second-line drugs on the WHO Essential Drugs List

Previous efforts to lower the prices of second-line drugs have yielded few results [46]. New approaches are clearly in order, since the cost of treating MDRTB in resource-poor settings is spent primarily on drugs. National TB programs that have undertaken the treatment of MDRTB may see a majority of drug disbursements go to purchase second-line drugs.

Lowering the costs of second-line antituberculous medications is a priority, but other steps must be taken in order to ensure the success of DOTS-Plus projects. In addition to affordability, drugs must be of sufficiently high quality to ensure that further resistance is not inadvertently generated. Thus quality control and good manufacturing practices are critical to the success of any such efforts [47-49]. One of the key desiderata for DOTS-Plus programs will be the enforcement of and adherence to quality standards for all second-line antituberculous agents by all DOTS-Plus participants.

Recent advocacy efforts have focused on pooled procurement and consideration of inclusion of these drugs in the WHO Essential Drugs List. Inclusion of second-line drugs in the WHO Essential Drugs List may serve efforts to combat MDRTB in several ways:

1. legal registration of drugs could be facilitated in countries with a high MDRTB burden;
2. costs could be decreased;
3. controlled and rational use of second-line antituberculous medications may be promoted; and
4. quality control and good manufacturing practices could be more readily applied to these agents, regardless of manufacturer.

The concept of "essential drugs" arose in the 1960s, with the goal of providing safe, affordable access to a variety of medications used to treat common and life-threatening illnesses [47]. With the exception of the fluoroquinolones, second-line antituberculous medications are not listed as essential drugs [50]. Given the public health impact of MDRTB and the need to respond promptly to this global threat, consideration is now being given to the addition of these drugs to the WHO's Essential Drugs List (EDL). Incorporation of second-line agents on the EDL poses the theoretical risk of increasing the uncontrolled use of these drugs. When second-line antituberculous agents are available on open markets, patients with drug-resistant TB often obtain these drugs from private physicians and local pharmacies. Because these drugs are expensive, therapy is often irregular, leading to acquired resistance. High prices are no protection against inappropriate use of these agents and may in fact heighten risk for acquiring resistance to these agents [20]. Thus, use of second-line antituberculous agents is best reserved for countries with DOTS-based TB-control programs in place and with adequate infrastructure and regulatory capacity. Strict control of these agents and their provision, free of cost to patients, should be the rule in DOTS-Plus programs, since poorly-executed DOTS-Plus programs will be one of the quickest ways to engender "MDRTB-Plus"[27]. One rational way to prevent misuse of these drugs is to advocate national regulations restricting their use to within national TB control programs. National regulations controlling the use of first-line antituberculosis drugs already exist in countries as disparate as Brazil, Norway, and Syria [51].

5.2   Pooled procurement of second-line drugs

Pooled procurement affords a means by which purchasers of small quantities of drugs can secure high-quality drugs at decreased cost by increasing bulk orders and streamlining payment procedures. DOTS-Plus programs would therefore gain numerous benefits from pooled procurement:
1. economies of scale through joint orders;
2. selection of drugs based on common formularies;
3. shared monitoring and quality assurance standards;
4. centralized payment mechanisms;
5. policed sole-source commitment; and
6. competitive bidding from multiple suppliers.

Pooled procurement has been shown to have salutary effects whether joint orders are based on regional consortia [52], according to disease category [43], or in keeping with shared health priorities [53]. It is increasingly clear that DOTS-Plus efforts would benefit significantly from the pooled procurement of second-line drugs. In order to be successful, pooled-procurement efforts require political will, strong institutional alliances, financial security requisite for prompt payment, and shared quality standards [52]. Currently, most countries need relatively small amounts of these medications, and pooling procurement will allow for economies of scale through joint orders. Procuring second-line antituberculosis drugs through a centralized system would uphold quality standards while helping to prevent the sale of these agents on the open market. Furthermore, pooled procurement would strengthen ties between the multiple groups currently addressing MDRTB, enhancing exchange of information and improved management of DOTS-Plus programs. Steps towards pooled purchasing for second-line antituberculosis medications are underway.

As efforts to contain MDR-TB are initiated, the need for new antituberculous drugs becomes increasingly urgent. Resistance to second-line drugs has already been documented in a number of settings. With the exception of the fluoroquinolones, no new clinically significant antituberculous agent has been developed since the 1970s. Thus, efforts to secure second-line drug supplies must proceed in parallel with investment into the development of effective new drugs. This endeavour will require the establishment of new public-private partnerships and high levels of political commitment on the part of countries and intergovernmental organizations.

In summary, the provision of high-quality second-line drugs has proven to be a major stumbling block in efforts to treat MDRTB. But the DOTS-Plus approach could help improve both access to and control over second-line drugs. In the early 1970s, RIF was widely considered "too expensive" to use on a global scale [54], yet it is now considered both indispensable and inexpensive; in some countries, legislation to prevent the sale of RIF on the open market is now being considered. With sufficient political will and advocacy efforts, we may aspire to similar outcomes regarding second-line antituberculosis drugs currently considered too costly to use in poor countries.

6. THE IMPORTANCE OF DIRECTLY OBSERVED THERAPY

DOTS-Plus is best implemented as an extension of national TB programs already committed to DOTS. DOTS-Plus builds on the strengths of DOTS, incorporating each of its basic components except one: it does not rely solely on fixed-dose, short-course chemotherapy. As noted above, DOTS-Plus strategies require political commitment at the highest national level and, at times, at supranational levels. DOTS-Plus also incorporates the methods of standardized case finding and reporting, as well as the financing and supply advantages inherent to DOTS programs. Most fundamentally, DOTS-Plus builds upon DOTS in its requirement that every dose of therapy be supervised.

Although directly observed therapy for TB has been official policy at the global level for a mere five years, the idea is over 40 years old [55,56]. In the United States, the Centers for Disease Control (CDC) established DOT as a cornerstone of federal TB policy in 1993 [55]. WHO adopted universal DOT a year later as part of a five-point policy package including (1) political commitment, (2) case finding using smear microscopy among symptomatic patients, (3) standardized short-course therapy for all sputum smear-positive cases, (4) a regular supply of essential anti-TB drugs, and (5) a standardized program monitoring and evaluation system [17].

One key reason DOT is so important in treating patients with MDRTB is that the second-line antituberculous agents often have more adverse effects than do first-line drugs. The potential adverse effects associated with antituberculous medications have been reviewed extensively by others [35,57-84]. Although some clinicians regard these adverse effects as reasons to avoid or interrupt the treatment of patients with MDRTB, emerging data suggest that in young cohorts with few co-morbidities, the occurrence of serious adverse effects is rare and does not compromise treatment outcomes [85]. Nonetheless, mild side effects to MDRTB regimens occur frequently, and close surveillance for rare but serious side effects is recommended. Because DOT requires daily contact between patients and supervising health workers, DOT allows health workers to identify promptly and manage adverse effects. Effective side effect management allows acceptable treatment tolerance; fewer drugs are sacrificed, default rates are minimized, and treatment outcome is improved [86].

In DOTS-Plus programs, therapy is best supervised by individuals trained in the use of second-line drugs. It is important to note, however, that a broad variety of health workers can be trained to administer these agents in an effective manner. A number of studies have demonstrated the effectiveness of community-health workers in responding to serious challenges to health [87-97]. In Peru, local community residents have been trained to serve as DOTS-Plus outreach workers. Their role includes supervision of DOT, management of common adverse effects, communication with other health providers, and provision of social and emotional support [86].

7.   EVALUATING DOTS-PLUS EFFORTS

A number of DOTS-based approaches to the treatment and control of drug-resistant tuberculosis have been proposed. Careful assessment of each DOTS-Plus program must be performed so that strengths may be identified and reinforced while weaknesses are eliminated. Comparative analyses should evaluate both clinical and programmatic components.

Several parameters may be used to assess the clinical effectiveness of an MDRTB treatment program [86]. Smear microscopy, including time to smear conversion, is an important index of response to therapy. Other relevant parameters include culture, radiography, and clinical response. These parameters should be followed regularly throughout therapy to identify potential treatment failures [86]. Each of these variables should be monitored and reported though operational-research protocols designed to evaluate DOTS-Plus programs.

In addition to using individual clinical outcomes as a measure of the efficacy of DOTS-Plus programs, a number of programmatic variables should be assessed as well. Among these are: ease of program implementation, reliability of DOT, rates of abandonment, enhancement of local capacity through training, quality control of all aspects of program operations, and short-term and long-term program costs. Cost-efficacy analyses should incorporate often-overlooked variables: the cost of failed treatments prior to initiation of MDRTB treatment; the use of medications to which patients' infecting strains are resistant; and the rate of MDRTB transmission during ineffective therapy.

Another phenomenon to be considered when calculating cost effectiveness is termed the "amplifier effect of short-course chemotherapy" [4]. This term describes the process by which patients infected with strains resistant to at least one drug not only fail short-course chemotherapy, but in the process may recruit additional resistance to other drugs. If these patients subsequently receive empiric re-treatment (commonly consisting of these same four drugs plus streptomycin), their infecting strain may only be susceptible to one or two of the drugs they receive, placing them at considerable risk of re-treatment failure and even further resistance (Figure 2).

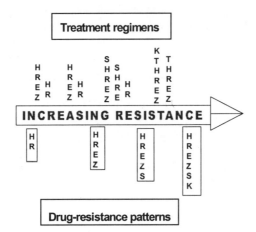

Figure 2. The amplifier effect of short-course chemotherapy. The figure depicts the chronological development of additional drug resistance in one patient after successive failed treatment regimens [20]. The boxes (bottom) contain the resistance profiles of sequential isolates demonstrating the amplifier effect of short-course chemotherapy. H, isoniazid; R, rifampicin; E, ethambutol; Z, pyrazinamide; S, streptomycin; K, kanamycin; T, thioacetazone.

What is the evidence for the amplifier effect of short-course chemotherapy? Conditions are such that it is difficult to obtain data, since studies would require serial cultures taken at two points during therapy, or before and after therapy. In most settings in which cultures are routinely performed, standards of care call for prompt alteration in treatment regimens based on the results of drug-susceptibility testing. But some studies do speak to this phenomenon. Mitchison and Nunn reviewed 12 controlled trials in Africa, Hong Kong, and Singapore, and found that only 2% of 246 patients with initial resistance to either INH, SM, or both, failed treatment after receiving six-month regimens comprising four or five drugs including RIF. However, of 23 patients with these initial resistance patterns who failed treatment despite receiving RIF for four or more months, 17 (74%) acquired resistance to RIF [98].

More recently, in a study done in northern Lima, 117 individuals with drug-resistant TB, who had received one or more standardized antituberculous drug regimens, had two or more isolates collected over an interval of at least three months, which were then submitted for drug-susceptibility testing. Preliminary analyses of drug-susceptibility results show evidence of amplification to first- or second-line antituberculous agents in 57 (49%) of these patients [99]. The following tables present part of this data.

Table 2. Number of antituberculous drugs to which patients acquired additional resistance after exposure to empiric short-course chemotherapy regimens [99]

Number of drugs to which additional resistance developed	N	%
One drug	18	36%
Two drugs	20	40%
Three drugs	12	24%

Table 3. Antituberculous drugs to which patients acquired additional resistance after exposure to empiric short-course chemotherapy regimens [99]

Drugs to which additional resistance developed	N	%
INH	7	14%
RIF	6	13%
PZA	21	42%
EMB	33	66%
SM	26	52%

Data from the former Soviet Union also support the contention that the amplifier effect will have an impact on treatment outcomes and, subsequently, on the epidemiology of new infections [25,100,101]. For example, of patients in TB Colony 33 in Mariinsk, Siberia, Portaels and colleagues have reported that "several MDRTB patients who completed a fully-supervised short-course treatment regimen have apparently developed resistance to additional agents (e.g., ethambutol) when the resistance profiles of their pre-and post-treatment isolates are compared" [25]. The 'amplifier effect' therefore undoubtedly occurs though the true frequency of this phenomenon remains to be defined.

What then are the implications of the amplifier effect, in considering cost effectiveness? In Figure 3, we compare the cost of treating MDRTB patients before and after amplification. The time lost to empiric regimens doomed to fail also means the loss of lung parenchyma, further jeopardizing chances of cure even with appropriate chemotherapy. Thus the cost of treatment failure is even higher than is commonly assumed.

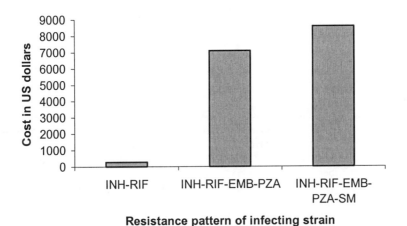

Figure 3. Cost for 18-month regimen for the treatment of two-, four-, and five-drug resistant TB (assuming six months with an injectable agent)[8]. INH, isoniazid; RIF, rifampicin; EMB, ethambutol; PZA, pyrazinamide; SM, streptomycin.

8. CONCLUSIONS: FROM DOTS TO DOTS-PLUS AND BACK AGAIN

The best way to work towards elimination of TB is to provide effective treatment of all cases of active disease. Had DOTS been established before the emergence of resistance to antituberculosis drugs, DOTS alone might have been sufficient for TB control. But MDRTB "hot spots" have been identified on four continents, and the transmission of drug-resistant strains of *M. tuberculosis* continues apace, as yet unchallenged by any coherent strategy. DOTS-Plus promises to build on the successes of international TB control while introducing innovations in response to a novel problem. It is a strategy that meets the demands imposed by complex epidemics in which both drug-susceptible and drug-resistant TB account for disease and new infections.

The long-term goal is of course to put MDRTB behind us, so that energies can once again focus on improving and replicating DOTS-based programs. But we are setting our sights too low in doing nothing in response to already existing epidemics. Antituberculosis drug resistance threatens, in some regions, to decrease the efficacy of DOTS just when the strategy is in need of massive reinforcement. If we do not make every effort to contain MDRTB, we may eventually reach a point at which expanded resources for DOTS will have limited efficacy.

REFERENCES

1. World Health Organization. Anti-tuberculosis drug resistance in the world: the WHO/IUATLD Global Project on Anti-tuberculosis Drug Resistance Surveillance 1994-1997 (WHO/TB/97.229). World Health Organization, Geneva, 1997.
2. Crofton J. The contribution of treatment to the prevention of tuberculosis. Bull Int Union Against Tuber 1962; 32: 643-653.
3. Iseman MD. Tailoring a time bomb: inadvertent genetic engineering. Am Rev Respir Dis 1985; 132: 735-736.
4. Farmer PE, Bayona J, Becerra M, et al. The dilemma of MDRTB in the global era. Int J Tuberc Lung Dis 1998; 2: 869-876.
5. Manalo F, Tan F, Sbarbaro JA, Iseman MD. Community-based short-course treatment of pulmonary tuberculosis in a developing nation. Initial report of an eight-month, largely intermittent regimen in a population with a high prevalence of drug resistance. Am Rev Respir Dis 1990; 142: 1301-1305.
6. Espinal MA, Kim SJ, Hong YP. Treatment outcome of multidrug resistant (MDR) tuberculosis (TB) cases under programme conditions. Int J Tuberc Lung Dis 1998; 2(Suppl. 2): S371.
7. Farmer PE, Kim JY. Community-based approaches to the control of multidrug-resistant tuberculosis: introducing "DOTS-plus". BMJ 1998; 317: 671-674.
8. Farmer PE, Timperi R, Mitnick C, Kim JY. Responding to outbreaks of MDRTB: Introducing "DOTS-Plus". In: Reichman LB, Hershfield ES (eds.), Tuberculosis: a comprehensive international approach, p. 447-469. Second edition. Marcel Dekker Inc., New York, 1999.
9. World Health Organization. Coordination of DOTS-Plus pilot projects for the management of MDR-TB (WHO/CDS/CBC/TB/99.262). World Health Organization, Geneva, 1999.
10. World Health Organization. Report: Basis for the development of an evidence-based case-management strategy for MDR TB within the WHO's DOTS strategy (WHO/TB/99.260). World Health Organization, Geneva, 1999.

11. Farmer PE, Furin J, Bayona J, et al. Management of MDR-TB in resource-poor countries. Int J Tuberc Lung Dis 1999; 3: 643-645.
12. Crofton J, Chaulet P, Maher D. Guidelines on the management of drug-resistant tuberculosis (WHO/TB/96.210). World Health Organization, Geneva, 1996.
13. Iseman MD. Treatment of multidrug-resistant tuberculosis. N Engl J Med 1993; 329: 784-791.
14. Frieden TR, Sherman LF, Maw KL. A multi-institutional outbreak of highly drug-resistant tuberculosis-- epidemiology and clinical outcomes. JAMA 1996; 276: 1229-1235.
15. Ministerio de Salud. Tuberculosis en el Peru- Informe 1996. Ministerio de Salud, Lima, Peru, 1997.
16. Weyer K, Fourie PB, Nardell EA. Multidrug-resistant tuberculosis in South Africa. In: The Global Impact of Drug-Resistant Tuberculosis. Program in Infectious Disease and Social Change, Harvard Medical School, Boston, MA, 1999.
17. World Health Organization. WHO Tuberculosis Programme: framework for effective tuberculosis control (WHO/TB/94.175). World Health Organization, Geneva, 1994.
18. Frieden TR, Fujiwara E, Washko R, Hamburg M. Tuberculosis in New York City: turning the tide. N Engl J Med 1995; 333: 229-233.
19. Garrett L. The coming plague. Farrar, Straus, and Giroux, New York, 1994.
20. Farmer PE, Bayona J, Becerra M, et al. Poverty, inequality, and drug resistance: meeting community needs, p. 88-102. In: Proceedings of the International Union Against Tuberculosis and Lung Disease North American Region Conference, Feb. 27-Mar. 2, 1997.
21. Coninx R, Eshaya-Chauvin B, Reyes H. Tuberculosis in prisons. Lancet 1995; 346: 1238-1239.
22. Farmer PE. Cruel and unusual: drug-resistant tuberculosis as punishment. In: Stern V, Jones R (eds.), Sentenced to Die? The problem of TB in prisons in East and Central Europe and Central Asia. London, Penal Reform International, 1999.
23. Reyes H, Coninx R. Pitfalls of tuberculosis programmes in prisons. BMJ 1997; 315: 1447-1450.
24. Akin M. Soros gives $12M for fight against TB in prisons. The Moscow Times March 20, 1999.
25. Portaels F, Rigouts L, Bastian I. Addressing multidrug-resistant tuberculosis in penitentiary hospitals and in the general population of the former Soviet Union. Int J Tuberc Lung Dis 1999; 3: 582-588.
26. Drobniewski F. Tuberculosis in prisons--forgotten plague. Lancet 1995; 346: 948-949.
27. Banatvala N, Matic S, Kimerling M, et al.. Tuberculosis in Russia. Lancet 1999; 354: 1036.
28. Goldfarb A, Kimerling ME. PHRI/Soros Russian TB program: an initiative of the International Center for Public Health. Submitted to the Gore-Primakov Commission edition. New York, NY: Public Health Research Institute, March 23, 1999.
29. Goldfarb A, Healing T, Kimerling ME. PHRI/MERLIN/WHO Tomsk TB project. New York, NY: Public Health Research Institute, July 5, 1999.
30. Coninx R, Mathieu C, Debacker M, et al. First-line tuberculosis therapy and drug-resistant *Mycobacterium tuberculosis* in prisons. Lancet 1999; 353: 969-973.
31. Heifets LB, Cangelosi GA. Drug susceptibility testing of *Mycobacterium tuberculosis*: a neglected problem at the turn of the century. Int J Tuberc Lung Dis 1999; 3: 564-581.
32. Grosset J. Systematic drug susceptibility testing: a necessary component of the 'DOTS Plus' strategy? Int J Tuberc Lung Dis 1999; 3: 549-550.

33. Collins C, Grange J, Yates M. Tuberculosis bacteriology: organization and practice. Reed Elsevier, Boston, 1997.

34. Vareldzis BP, Grosset J, de Kantor I, et al. Drug-resistant tuberculosis: laboratory issues. World Health Organization recommendations. Tuber Lung Dis 1994; 75: 1-7.

35. Goble M, Iseman MD, Madsen LA, et al. Treatment of 171 patients with pulmonary tuberculosis resistant to isoniazid and rifampin. N Engl J Med 1993; 328: 527-532.

36. Centers for Disease Control and Prevention. Management of persons exposed to multidrug-resistant tuberculosis. MMWR Morb Mortal Wkly Rep 1992; 41(RR-11): 59-71.

37. Rieder HL, Watson JM, Raviglione MC, et al. Surveillance of tuberculosis in Europe. Eur Respir J 1996; 9: 1097-1104.

38. Rieder HL, International Union Against Tuberculosis and Lung Disease, personal communication, September 1999.

39. Timperi R, Sloutsky A, Farmer PE. Global laboratory testing capacity for tuberculosis. Int J Tuberc Lung Dis 1998; 2: S290-S291.

40. Becerra MC, Freeman J, Bayona J, et al. Projections for an urban TB epidemic: The impact of control measures and emerging drug resistance in Lima's northern shantytowns. In: Becerra MC, Epidemiology of tuberculosis in the northern shantytowns of Lima, Peru. Sc.D. Thesis. Harvard University, Boston, MA, 1999.

41. Coninx R, Pfyffer GE, Mathieu C, et al. Drug resistant tuberculosis in prisons in Azerbaijan: case study. BMJ 1998; 316: 1423-1425.

42. Becerra MC, Freeman J, Bayona J, et al. Using treatment failure under effective directly observed short-course chemotherapy programs to identify patients with multidrug-resistant tuberculosis. Int J Tuberc Lung Dis (in press).

43. UNAIDS, World Health Organization. Access to drugs: UNAIDS technical update. UNAIDS, Geneva, 1998.

44. Kim JY, Furin JJ, Shakow AD, et al. Treatment of multidrug-resistant tuberculosis (MDR-TB): new strategies for procuring second- and third-line drugs. Int J Tuberc Lung Dis 1999; 3(Suppl. 1): S81.

45. Rieder HL. Socialization patterns are key to transmission dynamics of tuberculosis. Int J Tuberc Lung Dis 1999; 3: 177-178.

46. Chaulet P. The supply of antituberculosis drugs: price evolution. Tuber Lung Dis 1995; 76: 261-263.

47. Quick JD. Managing drug supply: the selection, procurement, distribution, and use of pharmaceuticals. Second edition. Kumarian Press, West Hartford, CT, 1997.

48. Chaulet P. The supply of antituberculosis drugs and national drug policies. Tuber Lung Dis 1992; 73: 295-304.

49. Weil DC. Drug supply: meeting a global need, p. 123-49. In: Porter JDH, McAdam KPWJ (eds.), Tuberculosis: Back to the Future. John Wiley and Sons, Ltd., New York, 1994.

50. World Health Organization. Tenth HWO model list of essential drugs. World Health Organization, Geneva, 1998.

51. Raviglione M, World Health Organization, personal communication, September 1999.

52. Burnett F. Pooled procurement of pharmaceuticals in the Caribbean. Proceedings from the Caricorn Health Ministers Conference, Trinidad July 15-18, 1996.

53. Fefer E, Pan American Health Organization, personal communication, May 1999.

54. Anonymous. Rifampicin or ethambutol in the routine treatment of tuberculosis. BMJ 1973; 4: 56.

55. Bayer R, Wilkinson D. Directly observed therapy for tuberculosis: history of an idea. Lancet 1995; 345: 1545-1548.

56. Iseman MD, Cohn DL, Sbarbaro JA. Directly observed treatment of tuberculosis: we can't afford not to try it. N Engl J Med 1993; 328: 576-578.
57. Peloquin CA. Controversies in the management of *Mycobacterium avium* complex infection in AIDS patients. Ann Pharmacother 1993; 27: 928-937.
58. Ormerod LP, Horsfield N. Frequency and type of reactions to antituberculosis drugs: observations in routine treatment. Tuber Lung Dis 1996; 77: 37-42.
59. Patel A, MCKeon J. Avoidance and management of adverse reactions to antituberculous drugs. Drug Safety 1995; 12: 1-25.
60. Ali J. Hepatotoxic effects of tuberculosis therapy. A practical approach to a tricky management problem. Postgrad Med 1996; 99: 217-220, 230-231, 235-236.
61. Holdiness, MR. Clinical pharmacokinetics of the antituberculosis drugs. Clin Pharmacokinet 1984; 9: 5115-44.
62. Gonzalez Montaner LJ, Dambrosi A, et al. Adverse effects of antituberculosis drugs causing changes in treatment. Tubercle 1982; 63: 291-294.
63. Zierski M, Bek E. Side-effects of drug regimens used in short course chemotherapy for pulmonary tuberculosis: a controlled clinical study. Tubercle 1980; 61: 41-49.
64. Newton R. Side effects of drugs used to treat tuberculosis. Scott Med J 1975; 20: 47-49.
65. Perez-Stable E, Hopewell P. Current tuberculosis treatment regimens: choosing the right one for your patient. Clin Chest Med 1989; 10: 323-339.
66. Nariman S. Advere reactions to the drugs used in the treatment of tuberculosis. Adverse Drug React Acute Poison Rev 1988; 7: 207-227.
67. Holdiness MR. Neurological manifestations and toxicities of the antituberculous drugs: a review. Med Toxicol 1987; 2: 33-51.
68. Yew WW, Wong CF, Wong PC, et al. Adverse neurological reactions in patients with multidrug-resistant pulmonary tuberculosis after co-administration of cycloserine and ofloxacin. Clin Infect Dis 1993; 17: 288-289.
69. Tack KJ, Smith JA. The safety profile of ofloxacin. Am J Med 1989; 87: 78S-81S.
70. Akhtar AJ, Crompton GK, Schonell MM. Para-aminosalicylic acid as a cause of intestinal malabsorption. Tubercle 1968; 49: 328-331.
71. Munkner T. Studies on goitre due to para-aminosalicylic acid. Scand J Repir Dis 1969; 50: 212-226.
72. Paaby P, Mnorvin E. The absorption of vitamin B12 during treatment with para-aminosalicylic acid. Acta Med Scand 1966; 180: 561-564.
73. Levine R. Steatorrhea induced by para-aminosalicylic acid. Ann Intern Med 1968; 68: 1265-1270.
74. Moore V. A review of side-effects experienced by patients taking clofazimine. Leprosy Rev 1983; 54: 327-335.
75. Ball P, Tillotson G. Tolerability of fluoroquinolone antibiotics: past, present, and future. Drug Safety 1995; 13: 343-358.
76. Lietman P. Fluroquinolone toxicities. An update. Drugs 1995; 49(Suppl. 2): 159-63.
77. Bucco T, Meligrana G, De Luca V. Neurotoxic effects of cycloserince therapy in pulmonary tuberculosis of adolescents and young adults. Scand J Respir Dis 1970; 71(Suppl.): 259-265.
78. Helmy B. Side effects of cycloserine. Scand J Respir Dis 1970; 71(Suppl.): 200-205.
79. Mattie H, Craig W, Pechere J. Determinants of efficacy and toxicity of aminoglycosides. J Antimicrobiol Chemother 1989; 24: 281-293.
80. Kahlmeter G, Dahlager J. Aminoglcoside toxicity – a review of clinical studies published between 1975 and 1982. *J Antimicrobiol Chemother* 1984; 13(Suppl. A): 9-22.

81. Kropp R, Jungbluth H, Radenbach K. Influence of capreomycin on renal function (preliminary results). Antibiotic Chemother 1970; 16: 59-68.
82. Devadatta S, Menon N, Nazareth O, et al. A double-blind study to determine the maximum tolerance dose of ethionamide when administered twice-weekly to patients with pulmonary tuberculosis. Tubercle 1970; 51: 263-269.
83. Combs DL, O'Brien RJ, Geiter LJ. USPHS tuberculosis short-course chemotherapy trial 21: effectiveness, toxicity, and acceptability. Ann Intern Med 1990; 112: 397-406.
84. Govindaraj M. Multiple-drug reactions to tuberculosis: an illustrative case. Tubercle 1968; 49: 416-418.
85. Furin JJ, Mitnick CD, Becerra M, et al. Absence of serious adverse effects in a cohort of Peruvian patients receiving community-based treatment for multidrug-resistant tuberculosis (MDR-TB). Int J Tuberc Lung Dis 1999; 3(Suppl. 1): S81.
86. Program in Infectious Disease and Social Change. Community-based treatment and control of multidrug-resistant tuberculosis: A DOTS-Plus handbook. Program in Infectious Disease and Social Change, Harvard Medical School, Boston, MA, 1999.
87. Quillian J. Community health workers and primary health care in Honduras. J Am Acad Nurse Pract 1993; 5: 219-225.
88. Ramprasad V. Community health workers—and evolving force. World Health Forum 1988; 9: 229-234.
89. Freeman P. A culturally oriented curriculum for aboriginal health workers. World Health Forum 1993; 14: 262-266.
90. Ronsmans C, Bennish M, Wierzba T. Diagnosis and management of dysentery by community health workers. Lancet 1998; 2: 552-555.
91. Christensen P, Karlqvst S. Community health workers in a Peruvian slum area: an evaluation of their impact on health behavior. Bull Pan Am Health Organ 1990; 24: 183-196.
92. Ghebreyesus T, Alemayehu T, Bosman A, et al. Community participation in malaria control in Tigray region Ethiopia. Acta Trop 1996; 61: 145-156.
93. Mburu F. Whither community health workers in the age of structural adjustment? Soc Sci Med 1994; 39: 883-885.
94. Rifkin S. Paradigms lost: toward a new understanding of community participation in health programs. Acta Trop 1996; 61: 79-92.
95. McCord C, Kleinman A. A successful program for para-professionals treating childhood diarrhea and pneumonia. Trop Doctor 1978; 8: 220-225.
96. Zeitz PS, Harrison LM, Lopez M, Cornale G. Community health worker competency in managing acute respiratory infections of childhood in Bolivia. Bull Pan Am Health Organ 1993; 27: 109-119.
97. Farmer PE, Robin S, Ramilus SL, Kim JY. Tuberculosis, poverty, and "compliance": lessons from rural Haiti. Semin Respir Infect 1991; 6: 373-379.
98. Mitchison DA, Nunn AJ. Influence of initial drug resistance on the response to short-course chemotherapy of pulmonary tuberculosis. Am Rev Respir Dis 1986; 133:423 30.
99. Mitnick CD, Freeman J, Bayona J, et al. Amplification of drug resistance by standardized short-course chemotherapy. Working Paper No. 7, Boston, MA: Program in Infectious Disease and Social Change, 1999.
100. Mirzoyev F, Leclerc A. Modification of resistance profiles to first line drugs among patients under standard, DOTS based treatment protocol. Int J Tuberc Lung Dis 1999;3(Suppl. 1): S123.
101. Matthys F. Treatment failure in Colony 33: causes for concern. Presentation at the 30th IUATLD World Conference on Lung Health, Madrid, Spain, September 14-18, 1999.

INDEX